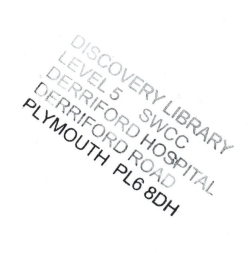
ESSENTIALS OF NURSING CRITICALLY ILL ADULTS

Sara Miller McCune founded SAGE Publishing in 1965 to support the dissemination of usable knowledge and educate a global community. SAGE publishes more than 1000 journals and over 800 new books each year, spanning a wide range of subject areas. Our growing selection of library products includes archives, data, case studies and video. SAGE remains majority owned by our founder and after her lifetime will become owned by a charitable trust that secures the company's continued independence.

Los Angeles | London | New Delhi | Singapore | Washington DC | Melbourne

ESSENTIALS OF NURSING CRITICALLY ILL ADULTS

SAMANTHA FREEMAN, COLIN STEEN AND GREGORY BLEAKLEY

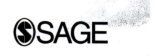

Los Angeles | London | New Delhi
Singapore | Washington DC | Melbourne

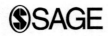

Los Angeles | London | New Delhi
Singapore | Washington DC | Melbourne

SAGE Publications Ltd
1 Oliver's Yard
55 City Road
London EC1Y 1SP

SAGE Publications Inc.
2455 Teller Road
Thousand Oaks, California 91320

SAGE Publications India Pvt Ltd
B 1/I 1 Mohan Cooperative Industrial Area
Mathura Road
New Delhi 110 044

SAGE Publications Asia-Pacific Pte Ltd
3 Church Street
#10-04 Samsung Hub
Singapore 049483

Editor: Alex Clabburn
Assistant editor: Ruth Lilly
Production editor: Tanya Szwarnowska
Copyeditor: Catja Pafort
Proofreader: Tom Bedford
Indexer: Melanie Gee
Marketing manager: George Kimble
Cover design: Sheila Tong
Typeset by: C&M Digitals (P) Ltd, Chennai, India
Printed in the UK

Library of Congress Control Number: 2020949214

British Library Cataloguing in Publication data

A catalogue record for this book is available from the British Library

ISBN 978-1-5264-9131-2
ISBN 978-1-5264-9130-5 (pbk)

At SAGE we take sustainability seriously. Most of our products are printed in the UK using responsibly sourced papers and boards. When we print overseas we ensure sustainable papers are used as measured by the PREPS grading system. We undertake an annual audit to monitor our sustainability.

CONTENTS

THE SAGE ESSENTIALS OF NURSING COLLECTION

Understand the fundamentals and build your knowledge

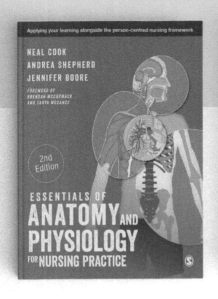

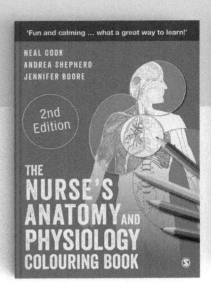

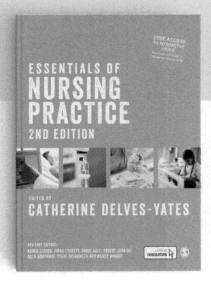

Prepare for practice through specialised learning

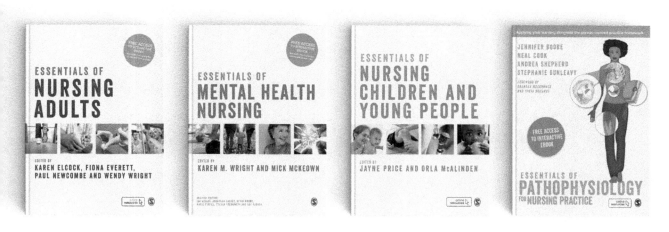

Look up key terms and procedures on the go

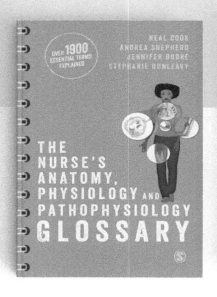

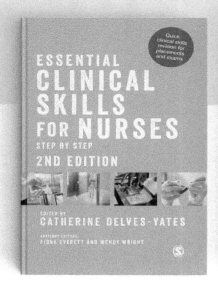

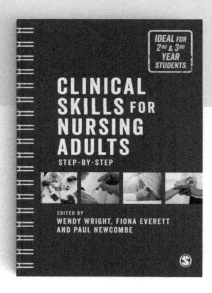

To find which Essentials of Nursing textbook is right for you, simply visit:
www.sagepub.co.uk/nursing-essentials

ABOUT THE AUTHORS

Dr Samantha Freeman, RN, Phd MSc, BSc (Hons), PGCE, SFHEA, RNT.

Sam Freeman is a senior lecturer in adult nursing and the Director of Postgraduate Taught Education for Division of Nursing, Midwifery and Social Work at the University of Manchester. Sam has nearly 30 years' experience in critical care and nurse education. Clinically, she worked in adult critical care where she was the department's lead on clinical audit. As an Advanced Life Support Instructor, she supported the education of the team via a bespoke intermediate life support programme. Sam has a particular interest in exploring how we best support those waking in the critical care environment. Sam's doctoral research explored the patient, family, and multidisciplinary team members' experiences and perspectives of agitation and its management in the adult critical care environment. As a nurse educator she is passionate about ensuring critical care education is championed across both under-graduate and postgraduate education.

Colin Steen, RN, MSc., PGCertEd., SFHEA, RNT.

Colin Steen is a Lecturer in Nursing at the University of Manchester and has specialised in acute and critical care for over 35 years. He has a wide experience of general, paediatric and neonatal intensive care but specialises in adult cardiothoracic critical care including heart, lung and heart/lung transplantation, ECMO and differential lung ventilation. He has worked as a research nurse in the development of drugs to control sepsis. He has a Masters degree in Health Sciences, holds a PGCert in higher education and is a Senior Fellow of the Higher Education Academy. He has collaborated with the Royal College of Nursing Critical Care and Inflight Forum on national transfer guidelines as well as the British Association of Critical Care Nursing and the CC3N on the early developments of the Step Competency Framework.

Dr Gregory Bleakley RN, D.Prof, PGCE, BSc (Hons), DipN, Adv.Cert (Critical Care), RNT, FHEA.

Greg started training as an adult nurse during the 1990s. Clinically, he worked in acute areas of nursing including Critical Care. He has a diploma, bachelor's degree, and doctorate in nursing. Greg also completed the university advanced certificate in critical care nursing as part of his first degree. In 2007, Greg was appointed as a Band 8a Regional Donor Transplant Co-ordinator/Specialist Nurse – Organ Donation. Greg started his clinically focused doctorate in 2012 whilst working in practice, graduating in 2018 with a thesis entitled 'A grounded theory study exploring critical care staff experiences of approaching relatives for organ donation'. Dr Bleakley commenced in post as a lecturer in adult nursing at the University of Manchester in 2016. He facilitates teaching, learning and assessment of undergraduate and postgraduate students. He holds a postgraduate certificate in education (PGCE), is a registered nurse teacher and a Fellow of the Higher Education Academy.

ABOUT THE CONTRIBUTORS

Mark Cole

Dr Mark Cole is a Senior Lecturer with the University of Manchester. He has extensive experience of working within Infection Prevention and control and delivering postgraduate educational units in the specialism.

Claire Burns

Claire Burns is a registered adult nurse and a lecturer in nursing at the University of Manchester where she teaches undergraduate nursing students. Claire's background is in critical care, she is currently involved in teaching the principles of critical care along with clinical skills teaching and the delivery of simulation-based education.

Sally Moore

Sally Moore is a Senior Critical Care Outreach Nurse with over 20 years' experience caring for critically ill adults.

Karen Heggs

Karen Heggs is a Senior Lecturer in Adult Nursing at The University of Manchester, joining the department of Nursing, Midwifery and Social Work in 2015. She qualified as a registered nurse in 1998 and has worked across a range of specialities throughout her career, most significantly in specialist palliative care in both hospice and acute care settings. She completed an MA in Ethics of Cancer and Palliative Care and has an interest in advance care planning and palliative care for people living with long term conditions and teaches on this subject in both undergraduate and postgraduate programmes.

Gillian Singleton

Gillian Singleton has been a Midwifery Lecturer at the University of Manchester since 2017. She qualified as a registered midwife in 1999. She worked as a Delivery Suite Coordinator for 8 years. Subsequently, she became the Delivery Suite Manager and Matron for Inpatient Services. Her area of expertise is intrapartum care and she has a Masters in Clinical Research.

Kim Wilcock

Kim Wilcock is a Midwifery Lecturer University of Manchester.

Emily Brennan

Emily graduated from the University of Manchester and commenced her first Staff Nurse role in Critical Care and Manchester Foundation Trust. She is now a trainee Advanced Critical Care Practitioner.

ACKNOWLEDGEMENTS

We would like to acknowledge the support provided by our clinical colleagues working with in critical care services at the University of Manchester NHS Foundation Trust, with particular thanks to Sally Moore, Emily Brennan, and Caitlin Mitchell.

INTRODUCTION

This book has been written for nursing students prior to or during a practice placement in critical care.

While the book is primarily aimed at nursing students in critical care, it also presents a solid foundation of relevant material for any nurse new to a critical care environment.

This book was developed by a dedicated team of lecturers and practitioners with a background and interest in critical care nursing. All have been keen to be involved because they understand the importance of person-centred, evidence-based nursing care and are aware of the challenges you may face when new to a highly technical environment that is critical care.

To further help your professional development, throughout the book, there is a consistent focus on the person-centred approach required to care for those experiencing critical illness. This book explores the pathway into and out of critical care service as well as the impact this can have on the person and their family.

The book will relate to the key elements of anatomy and physiology and point you towards resources to develop your knowledge further as needed. The threads of evidence-based practice and person-centred care are weaved throughout each chapter. The use of clinical scenarios and reflective activities will allow you to apply the theoretical knowledge gained in order to develop your clinical professional practice.

Self-care and developing yourself is key to achieving the first principle of **holistic** person-centred care. Good communication and compassion occur when you understand yourself and your motivations as well as the person or people you are communicating with, and part of that is valuing your own mental and physical health.

We have made the book as interactive as possible, with lots of different forms of learning to keep you excited and interested.

Everyone involved in this book is passionate about providing you with the knowledge, skills, and confidence to support your development in becoming a nurse who will create and sustain a humanised approach to critical care delivery.

NOTE TO LECTURERS: ACCESS TO ADDITIONAL TEACHING RESOURCES

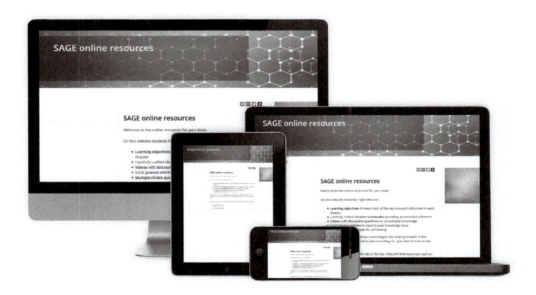

A collection of additional resources are available to lecturers and educators using this book:

- A testbank containing multiple choice questions suitable for either formative or summative assessment
- Selected links to relevant YouTube videos for each chapter
- Supporting PowerPoint slides for each chapter

You can easily upload all the resources into your institution's learning management system (i.e. Blackboard or Moodle), and customise the content to suit your teaching needs.

To access the resources go to the SAGE website https://study.sagepub.com/essentialcriticallyill and follow the onscreen instructions.

THE HISTORY AND DEVELOPMENT OF CRITICAL CARE NURSING

SAMANTHA FREEMAN

> " Critical care nursing is an area of adult nursing with a focus on the care of a person experiencing critical illness. As a critical care nurse, you are the linchpin, coordinating the team and ensuring compassionate, person-centred care is provided for those most to seriously ill along with caring for their families, it is an amazingly rewarding place to nurse.
>
> **Orla, Staff Nurse who has worked in critical care for 9 years** "

> " I was completely awestruck by the nurses on my first week of placement on the critical care department. I then researched all about critical care services and it's fascinating to read about how critical care and care nursing has evolved over the years. I can't wait to apply once I qualify!
>
> **Hadi, 3rd Year Student Nurse** "

LEARNING OUTCOMES

When you have finished studying this chapter you will be able to understand:

- The history and development of critical care
- Critical care environment
- The development of evidence-based practice and care bundles
- Working with the Critical Care team
- The importance of reflection and self care

INTRODUCTION

This chapter aims to provide you with some of the historical context of critical care and how critical care nursing has developed. The chapter will explore the nature of current critical care services and the configuration of care delivery. We will discuss contemporary critical care nursing and how evidence-based nursing in the area is progressing. In this chapter, the importance of professional issues in critical care and multi-professional team working – both of which are vital in this clinical setting – will be explored. The use of evidence-based **care bundles** are common and therefore the concepts of delivering care in this way will be introduced. The chapter will highlight some of the potential political, legal, ethical and moral dilemmas which you may meet. The notion of reflective practice and the importance of your personal self-care will also be incorporated.

THE HISTORY AND DEVELOPMENT OF CRITICAL CARE

First let's look back. Considering the establishment of critical care from a historical perspective may help us appreciate the important role nursing has within this environment.

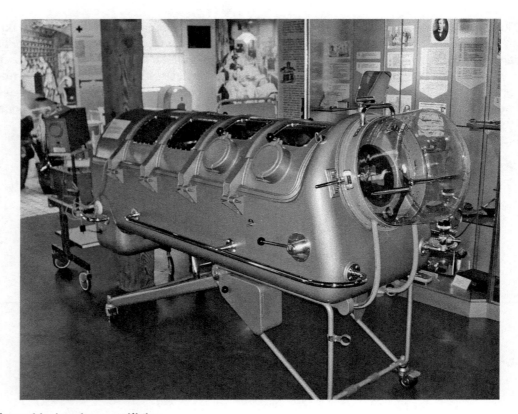

Figure 1.1   Iron lung ventilator

Source: Wikimedia Commons, URL: https://commons.wikimedia.org/wiki/File:Museum-gt-eiserne-lunge.jpg (accessed October 28, 2020). Reproduced under the Creative Commons Attribution 3.0 Unported License (CC BY 3.0), https://creativecommons.org/licenses/by/3.0/deed.en

Organising care, so that groups of the most unwell patients are nursed together, started during the 1940s and 1950s (Fairman, 1992), though it could be argued that there were several key events before this that shaped the development of critical care. Florence Nightingale in the 1850s demanded that those most seriously ill, as a result of fighting in the Crimean war, were placed near to the nurses station (Vincent, 2013).

As with a lot of medical development, many advances are due to activity during wartime and, over the early 1900s, medical and surgical technology was developing rapidly. However, one of the most significant groupings of seriously unwell patients was in the 1950s. This was as a result of several large polio epidemics, the most famous one being in Copenhagen. Within weeks, more than 300 patients developed respiratory paralysis and the ventilator facilities within the hospital were completely overwhelmed (West, 2005). The solution to the crisis was manual ventilation using a rubber bag attached to a tracheostomy tube. Around 200 medical students delivered the patients' ventilation around the clock and some patients were ventilated in this way for several weeks. Respiratory failure experienced by those who contracted polio resulted in the development and increased use of the iron lung ventilator (See Figure 1.1).

Over the next decade intensive care units were created in hospitals across America, Europe and Australia. Advances in medical technology, such as ventilation and monitoring, drove all of this development. The most recent significant change to UK critical care services began with the publication of *Critical to Success* (Audit Commission, 1999) and *Comprehensive Critical Care* (Department of Health, 2000). Both of these publications influenced care delivery and how critical care as a service was viewed. This development will be explored in more detail in Chapter 3.

There are very few accounts of the historical development of critical care nursing. Yet during the development of critical care there has been a reliance on nurses to closely monitor vital signs and provide continuous bedside **interventions**. As technology and treatments have advanced, so have the knowledge and skills of the nurses who work in critical care. As the care became more complex, so has the role, requiring the nurse to have in-depth knowledge of the speciality and the ability to apply that knowledge in line with professional standards. Changes in educational provision and concern about variation across the UK resulted in the development of the *Steps Framework for Adult Critical Care Nurses* (Critical Care Network – National Nurse Leads (CC3N), 2018) which focuses on the development of a competent critical care nurse.

THIS TOPIC IS ALSO COVERED IN CHAPTER 3

Based on a series of competency statements it describes an ability or level of knowledge considered to be a requirement of a particular role. The step competencies provide a national framework for nurses to ensure care delivery is consistent, safe and of a high standard (Deacon et al., 2017). The framework for critical care nursing currently has four steps; Step 1 covers core skills for those new to the environment, Steps 2 and 3 encompass more advanced skills alongside academic development and Step 4 provides a competency structure for the development of senior leaders within critical care nursing (CC3N, 2018). There are also competencies for specialist areas such as neurological, trauma and burns critical care specialities. Although England has introduced national standards for critical care competence, there is some variation, for example, Wales have their own adapted version with similar principles and requirements. The steps and how they link together can be seen in Figure 1.2.

It has been argued that the advancement of technology in nursing somehow limits our care and compassion. We have a professional responsibility to maintain our competence and knowledge base as well as to deliver compassionate care; these are not mutually exclusive activities. When people and their families require medical intervention, it is the level of empathy and compassion they experience

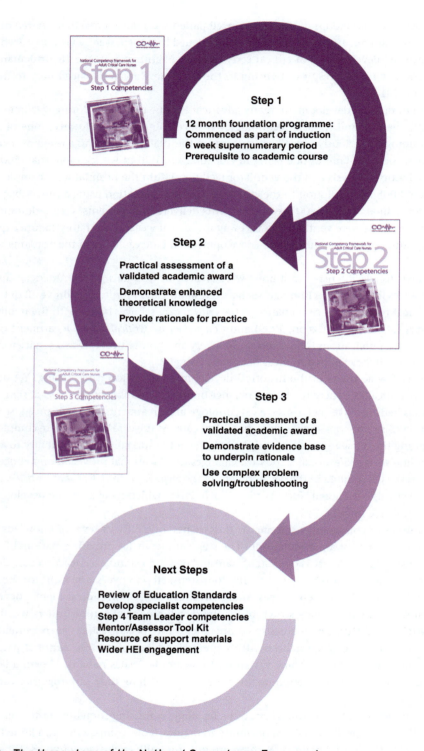

Step 1

12 month foundation programme:
Commenced as part of induction
6 week supernumerary period
Prerequisite to academic course

Step 2

Practical assessment of a
validated academic award

Demonstrate enhanced
theoretical knowledge

Provide rationale for practice

Step 3

Practical assessment of a
validated academic award

Demonstrate evidence base
to underpin rationale

Use complex problem
solving/troubleshooting

Next Steps

Review of Education Standards
Develop specialist competencies
Step 4 Team Leader competencies
Mentor/Assessor Tool Kit
Resource of support materials
Wider HEI engagement

Figure 1.2 The three steps of the National Competency Framework.

Source: Reproduced with permission from Critical Care Network National Nurse Leads, CC3N (2016).

which make the difference between the care being viewed as 'good' or bad' (Timpson et al., 2019). A career in critical care nursing will allow you to develop into a highly skilled, knowledgeable and compassionate practitioner. You may not be considering this just yet, but as an established critical care nurse, your future can expand into education roles, research or leadership roles; there are also Advanced Nurse Practitioner positions within critical care and maybe roles we have not even considered yet!

CRITICAL CARE ENVIRONMENT

Critical care is the care provided to patients who require intensive monitoring and/or the support of failing organs. Just to make this more complex, critical care can be referred to by different names, which really mean the same thing, for example Intensive Care Unit (ICU) or Intensive Therapy Unit (ITU). This terminology is different across the UK and internationally. If this confuses us as nurses, consider how confusing this is for those in our care or visiting. Whatever the name, the department cares for those with acute illness or injury who require specialised procedures and treatments by specialised staff. A classification of where people are cared for has been developed and now is employed in a number of healthcare institutions. This is shown in Table 1.1. However, it is vital that nurses are aware that people can deteriorate in any clinical setting. The Nursing and Midwifery Council (NMC) state that for entry to the register the student nurse must be able to respond proactively and promptly to signs of deterioration (NMC, 2018).

Table 1.1 The classification of care delivery

LEVEL	STANDARD
Level 0	Patients whose needs can be met through normal ward care in an acute hospital.
Level 1	Patients at risk of their condition deteriorating, or those recently relocated from higher levels of care, whose needs can be met on an acute ward with additional advice and support from the critical care team.
Level 2	Patients requiring more detailed observation or intervention, including support for a single failing organ system or post-operative care and those 'stepping down' from higher levels of care.
Level 3	Patients requiring advanced respiratory support alone or basic respiratory support together with support of at least two organ systems. This level includes all complex patients requiring support for multi-organ failure.

Source: Guidelines for the Provision of Intensive Care Services (2015: 11). Reproduced by kind permission of the Faculty of Intensive Care Medicine.

THIS TOPIC IS ALSO COVERED IN CHAPTER 3

The wider impact and responsibility of critical care will be discussed in Chapter 3.

PERSON-CENTRED CARE

If you look at images of critical care, they typically show a lot of equipment, monitoring, ventilation, and the person receiving the care can often be lost. The World Health Organisation (WHO, 2014) states that care should be 'people-centred' not 'disease-centred'. This goal can be more challenging in the critical care environment. This is mainly because of the nature of the admission to critical care requires an immediate biomedical intervention in a highly technical environment, and because of the intervention, the person loses the ability to communicate (Jakimowicz and Perry, 2015). No matter how challenging, it is vital that the team strives to promote a person-centred approach to care delivery. A person-centred approach can support the person in their recovery phase and during weaning from treatment as well as promoting a sense of control of decision-making about their own health (Bolster and Manias, 2010; Rose et al., 2014). There could be an increased risk that the critical care team reduces the person to an illness, disease, bed number or the type of surrounding technology (Jakimowicz and Perry, 2015). It is important that we get to know the person behind the illness, and, as we do not know the person prior to admission to critical care, family members can play an active role in this (Cederwall et al., 2018). To reinforce the notion of person-centred care, in this book, where possible, we have used the term, 'person' instead of 'patient', and the ways in which we can support person-centred care are explored in Chapter 2.

THIS TOPIC IS ALSO COVERED IN CHAPTER 2

THE DEVELOPMENT OF EVIDENCE-BASED PRACTICE

There are many reasons why someone may require support in a specialist critical care unit. Irrespective of the reason for their admission, the care they receive needs to be underpinned by the best available evidence.

The first documented use of the term 'evidence-based' is credited to Gordon Guyatt and the evidence-based working group in 1992. They described evidence-based medicine as a 'new paradigm for medical practice, in which evidence from clinical research should be promoted over intuition, unsystematic clinical experience, and pathophysiology' (Evidence-Based Medicine Working Group, 1992).

We all would want our practice to be effective and based on clinical research, however, evidence-based practice is much more than this. In Activity 1.1 you will critically consider the type of evidence you access to support the care delivery decisions you make.

ACTIVITY 1.1: CRITICAL THINKING

Consider a nursing intervention you have recently carried out. List all the types of 'evidence' you used to understand this activity; what it is, how to do it correctly and how to assess its impact.

1. How do you judge whether the evidence is correct or of value?
2. Write a list of the thing that may make you question the validity of a piece of evidence.

To support the review of the quality of evidence you can use assessment tools. There are many of these available but the Critical Appraisal Skill Programme (CASP) provides some good simple guidance. Further information can be found on their website https://casp-uk.net/ (accessed October 29, 2020).

Evidence-based practice is the conscientious use of current best evidence to inform decision making about a patient's care (Sackett et al., 2000). Research evidence tells us what does and does not work, and evidence-based practice is the process of collecting, processing, and implementing research findings to improve clinical practice, the work environment, or the person's outcome.

Hierarchy of evidence

The evidence we use to support care delivery has a hierarchy, which really relates to how robust or non-biased a particular study appears to be. Figure 1.3 shows this hierarchy in the form of a pyramid: types of evidence at the top of the pyramid are considered to have more robust procedures than those at the bottom.

Reflecting on Figure 1.3, what we as nurses need to remember is that not every clinical question can be answered by a randomised controlled trial. What we should be considering is, was the right research approach taken to answer the research question? Some of the complex issues within critical care need

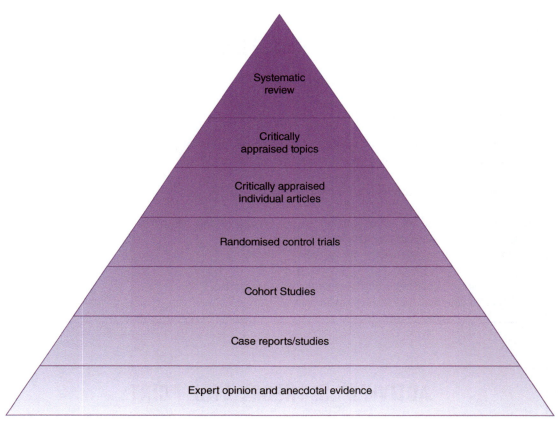

Figure 1.3   Hierarchy of evidence

multiple approaches to generate the evidence base, and at the moment some practice is based on the lower 'expert opinion', as there is nothing else available to clinical teams.

CARE BUNDLES

THIS TOPIC IS ALSO COVERED IN CHAPTER 7

Delivering evidence-based care via **care bundles** is a popular approach in critical care. Providing care in this way aims to improve the quality of very complex care and reduce variation in care delivery (Lavallée et al., 2017). The bundles contain three to five evidence-informed practices (Resar et al., 2012), which are to be delivered collectively and consistently with the aim of improving the person's outcome (Lavallée et al., 2017). Much of the evidence supporting the elements within care bundles could be viewed as 'lower level' evidence, based on small studies or observational data. It is the combination of measures together that result in a positive impact (Horner and Bellamy, 2012). Two of the common care bundles you will encounter in critical care are the ventilator care bundle and central line care bundle. One of the best-known examples of a care bundle is the surviving **sepsis** campaign. In Activity 1.2 you will be exploring the bundle and reflecting on your practice.

ACTIVITY 1.2: RESEARCH AND EVIDENCE-BASED PRACTICE

Take a look at the Surviving Sepsis campaign:

www.survivingsepsis.org

You can also access this short film clip of Ron Daniels, who led the development of guidelines to manage sepsis and the implementation of these into practice:

www.youtube.com/watch?v=vYQcnUl3k3U

On this website you can access educational material, protocols and checklists to support your practice and increase your understanding of sepsis.
    Reflect on your experiences of the managing of sepsis.

1. What are the challenges of implementing this care bundle?
2. How do you think they could be overcome?

ACTIVITY 1.3: THEORY STOP POINT

1. What do you think the barriers are when trying to implement a care bundle in a practice area?
2. What could be the negatives of using care bundles?
3. How do you think the effectiveness of care bundles is assessed?

CLINICAL DECISION-MAKING

The assessment of an individual's health status, in any clinical setting, requires critical thinking and clinical decision-making skills.

Critical thinking requires you to have the capacity to consider your thought process, then actively assess and regulate it (Hayes et al., 2017). When health care staff fail to think critically, commonly when under high pressure or in a rushed situation, they can fall foul of cognitive bias. This can be the result of lack of situational awareness or confirmation bias. Situational awareness describes a person's perception, comprehension and subsequent projection of what is going on in the environment around them (Graafland et al., 2015). In Activity 1.4 you will be considering your own perception of situations and how this may impact on your practice.

ACTIVITY 1.4: CRITICAL THINKING

Our perceptions are easily influenced by the elements outlined above. Watch this clip called 'The Monkey Business Illusion' www.youtube.com/watch?v=IGQmdoK_ZfY (accessed October 29, 2020).

1. In practice, what factors do you think influence your perception of a situation?
2. How do you think our perceptions of situations could help our practice or potentially be harmful to our practice?

Your perception of a situation can lead to confirmation bias. This is when we put more significance on a particular bit of evidence because it supports our viewpoint. It is acknowledged that in highly technical areas non-technical skills, which support our situational awareness and potentially minimise our biases, can be as important as our technical abilities.

Additionally, we all have unconscious bias that can impact on our assessment of a situation and our decision-making. Our views and any possible bias we have will be influenced by our background, our experiences and any social stereotypes we may choose to believe. Unconscious bias happens when we make quick judgments and assessments of people and situations without realising. Activity 1.5 asks you to consider your own unconscious bias and its impact.

ACTIVITY 1.5: REFLECTIVE PRACTICE

Consider you own unconscious biases (we all have them) and write these down.

1. Reflecting on your own experience, can you recall a time or occasion when you let your unconscious bias impact on your behaviour or judgement?
2. How might you handle this differently in the future?

There is no template answer to this activity, as it is based on your own reflection.

Being aware of all these potential sources of bias in our assessment of situations is important in ensuring we provide safe, high-quality care. One educational approach to support this is referred to as 'Human Factors' and is linked to improvements in safety. In relation to health care, it looks at how we interact with our environment with the aim of developing our cognitive and interpersonal skills to be effective in team-based, high-risk activity (Henriksen et al., 2008). In Activity 1.6 you will be asked to watch a short film and then reflect on what you have seen.

ACTIVITY 1.6: CRITICAL THINKING

Watch this clip called 'Just a Routine Operation'

www.youtube.com/watch?v=JzlvgtPlof4 (accessed October 29, 2020)

Reflect on what you have seen.

1. Why do you think the nurse's opinion was not heard?
2. What strategy could have helped the nurse vocalise her concern?

There is a raft of assessment tools available to you to support your decision-making in critical care, and these will be explored in more detail in each relevant chapter. Clinical decisions should be based on all the information gathered via these assessments to then determine the best course of action. Unfortunately, it is not as easy as that and a more complex process is undertaken. Standing (2005: 34, cited in Standing, 2010: 7) suggests that clinical decision making involves '…information processing, critical thinking, evaluating evidence, applying relevant knowledge, problem solving skills, reflection and clinical judgement'. Following this we decide one course of action over another.

CLINICAL DECISION-MAKING IN CRITICAL CARE

The nurse does not make clinical decisions in isolation in critical care. What you will experience in a critical care environment is excellent multi-professional team working.

THE CRITICAL CARE TEAM

Due to the many diverse requirements needed to support someone during critical illness, a multi-professional team approach to care is required, and quite often the nurse is central to the coordination of care provision (Freeman et al., 2018). **Multi-professional team working** is key; due to the complex nature of critical care not one professional has all the knowledge or skills to respond (Rose, 2011). The team within critical care is comprised of staff from many different professional groups: doctors, nurses, advanced critical care practitioners, physiotherapists, radiographers, **dieticians**, infection control and microbiology, and pharmacists, with further input by occupational therapy, **speech and language therapy**, and clinical psychology. Domestic staff, porters, administration staff and technicians also have a vital role to play in supporting care delivery. You may need to link with social workers or family liaison officers and leaders from various faiths. Research has shown the importance of effective teamwork for ensuring positive outcomes in the care of this in the critical care environment (Reader and Cuthbertson, 2011). Effective team working is prevalent in most critical care departments, however sometimes this can be challenging especially for more junior members of the team.

Group reflection can strengthen the team and is vital when dealing with stressful and distressing situations. The use of the 'Schwartz round' approach has become more commonplace, generating a positive evidence base around team effectiveness. Schwartz rounds were the idea of Ken Schwartz in 1994 who was diagnosed with a terminal illness. He devised a structured forum to allow staff both clinical and non-clinical to discuss the emotional aspect of healthcare provision. The idea was brought and supported in the UK by the Point of Care Foundation. In Activity 1.7 you will reflect on a team you have worked within and explore how well this team worked together.

ACTIVITY 1.7: REFLECTIVE PRACTICE

Reflect on a team you have worked within.

1. Did the team work well together or not? Why was this?
2. What do you think the barriers were to effective team working?
3. How could these barriers have been overcome?

MORAL CHALLENGES FOR THE CRITICAL CARE NURSE

The team of staff working within critical care can be faced with political, legal, ethical and moral dilemmas. As these issues arise throughout this book, we will explore the impact on the person, the family and the staff involved in more detail. In summary, these issues could be seen as lower level issues, such as the movement of critical care staff to help nurse in other areas outside of their speciality. They could also be more challenging issues relating to the allocation of finite resources, for example two patients needing the one critical care bed available. Having a critical care illness can impact on the decision-making ability of the individual and there can be legal interventions to consider, such as lasting power of attorney or advanced directives. There can be numerous legal and ethical issues around supporting the individual at the end of their life including withdrawing treatment, and how this is managed. The person experiencing critical care often has their physical movement restricted either pharmacologically, or due to the presence of equipment and monitoring, or sometimes via the application of physical restraints. The above scenarios make demands on the critical care team to undertake a moral decision-making approach.

It's vital that we focus on the person we are treating and that all the care we deliver is always for their benefit. It can be challenging with all the technology we have, but just because we can do something it doesn't mean we should.

Peter, Critical Care Matron

ACTIVITY 1.8: CASE STUDY

THIS TOPIC
IS ALSO
COVERED IN
CHAPTER 15

Imrana is a 68-year-old woman who experienced complications following her cardiac surgery. This resulted in her being cared for in critical care for longer than planned. There have been several attempts to wake her but each time she wakes she tries to pull her airway out or get out of the bed. So far this has resulted in the use of **sedation** to keep her safe. Her husband asks you, 'why can't you put something on her arms to stop her pulling her airway when she wakes up?'

1. What is your initial response?
2. Do you think restraining her movement with medications is better or worse than using wrist restraints?
3. What other strategies could you also try?

Take some time to read the three journals articles below:

Burk, R.S., Grap, M.J., Munro, C.L., Schubert, C.M. and Sessler, C.N. (2014) 'Agitation onset, frequency, and associated temporal factors in critically Ill adults', *American Journal of Critical Care*, 23 (4): 296–304. https://www.ncbi.nlm.nih.gov/pmc/articles/PMC4451814/ (accessed October 29, 2020).

Chang, L.-Y., Wang, K.-W.K. and Chao, Y.-F. (2008) 'Influence of physical restraint on unplanned extubation of adult intensive care patients: A case-control study', *American Journal of Critical Care*, 17: 408–16. Available from https://www.researchgate.net/publication/23241967_Influence_of_physical_restraint_on_unplanned_extubation_of_adult_intensive_care_patients (accessed October 29, 2020).

Curry et al. (2008) 'Characteristics associated with unplanned extubations in a surgical intensive care unit', *American Journal of Critical Care*, 17 (1): 45–51. Available from https://www.research-gate.net/publication/5691697_Characteristics_Associated_With_Unplanned_Extubations_in_a_Surgical_Intensive_Care_Unit (accessed October 29, 2020).

4. Have you changed your view?

Discuss this case with colleagues and see what they think. There are no template answers to Questions 1, 2 and 4 as these are based on your own views. An answer to Question 3 has been provided.

WHAT'S THE EVIDENCE?

The issue outlined in the case study above can be common in critical care and the teams have minimal evidence on which to base their decision. This can lead to feelings of anxiety and distress within the team and particularly the nursing staff. Read the article below which looks at the views and opinions from the multi-disciplinary team in relation to the management of acute agitation in adult critical care.

Freeman. S., Yorke. J. and Dark. P. (2019) 'The management of agitation in adult critical care: Views and opinions from the multi-disciplinary team using a survey approach', *Intensive and Critical Care Nursing* 54: 23–8. doi.org/10.1016/j.iccn.2019.05.004

REFLECTIVE PRACTICE AND SELF-CARE

> At first, I found reflection a bit strange, I mean we all think about what we have done, but actually to properly reflect on my practice I did need some structure and space. Once is got my head round that I found it vital to help with challenges I faced throughout my degree, both good and bad!
>
> **Beth, 3rd year student nurse**

During a placement or the first few weeks working in a critical care environment you are exposed to so many clinical scenarios where the individual and the family have suffered a significant level of stress and shock. Your learning will be accelerated as you are exposed to new treatments, different interventions and thought-provoking situations. As rewarding as this experience is, it can be demanding both physically and psychologically and its important that this is acknowledged, and you consider strategies that may help you.

Reflection can be described as an activity where you consider your knowledge and understanding of your practice, learning from your experience, which in turn improves the care you provide (Timpson et al., 2018).

Boud et al. (1985: 19) offer the definition:

Reflection is an important human activity in which people recapture their experience, think about it, mull over and evaluate it. It is this working with experience that is important in learning.

There are many different models of reflection to support you and you can select the model that suits you and your learning style. In Activity 1.9 you will look at different reflective models and select the one most suited to your own learning style.

ACTIVITY 1.9: REFLECTIVE PRACTICE

Consider an event you have experienced in your practice. Look up the three reflective models listed below. Reflect on the event using the three models suggested. Once you have completed this, consider which model you feel supports your reflective activity in the best way. You will be asked to reflect again, and you can then apply the model you like the most.

- Gibbs (1988): Reflective Cycle
- Johns (2000): Model for Structured Reflection
- Rolfe et al. (2001): Model What, So What, Now What

There is no template answer to this activity as it is based on your own reflection.

Seeking the support of others is a really important self-care approach. Everyone will be able to remember when they started working in critical care, so find someone in the team you can talk to. Some departments have formal support, buddy systems or clinical supervision. Clinical supervision is when you reflect with a colleague or independent professional (Heggs and Freeman, 2018).

The activity can be one-to-one or as a group and has been acknowledged as a positive step in improving working relationships and increasing feelings of job satisfaction (Bifarin and Stonehouse, 2017). In Activity 1.10 you will be asked to consider your own approaches to stress management.

ACTIVITY 1.10: REFLECTIVE PRACTICE

Consider the ways in which you keep yourself healthy and manage your stress. Discuss these strategies with your friends or colleagues.

1. Are there any common approaches?
2. What do you think works and what doesn't work?
3. Can you use any different approaches next time you are feeling stressed?

The Royal College of Nursing (2018) has published some guidance on self-care, which you may want to look at: www.rcn.org.uk/professional-development/publications/pub-006703 (accessed October 29, 2020).

There is no template answer to this activity as it is based on your own reflection.

YOUR DEVELOPMENT

As highlighted so far, there is a lot to learn and experience when you are in a critical care environment. There are many skills which are transferable to other care environments, or you may (hopefully) stay within critical care. Wherever your career takes you, the knowledge gained and professional development during your time in critical care will be invaluable. You will develop skills that relate to leadership and clinical decision-making. You might think it surprising to mention leadership when you are at the beginning of your professional development; however, leadership is mostly about behaviour and is necessary at all clinical levels (Burns, 2018). Leadership does not need to be linked to a position of authority and is different to a manager. There is a raft of leadership theory, which is not the focus of this book, but developing yourself and your leadership ability requires self-awareness and personal reflection. In Activity 1.11, you will think of a leader you have worked alongside and what you feel were positive and not so positive attributes.

ACTIVITY 1.11: CRITICAL THINKING

Consider the leaders you have encountered who were good, and who were not so good.

1. Consider what made them different; was it their skills and knowledge, personality or the position within the team?
2. What are the barriers to effective teamwork?
3. How do you overcome these?

There is no template answer to Question 1 as this is based on your own experience. Answers to Questions 2 and 3 have been provided.

CHAPTER SUMMARY

This chapter has supported your understanding of the following topics:

- The development of critical care and critical care nursing
- The importance of evidence-based practice
- The importance of person-centred care
- The importance of and challenges of team working
- The importance of self-care, reflective practice and your personal development

---

GO FURTHER

Books

Bolton, G. and Delderfiled, R. (2018) *Reflective Practice: Writing and Profession Development* (5th edition). London: Sage.

- This text will give you a deeper understanding of how to reflect and capture your reflections. It will help you start to think about reflective practice and support the development of your professional reflective skills.

Burns, D. (2018) 'Leadership and Management', in D. Burns (ed.) *Foundations of Adult Nursing*, (2nd edition). London: Sage. pp. 187–220.

- If you want to understand more about leadership theory this is an excellent introduction. Is easy to read and explores traditional leadership theory as well as the newer emerging theories such as ethical leadership.

Cullum. N., Ciliska, D., Haynes, B. and Marks, S. (2008) *Evidence-based Nursing: An Introduction*. Oxford: Wiley-Blackwell.

- To understand more about evidence-based practice in healthcare the above text gives a good overview.

Greenhalgh, T. (2014) *How to Read a Paper: The Basics of Evidence-based Medicine* (5th edition). Chichester: Wiley.

- This is a book which will support you in understanding the quality of the papers you are reading. It will help you unpick the quality of different types of evidence.

Useful websites

https://conjointly.com/kb/ (accessed November 14, 2020).

- This website is a good starter resource when looking at different type of evidence, particularly if you are unsure of what some of the research terminology means.

www.cc3n.org.uk/step-competency-framework.html (accessed November 14, 2020).

- This website will take you to look at the Step one competencies, which are aimed at those new to critical care, their learning and development over the first 12 months.

www.pointofcarefoundation.org.uk/our-work/schwartz-rounds/about-schwartz-rounds/ (accessed November 14, 2020).

- This website contains more information and some short film clips on how Schwartz rounds are supported.

Journal articles

Baker, D., Day, R. and Salas, E. (2006) 'Teamwork as an essential component of high reliability organisations', *Health Service Research*, 41 (4): 1576–98.

- This article will give you a deeper understanding of the importance of teamworking.

REFERENCES

Audit Commission (ed.) (1999) *Critical to Success*. London: Audit Commission for Local Authorities and the National Health Service in England and Wales. Available from http://www.wales.nhs.uk/sites3/documents/768/CriticalToSuccess.pdf (accessed October 28, 2020).

Bifarin, O. and Stonehouse, D. (2017) 'Clinical Supervision: An important part of every nurse's practice', *British Journal of Nursing*, 26 (6): 331–5.

Bolster, D., and Manias, E. (2010) 'Person-centred interactions between nurses and patients during medication activities in an acute hospital setting: Qualitative observation and interview study', *International Journal of Nursing Studies*, 47: 154–65.

Boud, D., Keogh, R., and Walker, D. (1985) *Reflection: Turning Experience into Learning*. London: Kogan Page.

Burns (2018) 'Leadership and Management', in D. Burns (ed.) *Foundations of Adult Nursing*, (2nd edition). London: Sage. pp. 187–220.

Cederwall, C.J., Olausson, S., Rose, L., Naredi, S. and Ringdal, M. (2018) 'Person-centred care during prolonged weaning from mechanical ventilation, nurses' views: An interview study', *Intensive and Critical Care Nursing*, 46: 32–7. https://doi.org/10.1016/j.iccn.2017.11.004

Critical Care National Network Nurse Leads (CC3N) (2018) 'Steps Framework for Adult Critical Care Nurses', *Critical Care National Network Nurse Leads Forum*. Available from https://www.cc3n.org.uk/step-competency-framework.html (accessed October 28, 2020).

Deacon, K.S., Baldwin, A., Donnelly, K.A., Freeman, P., Himsworth, A.P., Kinoulty, S.M., Kynaston, M., Platten, J., Price, A.M., Rumsby, N. and Witton, N. (2017) 'The National Competency Framework for Registered Nurses in Adult Critical Care: An overview', *Journal of the Intensive Care Society*, 18 (2): 149–56.

Department of Health (ed.) (2000) *Comprehensive Critical Care: A Review of Adult Critical Care Services*. London: Department of Health. Available from http://webarchive.nationalarchives.gov.uk/20130107105354/http://www.dh.gov.uk/prod_consum_dh/groups/dh_digitalassets/@dh/@en/documents/digitalasset/dh_4082872.pdf (accessed 28 October 2020).

Evidence-Based Medicine Working Group (1992) 'Evidence-based medicine: A new approach to teaching the practice of medicine', *Jama*, 268 (17): 2420–5. www.cebma.org/wp-content/uploads/EBM-A-New-Approach-to-Teaching-the-Practice-of-Medicine.pdf (accessed October 29, 2020).

Fairman, J. (1992) 'Watchful vigilance: Nursing care, technology, and the development of intensive care units', *Nursing Research*, 41 (1): 56–60.

Freeman, S., Yorke, J. and Dark, P. (2018) 'Patient agitation and its management in adult critical care: A integrative review and narrative synthesis', *Journal of Clinical Nursing*, 27 (7–8): e1284-e1308.

Freeman, S., Yorke, J. and Dark, P. (2019) 'The management of agitation in adult critical care: Views and opinions from the multi-disciplinary team using a survey approach', *Intensive and Critical Care Nursing*, 54: 23–8. doi.org/10.1016/j.iccn.2019.05.004

Gibbs, G., (1988) *Learning by Doing: A Guide to a Teaching And Learning Methods*. Oxford. Oxford Brooks Further Educational Unit.

Graafland, M., Schraagen, J.M.C., Boermeester, M.A., Bemelman, W.A. and Schijven, M.P. (2015) 'Training situational awareness to reduce surgical errors in the operating room', *British Journal of Surgery*, 102 (1): 16–23.

Hayes, M.M., Chatterjee, S. and Schwartzstein, R.M. (2017) 'Critical thinking in critical care: Five strategies to improve teaching and learning in the intensive care unit', *Annals of the American Thoracic Society*, 14 (4): 569–75.

Heggs, K. and Freeman, S., (2019) 'Managing the Transition to Registered Nursing Practice', in D. Burns (ed.) *Foundations of Adult Nursing* (2nd edition). London: Sage. pp. 459–83.

Henriksen, K., Dayton, E., Keyes, M.A., Carayon, P. and Hughes, R. (2008) 'Understanding adverse events: A human factors framework', in R.G. Hughes (ed.) *Patient Safety and Quality: An Evidence-Based Handbook for Nurses*. Rockville, MD: Agency for Healthcare Research and Quality (US). pp. 67–86. Available from: www.ncbi.nlm.nih.gov/books/NBK2651/ (accessed October 19, 2020).

Horner, D.L. and Bellamy, M.C. (2012) 'Care bundles in intensive care', *Continuing Education in Anaesthesia, Critical Care and Pain*, 12 (4): 199–202.

Jakimowicz, S. and Perry, L. (2015) 'A concept analysis of patient-centred nursing in the intensive care unit', *Journal of Advanced Nursing*, 71 (7): 1499–517.

Johns C. (2000) Becoming a reflective practitioner: a reflective and holistic approach to clinical nursing practice, development and clinical supervision. Oxford: Blackwell Science.

Lavallée, J.F., Gray, T.A., Dumville, J., Russell, W. and Cullum, N. (2017) 'The effects of care bundles on patient outcomes: A systematic review and meta-analysis', *Implementation Science*, 12 (1): 1–13.

Nursing and Midwifery Council (NMC) (2018) *Future Nurse: Standards of Proficiency for Registered Nurses*. London. Nursing and Midwifery Council. Available from https://www.nmc.org.uk/globalassets/sitedocuments/education-standards/future-nurse-proficiencies.pdf (accessed January 7, 2021).

Reader, T.W. and Cuthbertson, B.H. (2011) 'Teamwork and team training in the ICU: Where do the similarities with aviation end?', *Critical Care*, 15 (6): 1–6.

Resar, R., Griffin, F.A., Haraden, C., Nolan, T.W. (2012) *Using Care Bundles to Improve Health Care Quality*. IHI Innovation Series white paper. Cambridge, MA: Institute for Healthcare Improvement. Available from http://www.ihi.org/resources/Pages/IHIWhitePapers/UsingCareBundles.aspx (accessed October 28, 2020).

Rolfe, G., Freshwater, D., & Jasper, M. (2001) *Critical reflection for nursing and the helping professions: A user's guide*. Basingstoke: Palgrave.

Rose, L. (2011) 'Interprofessional collaboration in the ICU: How to define?', *Nursing in Critical Care*, 16 (1): 5–10.

Rose L., Dainty KN., Jordan J., Blackwood B. (2014) 'Weaning from mechanical ventilation: A scoping review of qualitative studies', *American Journal of Critical Care*, 23(5): e54–70. doi: 10.4037/ajcc2014539. PMID: 25179040 (accessed January 7, 2021).

Sackett, D.L., Straus, S.E., Richardson, W.S., Rosenberg, W.M.C. and Haynes, R.B. (2000) *Evidence-based Medicine: How to Teach and Practice EBM* (2nd edition). Edinburgh: Churchill Livingstone.

Standing, M. (2010) 'Perceptions of clinical decision-making: A matrix model', in M. Standing (ed.) *Clinical Judgement and Decision-Making in Nursing and Interprofessional Healthcare*. Maidenhead: Open University Press. pp. 1–27.

Timpson, J., Lee-Woolf, E., and Brooks, J., (2019) 'Essentials of nursing: Values, knowledge, skills and practice', in D. Burns (ed.) *Foundations of Adult Nursing* (2nd edition). London: Sage. pp. 3–32.

Vincent, J. (2013) 'Critical care – where have we been and where are we going?', *Critical Care* 17: 1.

West, J.B. (2005) 'The physiological challenges of the 1952 Copenhagen poliomyelitis epidemic and a renaissance in clinical respiratory physiology', *Journal of Applied Physiology*, 99 (2): 424–32. http://jap.physiology.org/cgi/doi/10.1152/japplphysiol.00184.2005 (accessed October 28, 2020).

WHO (2014) *WHO Global Strategy on People-centred and Integrated Health Services*. Copenhagen: World Health Organisation.

HUMANISING CRITICAL CARE

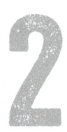

SAMANTHA FREEMAN

> " Patients are not just a collection of symptoms, defined by their illness [...] it can be quite intimidating. Don't forget to say hello, reassure us, update us and include us.
>
> **Elizabeth Edwards, was in the ICU following treatment for Stage IV metastatic melanoma.** "

LEARNING OUTCOMES

When you have finished studying this chapter you will be able to understand:

- What humanising critical care means
- Strategy to promote humanised care
- Importance of communication
- How we can promote comfort in critical care
- The role the family can play in care

INTRODUCTION

This chapter will explore what humanising critical care means and why it's important. It will present the evidence base surrounding why and how alternative therapies and environmental factors can impact on the person experiencing critical illness and their families. The chapter will encourage you to explore ways in which you are able to see the person within such a highly technical clinical environment.

WHAT DOES HUMANISING CRITICAL CARE MEAN?

When a person is critically unwell, unconscious, and surrounded by lots of technical equipment, it is easy for busy practitioners to forget that there is a person at the centre of the care they are delivering. It is all too easy for a person's identity to become lost. We can exacerbate the problem by placing the person in a hospital gown or nursing them naked, not assisting them to wear their glasses or hearing aid and de-personalising them by using their bed number or condition to refer to them rather than their name. No matter how unwell the person is or how busy the department we must provide respectful and humane care. Approaches to ensure humanised care delivery in critical care may have benefits in boosting the person's engagement with their own well-being (Wilson et al., 2019). Table 2.1 illustrates some humanising and de-humanising activities. Some of the **interventions** sound quite simple but it is all too common in a busy environment to forget the basics. When people are labelled by their illness, even if unaware, they are not being treated with respect (Henry et al., 2015).

Table 2.1   Outline of some humanising and de-humanising behaviours

Humanising behaviours	De-humanising behaviours
• Unrestricted family visitation • Knowing the person (non-medical facts) • Physical touch (e.g. handholding) • Communicate with the person not just about or over them • Common courtesy communications (introduction, explanations of what is about to happen, permission to touch) • Attending promptly to the person's needs • Individualising communication modalities • Giving the person some locus of control of their environment • Use eyeglasses, hearing aids and dentures as feasible • Personal hygiene (hair care, oral care etc.)	• Loss of identity (and appearance) • Loss of ability to communicate • Loss of ability to advocate for one self • Loss of family presence • Loss of control • Loss of respect • Loss of modesty/privacy • Purposeful shaming/mocking • Purposeful exploitations (e.g. for research)

Source: Adapted from Wilson et al., *Humanizing the Intensive Care Unit* (2019) under the Creative Commons Attribution 4.0 International License: http://creativecommons.org/licenses/by/4.0/

IMPORTANCE OF COMMUNICATION

There are elements of communication that are the same across all care environments. However, there are some unique challenges which you will face due to the nature of critical care. The people you will be caring for will have a number of barriers that will affect the way you can communicate with them and they can communicate with you.

Not only are they critically unwell, they may be unable to verbalise their needs and concerns due to the placement of a **tracheostomy** or **endotracheal tube**, or the change to their level of consciousness. Their family and visitors will be in a high state of stress and anxiety, which can also affect communication.

A number of studies have been conducted exploring what it is like to be cared for in critical care. The predominating issue is communication, as the person feels voiceless. This can lead to a loss of identity (Karlsson et al., 2012) and feelings of frustration (Tate et al., 2012) and can become a major cause of distress (Alasad et al., 2015).

Supporting communication

We have already mentioned the importance of simple ways to humanise the care we deliver. Ensuring that someone who wears glasses has access to them, or if they use a hearing aid, that this is in place and working, will massively improve communication. There are a number of other ways to support communication, but you do need to be aware that these strategies will not work in all circumstances and can actually increase frustration if persistently used when ineffective. Providing a pen and paper for the person to write down what they want to communicate may be one way to support communication, however, there are considerations if you adopt this method. In Activity 2.1 you will be asked to consider these.

ACTIVITY 2.1: CASE STUDY

Moab is intubated but awake. He is agitated and desparately trying to speak but is prevented by the presence of the endotracheal tube. The nurse looking after him has given him a pen and paper to write down what he is trying to say.

1.   What assumptions have we made when providing a pen and paper to aid communication?
2.   List the possible issues with using this approach.

Non-verbal communication

To support communication most critical care departments use pointer boards or flash cards with common requests as images. This approach does not need some of the skills required to write but does limit the communication to the images available.

Many of the staff within critical care become expert lip readers. The way you can improve your lip reading is to ensure you face the person straight on and stand a little further away to improve your view. You need to remember that the way people speak can be altered by ill-fitting dentures or may be hampered by the presence of wire or tubes they are not used to. Additionally, our regional accents, if different, can impact on the ability to lip read.

Or you may just need more practice!

There has also been the development of apps to support communication. One you can download for free is the *Patient Communicator App* (https://www.sccm.org/MyICUCare/THRIVE/Patient-and-Family-Resources/Patient-and-Family), which can be adjusted for non-English speakers. Activity 2.2 asks you to consider the usefulness of apps in practice.

ACTIVITY 2.2: REFLECTIVE PRACTICE

Download the Patient Communicator App or similar and work through it.

1. How do you think this would work in a clinical setting?
2. What issues do you think there might be?

Verbal communication

It is easy to forget but sometimes the critically unwell person can still verbalise and communicate. They will be anxious as well as unwell so this can affect their ability to retain information and affect the way in which they communicate.

For those who have an artificial airway, more specifically a tracheostomy tube, there is a range of devices to allow speech. These may be fenestrated tracheostomy tubes, which is a tube with holes to allow air to flow and, therefore, speech or a one-way speaking valve.

Speech and language therapists have a key role to play in supporting the promotion of speech and you should consider their involvement in care as soon as possible.

Any strategy you select will need to be appropriate for the individual, and what may work on one day may not work the next, so you also need to remain flexible in your approach.

One major barrier to communication is the use of **sedation**. This is administered to ensure that treatments and interventions, which are often painful, are tolerated. The promotion of lighter sedation regimes enhances the person's capacity to communicate with both staff and their family (Vincent et al., 2016). The assessment, monitoring and titration of sedation are covered later in this chapter.

All the visitors and families you encounter in critical care will be experiencing varying degrees of anxiety and worry. You need to respect the person's pattern of communication and ways of dealing with stress as this may differ from yours. It can be worrying as a student or new member of the team, but humility and honesty are essential. If you do not know the answers to a question then say so, but always find someone else who can help.

When caring for someone in critical care what is useful for you to remember is you cannot change what is happening to these people. What you can do is provide timely, sensitively delivered information in an attempt to empower them to deal with the situation and make informed decisions.

PROMOTION OF COMFORT

Making someone feel comfortable may be ensuring they are frequently re-positioned and have their hygiene needs met. In critical care the nursing of someone in a particular position, such as in the prone position (this is the person laying face down), is considered a therapeutic intervention and is covered in more detail in Chapter 6. The assessment and management of the person's hygiene need, and maintenance of skin integrity is also covered elsewhere in Chapter 12.

However, although these topics are covered elsewhere you still need to consider these factors when promoting comfort.

THIS TOPIC IS
ALSO COVERED
IN CHAPTER 6
AND 12

Management of pain, agitation and anxiety

One way of promoting comfort is to manage the person's pain but, as you can imagine, this is complex in critical care. As sedation is used frequently to ensure the person can tolerate invasive treatments, such as ventilation, it maybe that some healthcare staff underestimate symptoms such as pain. It has been shown that those in critical care experience moderate to severe pain during rest as well as pain during procedures (Devlin et al., 2018). Following a critical care stay many people note that pain, agitation and anxiety are distressing symptoms they have experienced (Jeitziner et al., 2015). The American College of Critical Care Medicine (2013) published a set of clinical practice guidelines around the management of pain, agitation and **delirium** in critical care (Barr et al., 2013). The guidance outlines the importance of assessment, prevention and treatment and provides some management strategies. The guidance includes delirium, however, the assessment and management of delirium is covered in Chapter 15 as it is closely linked to sedation practice.

If we go back to look at pain management, the use of assessment tools has been shown to improve the quality of assessment of pain and effectiveness of any interventions. In Activity 2.3 you will be looking at the Critical Care Pain Observation Tool and comparing this to other tools you may have used.

THIS TOPIC
IS ALSO
COVERED IN
CHAPTER 15

ACTIVITY 2.3: CRITICAL THINKING

The assessment tool recommended by the above guidance is the Critical Care Pain Observation Tool (CCPOT) developed by Gélinas et al. (2006). It is considered the most valid and reliable tool to use when the person cannot self-report their pain. Take a look at this tool and consider the questions below. https://kpnursing.org/professionaldevelopment/CPOTHandout.pdf (accessed October 29, 2020).

1. How does this differ from the pain assessment tools you have used before?
2. Discuss this with a peer or your practice supervisor.

The assessment of the person and their pain needs to be ongoing. The management of pain, from a nurse perspective, follows the same principles as in any other setting. We need to act as an advocate to ensure effective pain control is prescribed, administer this, and monitor the effectiveness. Analgesia prescription and administration should follow the guidance provided by the World Health Organisation's Analgesic Ladder (WHO, 1986) (see Figure 2.1).

What is different in the critical care setting is the administration of analgesia alongside sedation.

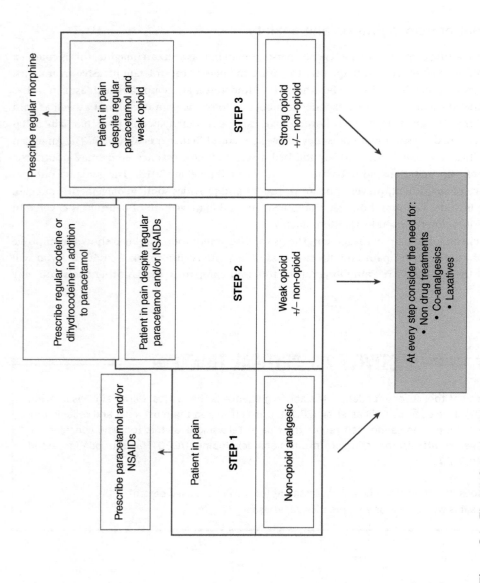

Figure 2.1 The WHO Analgesic Ladder

Source: Ashelford et al. (2019: 165).

SEDATION PRACTICE

The term 'sedation' as defined by the American Society of Anaesthesiologists (2018) comprises a **continuum** of states ranging from minimal sedation through to general anaesthesia. Sedation for those experiencing critical illness has evolved from an era of liberal use of sedatives to a much more restricted use (Porhomayon et al., 2015). The UK Intensive Care Society guidelines on the use of sedation acknowledge that the management of distress and agitation in critical care does not solely rest on the use of medication but requires an understanding of the causes of the distress and the creation of an environment that reduces stress. The specific indications for use of sedation are to alleviate pain, to facilitate the use of otherwise distressing treatments and to minimize discomfort so as to augment the effectiveness of a treatment (Whitehouse et al., 2014). Sedation can be viewed as a treatment in its own right, for example to control seizures or management of **intracranial** pressure.

It can also be administered:

- To reduce anxiety
- To control agitation
- For amnesia during neuromuscular blockade

(Whitehouse et al., 2014: 10)

The administration of sedation in critical care is predominantly via the **intravenous** (IV) route. This route has the benefit of faster onset of action and the effect of the sedative is easily titratable (Narayanan et al., 2016). A variety of medications may be used for sedation including opioids, benzodiazepines, intravenous and inhaled general anaesthetic agents, neuroleptic drugs, phencyclidine derivatives, phenothiazines, a-agonists (drugs that stimulate alpha receptors in the body, for example adrenergic receptors such as sedatives) and barbiturates (Whitehouse et al., 2014).

THIS TOPIC IS ALSO COVERED IN CHAPTER 15

ACTIVITY 2.4: THEORY STOP POINT

Understanding the administration and monitoring of sedation can be overwhelming when you are new. The practice can be different to administration you have seen, and you will be normally administering the medication via an intravenous route, which again may be new to you. Two useful resources to start reading to support your understanding of analgesia are:

a. Whitehouse, T. et al. (eds) (2014) *Intensive Care Society Review of Best Practice for Analgesia and Sedation in the Critical Care.*

To access the above, follow this link: www.ics.ac.uk/ICS/GuidelinesAndStandards/StandardsAndGuidelines.aspx. Find 'Sedation for Patients in ICU' under ICS Guidelines.

b. Narayanan, M. et al. (2016) 'Analgesia in intensive care: Part 1', *BJA Education*, 16 (2): 72–8. https://doi.org/10.1093/bjaceaccp/mkv018

1. Why do you think sedation practice is so variable?
2. List some of the factors that could affect the decision-making when selecting a sedative to prescribe and administer

Assessment of sedation

The use of clinically validated scales to support the monitoring and titration of sedation is recommended (Vincent et al., 2016). There are various assessment tools used to evaluate levels of sedation. The Ramsay scale, developed in 1974, was the first tool to assess levels of sedation (Whitehouse et al., 2014). Subsequently, numerous sedation scoring tools have been developed. In a systematic review conducted by De Jonghe et al. in 2000, 25 scoring tools were identified. The instruments include descriptions of the level of consciousness, and often descriptions of agitation, pain, or synchrony with the ventilator. Tools of high reliability in adult critical care were the Ramsay scale (1974), the Sedation-Agitation Scale (Riker et al., 1999) and the Motor Activity Assessment Scale (De Jonghe et al., 2000). Since this review, the Richmond Agitation-Sedation Scale (RASS) (Sessler et al., 2002) was published and has demonstrated excellent performance with inter-rater reliability and validity and has been the first score to detect changes over time in the critically ill (Reschreiter et al., 2008).

The Richmond Agitation and Sedation Scale (RASS) is a validated diagnostic tool for use in critical care. The scores are from comatose (score of −5) to combative (score of +4). Further details of the RASS tool are given in Table 2.2. The ten-point scale assesses both the level of sedation and the degree of agitation (Whitehouse et al., 2014). The tool has been validated against the bispectral index (BIS) monitor which is an objective device to assess the depth of anaesthesia (Karamchandani et al., 2010). The tool also integrates with other assessment tools for delirium such as the CAM-ICU tool.

Table 2.2 Richmond Agitation and Sedation Scale (Sessler., et al. 2001)

Score	Description
+4	Violent and aggressive
+3	Very agitated, pulling at tubes and lines
+2	Agitated, intolerant of ventilator and very restless
+1	Restless, anxious but not aggressive
0	Alert and calm, awake and settled
−1	Drowsy, not fully alert but eyes opened spontaneously
−2	Light sedation, rousable and responsive but only briefly.
−3	Moderate sedation, movement or eye open to voice
−4	Deep sedation, no response to voice but responds to pain
−5	Unrousable, no response to voice or painful stimuli

The use of an assessment tool only supports one element of care and is part of a wider clinical picture. Using the RASS or equivalent requires a sedation target to be set and then someone, usually the nursing staff, will titrate, or change, the sedation to reach or maintain the agreed target.

However, the assessment and management of the person's sedation requires several decisions that incorporate appropriate assessment using the tool together with more iterative processes (Aitken et al., 2009). This could encompass the consideration of how the individual responded to previous sedation changes to wider clinical issues relating to other events within the department. In addition to this, the individual clinician's own biases can determine their perspectives on care and treatment (Palacios-Ceña et al., 2016).

The Pain, Agitation and Delirium (PAD) guidance also notes the importance of ensuring comfort, frequent re-orientation, and maintenance of normal sleep pattern (Barr et al., 2013). A concept offered by Vincent et al. (2016) is the comfort and person-centred care without excessive sedation: eCASH, which stands for *early Comfort using Analgesia, minimal Sedation and maximal Humane care*, illustrated in Figure 2.2.

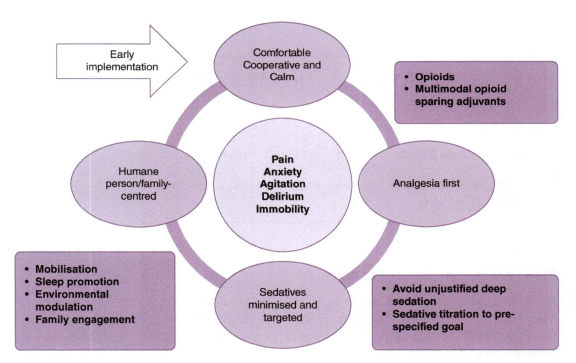

Figure 2.2   Diagram of the eCASH concept

Source: Adapted and reproduced by kind permission of Springer Nature. Vincent et al. (2016).

PROMOTION OF SLEEP

Sleep is a complex process affected by physiological, psychological and environmental factors. As we all know when we have a lack of sleep we can feel unwell but sleep deprivation can impact on the person's ability to think clearly and, in the critically ill, this can lead to the development of delirium (Pulak and Jensen, 2016). Sleep and sleep deprivation in the critically ill have been researched over a number of years and yet are still challenging to promote. Those who have a critical care admission can experience disruption to their sleep during all stages of their illness and following discharge (Tembo et al., 2013).

Circadian rhythm disruption

Our sleeping and wakefulness pattern over the course of 24 hours is defined as our circadian rhythm. The circadian pacemaker drives the circadian rhythm. This 'pacemaker' is situated in the anterior hypothalamus, within the brain. The circadian rhythm or pattern is described as 'inbuilt', however, external factors such as light can upset the pattern of our sleep and wakefulness.

As critical care departments tend to be well or brightly lit most of the time, and increased light is required during procedures, the circadian rhythm of those admitted is affected. This persistent exposure to light may also contribute to reduction in melatonin levels. Melatonin is a hormone that aids sleep, produced when light is reduced. In addition to this we administer sedatives and other medications that alter the person's sleep pattern.

ACTIVITY 2.5: THEORY STOP POINT

The maintenance of sleep and the physiological effects of sleep deprivation are complex. Please read the following paper:

Telias, I. and Wilcox, E. (2019) 'Sleep and circadian rhythm in critical care', *Critical Care*, 23: 82.

1. When caring for some in critical care, what changes do you think you can make to promote a healthy sleep pattern?

Sleep promotion via care bundles

Across the current literature the use of sleep bundles has been proposed as a method for promoting sleep. The sleep bundle would include the promotion of a regular sleep/wake cycle, ensuring a reduction in noise and light during the night as well as reduction the number of 'care episodes', such as position changing or mouth care, when the person is sleeping (Vincent et al., 2016).

Reduction of noise

The World Health Organization (WHO) suggest that the average hospital should have sound levels that do not exceed 35 decibels (dB) with a maximum of 40 dB overnight. One study investigating the level of sound in critical care departments found that sound levels are consistently above the WHO recommendations (Darbyshire and Young, 2013). This study was only conducted in the UK and dates back to care provision in 2013, however the level of noise still remains an issue. The main sources of noise are staff activity and the noise from the equipment. A review of noise and possible reduction of noise in critical care departments suggested that some changes in staff behaviour may help, such as reducing the volume of conversations and moving away from the bedside

(Delaney et al., 2019). Other strategies suggested were reducing alarm volumes and the use of earplugs or noise cancelling headsets.

It has also been suggested that eye masks and earplugs would help promote sleep, and this seems reasonable, however it is difficult to measure the effectiveness of these strategies due to the complex reasons sleep is disturbed in critical care. Activity 2.6 will ask you to reflect on your own sleep and what can affect it.

ACTIVITY 2.6: REFLECTION

1. What strategies do you use to help you sleep?
2. How many of these strategies could you offer to someone in a critical care environment?

Try to consider yourself in critical care.

3. Would you like to wear earplugs and an eye mask?
4. What do you think we need to consider if we are to use these strategies?

There is no template answer to this activity as it is based on your own reflection.

Another way of promoting sleep and a day/night cycle is having access to natural light. This is something that is perhaps now considered more in newer designs of critical care departments, but not something all critical care areas have access to. What should be available is a clock the person can see and some way of them knowing the date. Offering reassurance and reorientation when caring for someone in critical care is key to ensuring the day/night cycle is reinforced. Another bundle of care to consider is the ABCDEF bundle (Marra et al., 2017), which is not to be confused with the ABCDE assessment (Resuscitation Guidelines)! This bundle includes six elements, which, if delivered together, work to improve the person's recovery and outcome. The elements of the whole **care bundle** are in the box below, but the section most relevant to sleep is: *Early mobility and Exercise.*

ELEMENTS OF THE ABCDEF BUNDLE

Assess, prevent, and manage pain
Both Spontaneous Awakening Trials (SAT) and Spontaneous Breathing Trials (SBT)
Choice of analgesia and sedation
Delirium: Assess, prevent, and manage
Early mobility and exercise
Family engagement and empowerment

Source: Marra et al., 2017

Exercise and stimulation during the day is one way of encouraging daytime activity, marking out to the person the differences between the day and night. In Activity 2.7 you will consider the barriers to mobility in critical care and think of ways in which they may be overcome.

ACTIVITY 2.7: CRITICAL THINKING

Considering the need to promote early mobility and exercise in critical care, this is still not always achieved. Jot down the reasons you think early mobility and exercise is not achieved. Then consider how you could overcome these issues.

1. Who should be included in planning and supporting activities?

Some level of physical activity has been shown to be possible and safe, even in complex situations (Marra et al., 2017). What is needed is a **multi-professional team** approach to lessen fear felt by staff. This was made clear in a study performed by Chohan et al. (2018) who showed an increase from 0% to 87% of patients sitting on the side of the bed referred to in the study as, having a 'daily dangle'. The case study below about Michelle asks you to consider strategies to aid sleep but also how family members can impact or assist.

ACTIVITY 2.8: CASE STUDY

You are looking after Michelle on the early shift. At handover you were informed that she had been agitated and restless all night and at times aggressive to the staff. She is 55 years old and had been cared for in the critical care environment for over a week following complications of a chest infection post a routine operation. Over your shift she is drowsy and drifts off to sleep when she is left alone and the nurse you are working with advises that you don't wake her. Her husband, Darren, and teenage daughter, Melissa, visit every day. Today Melissa becomes tearful, as her mum appears to not want her there. Darren start to express that he feels angry and useless as he is traveling in only to find Michelle asleep and uninterested in them. Darren cannot understand the reports that Michele has been aggressive over night as this is not in her nature and thinks it must be something to do with the care.

1. What is your initial communication strategy to reassure Darren and Melissa?
2. Plan an outline of interventions that may help the situation. Are there any interventions the family could be involved with if they wish?

Discuss the scenario with a colleague. Do you share the same opinion on how it should be managed?

PSYCHOLOGICAL SUPPORT

Given what we have covered so far, it is no surprise to find that 45-80% of those who have had an admission to critical care experience acute levels of stress (Wade et al., 2018). There has been an increase in the use of non-pharmacological interventions to minimise the stressors in critical care and support those experiencing extreme stress levels. These interventions could be the use of music, massage, relaxation techniques and even pet therapy. However, these interventions are under researched, and not supported with a clear evidence base as to their impact. Research into these interventions is challenging due to the many variables in delivery and the heterogeneous, or diverse, nature of the group of people who may be in critical care. When considering the use of non-pharmacological interventions, you should, where possible, involve the person and ask about their preferences. Can you imagine your most hated song playing as part of your music therapy? If asking the person is not possible, then consider involving the family.

FAMILY INVOLVEMENT IN CARE

Throughout this textbook we will be looking at the impact of critical care on the individual. However, we also need to consider the individual as part of a 'family'. We are using the term family, but this can mean different things to different people, so in this context it is whomever is significant to the person you are caring for. Supporting the involvement of the family in care delivery and decision-making is an important aspect of your role in critical care. There have been a number of studies exploring family involvement and it still remains the case that the nursing staff act as 'gatekeepers' to this activity, meaning the nurse at the bedside can influence how well (or not well) this is done. In Activity 2.9 you will reflect on your experience of family involvement in care delivery.

ACTIVITY 2.9: REFLECTION

Reflect on your experience so far in relation to the involvement of family in care.

1.   What has stopped you doing this and what has encouraged you?
2.   What have other nurses done to facilitate family involvement?

There is no template answer to this activity as it is based on your own reflection.

As with the person in your care, the family members need to be treated on an individual basis. Families may want to be involved at different levels and there will be family dynamics, which you are unaware of, which may prevent involvement in care. You also need to be aware of cultural barriers which may exist, preventing the family's involvement care. Already the involvement of the family may sound daunting to you but all you need to be is open and supportive and let the family guide you on what they would like or not like to do.

WHAT'S THE EVIDENCE?

One barrier to family involvement is the visiting hours. This subject is hotly debated across critical care literature and is inconsistent in practice. Find out the visiting hours of your department and research what the wider literature says about this. Discuss with a colleague why the department has opted for the visiting hours it has and what would be the pros and cons of changing.

In 2012 the British Association of Critical Care Nurses (BACCN) wrote a position statement on this matter, but family access to visiting is still variable.

ACTIVITY 2.10: REFLECTION

Considering what you have read so far reflect on the two questions below and maybe discuss them with peers or your practice supervisor.

1.   Why do you think some units restrict family visits?
2.   Consider the benefits of restricted and open visiting and who may or may not benefit in both instances.

If supported in an effective way, families can have a huge impact in reducing stress for the person in critical care as well as helping you get to know the person you are looking after. Often families can feel useless and a bit of a 'spare part' sat beside their loved one surrounded by all the technology. They may be fearful of touching the person in case they knock a wire or tubing. One way of encouraging family involvement is supporting their contribution to the 'patient diary'.

DIARIES

THIS TOPIC
IS ALSO
COVERED IN
CHAPTER 17

In recent years there has been an increased interest and development in using diaries as a way of documenting the person's stay in critical care. The use of this approach is variable across both the UK and internationally. Again, there is limited evidence, at the moment, regarding the effectiveness of diaries in the reduction of psychological distress post discharge. One positive aspect of the diary, which may be beneficial, is the contribution a family can make. In most departments the bedside nurse completes the events of the day in the diary but there are a number of places where you can encourage the family to contribute. The use of diaries will be explored in more detail in Chapter 17 as the chapter considers discharge and rehabilitation.

CHAPTER SUMMARY

This chapter has supported your understanding of the following topics:

- What humanised care is and some strategies for implementation
- The importance of the management of pain, agitation and anxiety
- The importance of sleep and sleep promotion
- The importance of the involvement of the family in care

GO FURTHER

Books

Case, M. (2019) *How to Treat People: A Nurse at Work*. London: Penguin.

- This book is written by a nurse and gives a different perspective on care.

Awdish, R. (2017) *In Shock*. New York, NY: St Martin's Press.

- This book is written by a doctor after her stay in critical care and how this has improved her practice.

Grant, A. and Goodman, B. (2018) *Communication and Interpersonal Skills in Nursing* (4th edition). London: Sage.

- This book will provide you with additional reading around communication and interpersonal skills

Useful websites

http://www.icusteps.org/ (accessed October 29, 2020).

- ICUsteps is a charity and support group set up for those who have had a critical care admission. You may want to point people to this in the future.

http://www.healthtalk.org/ (accessed October 29, 2020).

- This a website that has people talking about their experiences of their stay in critical care.

http://www.icu-diary.org/diary/Diary.html (accessed October 29, 2020).

- The website is the base of an informal network for all health care workers that are interested in the use of diaries in critical care.

Journal articles

The following journal articles will explore some of the chapter topic in more detail:

Freeman, S., Yorke, J. and Dark, P. (2018) 'Patient agitation and its management in adult critical care: An integrative review and narrative synthesis', *Journal of Clinical Nursing* 27 (7–8): e1284–e1308.

Wade, D., Als, N., Bell, V., Brewin, C., D'Antoni, D., Harrison, D.A […] and Rowan, K.M. (2018) 'Providing psychological support to people in intensive care: Development and feasibility study of a nurse-led intervention to prevent acute stress and long-term morbidity', *BMJ Open*, 8 (7): 1–12.

Ullman, A.J., Aitken, L.M., Rattray, J., Kenardy, J., Le Brocque, R., MacGillivray, S. and Hull, A.M. (2015) 'Intensive care diaries to promote recovery for patients and families after critical illness: A Cochrane Systematic Review', *International Journal of Nursing Studies*, 52 (7): 1243–53. doi. org/10.1016/j.ijnurstu.2015.03.020

Wøien, H. and Bjørk, I.T. (2013) 'Intensive care pain treatment and sedation: Nurses' experiences of the conflict between clinical judgement and standardised care: An explorative study', *Intensive and Critical Care Nursing*, 29 (3): 128–36. doi.org/10.1016/j.iccn.2012.11.003

REFERENCES

Aitken, L.M., Marshall, A.P., Elliott, R. and McKinley, S. (2009) 'Critical care nurses' decision making: Sedation assessment and management in intensive care', *Journal of Clinical Nursing*, 18 (1): 36–45.

Alasad, J.A., Tabar, N.A. and Ahmad, M.M. (2015) 'Patients' experience of being in intensive care units', *Journal of Critical Care*, 30 (40): 859.e7–11.

American Society of Anaesthesiologists (2018) 'Position on Monitored Anaesthesia Care', *American Society of Anaesthesiologists*. Available from https://www.asahq.org/standards-and-guidelines/position-on-monitored-anesthesia-care (accessed October 29, 2020).

Ashelford, S., Raynsford, and Taylor, V. (2019) *Pathophysiology and Pharmacology in Nursing* (2nd edition). London: Sage.

Barr, J., Fraser, G.L., Puntillo, K., Ely, E.W.., Gélinas, C., Dasta, J.F. […] and Jaeschke, R. (2013) 'Clinical practice guidelines for the management of pain, agitation, and delirium in adult patients in the Intensive Care Unit', *Critical Care Medicine*, 41 (1): 263–306. doi.org/10.1097/CCM.0b013e3182783b72

Chohan, S., Ash, S. and Senior, L. (2018) 'A team approach to the introduction of safe early mobilisation in an adult critical care unit', 7: e000339. http://dx.doi.org/10.1136/bmjoq-2018-000339

Darbyshire, J.L. and Young, J.D. (2013) 'An investigation of sound levels on intensive care units with reference to the WHO guidelines'. *Critical Care*, 17 (5): R187. Available from http://ccforum.com/content/17/5/R187 (accessed October 30, 2020).

De Jonghe, B., Cook, D.J. Appere-de-Vecchi, C. Guyatt, G., Meade, M. and Outin, H. (2000) 'Using and understanding sedation scoring systems: A systematic review', *Intensive Care Medicine*, 26 (3): 275–85.

Delaney, L., Litton, E. and Van Haren, F. (2019) 'The effectiveness of noise interventions in the ICU', *Current Opinion in Anaesthesiology*, 32 (2): 144–9.

Devlin, J.W., Skrobik, Y., Gélinas, C., Needham, D.M., Slooter, A.J.C., Pandharipande, P.P. […] and Alhazzani, W. (2018) 'Clinical practice guidelines for the prevention and management of pain, agitation/sedation, delirium, immobility, and sleep disruption in adult patients in the ICU', *Critical Care Medicine*, 46 (9): e825–e873. doi.org/10.1097/CCM.0000000000003299

Gélinas, C., Fillion, L., Puntillo, K., Viens, C. and Fortier, M. (2006) 'Validation of the critical-care pain observation tool in adult patients', *American Journal of Critical Care*, 15: 420–7.

Gibson, V., Plowright, C., Collins, T., Dawson, D., Evans, S., Gibb, P., Lynch, F., Mitchell, K., Page, P. and Sturmey, G. (2012) 'Position statement on visiting in adult critical care units in the UK', *Nursing in Critical Care, British Association of Critical Care Nurses*. https://doi.org/10.1111/j.1478-5153.2012.00513.x (accessed January 7, 2021).

Henry, L.M., Rushton, C., Beach, M.C. and Faden, R. (2015) 'Respect and dignity: A conceptual model for patients in the Intensive Care Unit', *Narrative Inquiry in Bioethics*, 5 (1A): 5A–14A. Available from https://muse.jhu.edu/content/crossref/journals/narrative_inquiry_in_bioethics/v005/5.1A.henry.html (accessed October 29, 2020).

Jeitziner, M.M., Hamers, J.P., Bürgin, R., Hantikainen, V. and Zwakhalen, S.M. (2015) 'Long-term consequences of pain, anxiety and agitation for critically ill older patients after an intensive care unit stay', *Journal of Clinical Nursing*, 24 (17/18): 2419–28.

Karamchandani, K., Rewari, V., Trikha, A. and Batra, R.K. (2010) 'Bispectral index correlates well with Richmond agitation sedation scale in mechanically ventilated critically ill patients', *Journal of Anesthesia*, 24 (3): 394–8.

Karlsson, V., Bergbom, I., and Forsberg, A. (2012) 'The lived experiences of adult intensive care patients who were conscious during mechanical ventilation: A phenomenological-hermeneutic study'. *Intensive & Critical Care Nursing*, 28 (1): 6–15. https://doi.org/10.1016/j.iccn.2011.11.002

Marra, A., Ely, W., Pandharipande, P. and Patel, M. (2017) 'The ABCDEF bundle in critical care', *Critical Care Clinics*, 33 (2): 225–43.

Narayanan, M., Venkataraju, A. and Jennings, J. (2016) 'Analgesia in intensive care: Part 1', *BJA Education*, 16 (2): 72–8.

Palacios-Ceña, D., Cachón-Pérez, J.M., Martínez-Piedrola, R., Gueita-Rodriguez, J., Perez-De-Heredia, M. and Fernández-De-Las-Peñas, C. (2016) 'How do doctors and nurses manage delirium in intensive care units? A qualitative study using focus groups', *BMJ Open*, 6: e009678. doi.org/10.1136/bmjopen-2015-009678

Porhomayon, J., Joude, P., Adlparvar, G., El-Solh, A.A. and Nader, N.D. (2015) 'The impact of high versus low sedation dosing strategy on cognitive dysfunction in survivors of intensive care units: A systematic review and meta-analysis', *Journal of Cardiovascular and Thoracic Research*, 7 (2): 43–8. http://dx.doi.org/10.15171/jcvtr.2015.10

Pulak, L. and Jensen, L. (2016) 'Sleep in the Intensive Care Unit: A review', *Journal of Intensive Care Medicine*, 31 (1): 14–23. https://doi.org/10.1177/0885066614538749

Reschreiter, H., Maiden, M. and Kapila, A. (2008) 'Sedation practice in the intensive care unit: A UK national survey', *Critical Care*, 12 (6): 1–8.

Riker, R.R., Picard, J.T. and Fraser, G.L. (1999) 'Prospective evaluation of the Sedation-Agitation Scale for adult critically ill patients', *Critical Care Medicine*, 27 (7): 1325–9. doi.org/10.1097/00003246-199907000-00022

Sessler, C.N., Gosnell, M.S., Grap, M.J., Brophy, G.M., O'Neal, P.V, Keane, K.A., Tesoro, E.P. and Elswick, R.K. (2002) 'The Richmond Agitation-Sedation Scale: Validity and reliability in adult intensive care unit patients', *American Journal of Respiratory and Critical Care Medicine*, 166 (10): 1338–44. www.atsjournals.org/doi/full/10.1164/rccm.2107138 (accessed October 30, 2020).

Tate, J.A., Devito Dabbs, A., Hoffman, L.A., Milbrandt, E. and Happ, M.B. (2012) 'Anxiety and agitation in mechanically ventilated patients', *Qualitative Health Research*, 22 (2): 157–73.

Tembo, A.C., Parker, V. and Higgins, I. (2013) 'The experience of sleep deprivation in intensive care patients: Findings from a larger hermeneutic phenomenological study', *Intensive and Critical Care Nursing*, 29 (6): 310–16. doi.org/10.1016/j.iccn.2013.05.003

Vincent, J.L., Shehabi, Y., Walsh, T.S., Pandharipande, P.P., Ball, J.A., Spronk, P., Longrois, D., Strøm, T., Conti, G., Funk, G.C., Badenes, R., Mantz, J., Spies, C. and Takala, J. (2016) 'Comfort and patient-centred care without excessive sedation: The eCASH concept', *Intensive Care Medicine*, 42 (6): 962–71.

Wade, D., Als, N., Bell, V., Brewin, C., D'Antoni, D., Harrison, D.A. [...] and Rowan, K.M. (2018) 'Providing psychological support to people in intensive care: Development and feasibility study of a nurse-led intervention to prevent acute stress and long-term morbidity', *BMJ Open*, 8 (7): 1–12.

Whitehouse, T., Snelson, C. and Grounds, M. (eds) (2014) *Intensive Care Society Review of Best Practice for Analgesia and Sedation in the Critical Care*. Available from https://www.ics.ac.uk/ICS/ICS/GuidelinesAndStandards/ICSGuidelines.aspx as 'Sedation for Patients in ICU' (accessed October 29, 2020).

Wilson, M., Beesley, S., Grow, A., Rubin, E., Hopkins, R., Hajizadeh, N. and Brown, S.M. (2019) 'Humanizing the intensive care unit', *Critical Care*, 23 (32): 2327–7. Available from https://ccforum.biomedcentral.com/articles/10.1186/s13054-019-2327-7 (accessed October 29, 2020).

THE CRITICAL CARE CONTINUUM

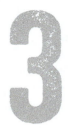

SALLY MOORE AND SAMANTHA FREEMAN

> " It's really hard on the ward when I've got someone sick, but when I ask for help and everyone turns up, I feel part of an amazing team.
>
> **Gemma, Staff Nurse, Medical Admissions Ward** "

> " I spent a day with the outreach team. Really enjoyed it and learned so much about assessment.
>
> **John, 2nd Year Student Nurse** "

LEARNING OUTCOMES

When you have finished studying this chapter you will be able to understand:

- The recent changes to what we understand as Critical Care
- The organisational approaches and some educational strategies to Critical Care services
- Critical Care for the person deteriorating on the ward
- The escalation and de-escalation of the level of care and intervention

INTRODUCTION

In this chapter, building on Chapters 1 and 2, we will review what is included in the critical services or continuum, how this approach has developed, and educational strategies for critical care nurses. We will also explore local, regional, and national organisational approaches, which help to ensure a high-quality care continuum. We will look at the notion of hospital-wide critical care services as well as the various referral pathways. The different models of critical care outreach are included, and the aims of the service will be discussed. The role of acute care teams in intervening in pre-critical care admission in the emergency recognition and response will be addressed. The assessment of the acutely unwell person will be briefly explored, and this will progress to the internal transfer of critically ill patients to the critical care unit.

We will also examine strategies for recognising and responding to those who are deteriorating and the complex needs of the people who are discharged from critical care to an area of lower dependency.

THE CRITICAL CARE CONTINUUM

Comprehensive Critical Care (CCC) (DOH 2000) stopped us from thinking of critical care as a geographical location within a hospital but rather a clinical need for the individual. This turn of the century document spoke of critical care as 'encompassing the whole of the patient's pathway' and was intended to explicitly meet 'the needs of the patient' and be 'patient focused'. This publication from an expert group in response to Critical to Success (Audit Commission, 1999) prompted clinicians to examine the pathway before and after a critical care admission which is referred to as the Critical Care continuum.

Pathways through critical care services

The reasons for a critical care admission are numerous and varied. Generally, admissions to the department come via four main routes, these being:

1. Following planned listed surgery
2. Following emergency surgery
3. From the emergency department
4. From the ward areas

In Activity 3.1 you will be exploring the data about admission in more detail and considering possible reasons for any differences observed.

ACTIVITY 3.1: CRITICAL THINKING

Nationally, approximately 23 percent of admissions are planned and the remainder of admissions arrived via an unplanned route. The Intensive Care National Audit and Research Centre (ICNARC) collect and collate vast amounts of data surrounding critical care, including admission and survival rates.

Access the ICNARC database via www.icnarc.org/Reporting (accessed October 30, 2020).

Look at each of the pathways above and access the most recent data on pathway-dependent admission and survival rate. Evaluate which pathway is the most common route into critical care. Then look at survival rates.

1. Why do you think this may be?

Those experiencing critical illness and their family also need to navigate lots of different services. The ICUsteps charity has created a roadmap illustrating the critical illness journey.

You can access the roadmap here: https://icusteps.org/assets/files/critical-illness-roadmap.pdf (accessed October 30, 2020).

Changes to what we understand as Critical Care

The Audit Commission's *Critical to Success* (1999) and the Department of Health's *Comprehensive Critical Care (CCC)* (2000) were pivotal in promoting the modernisation of Critical Care. CCC changed our focus from 'Intensive Care' being a specific ward, to Critical Care as a clinical need of an individual anywhere in the hospital and described this as being 'Critical Care without walls'. The paper acknowledged the importance of the pathway pre- and post-Critical Care admission, or the Critical Care Continuum. The CCC (DOH, 2000) review advocated a modernisation of Critical Care services, which was supported by 'The NHS Plan' later the same year. This promised a 30 per cent increase in adult critical care beds. Subsequent guidelines produced by the National Institute of Clinical Excellence continue to shape our Critical Care services. In Activity 3.2 you will be studying the differences between different sources of evidence.

ACTIVITY 3.2: RESEARCH AND EVIDENCE-BASED PRACTICE

Consider the differences between policies, guidelines, standard operating procedures, recommendations, mandated services and targets, and how they may impact your practice.

1. How are research and evidence used to guide them?
2. What is the mechanism of them being filtered through senior management teams and getting to the 'shop floor'?

WHAT'S THE EVIDENCE?

Given what we have covered so far, familiarise yourself with the following papers:

*   Department of Health (2000) *Comprehensive Critical Care: A Review of Adult Critical Care Services.* London: Department of Health. Available from https://webarchive.nationalarchives.gov.uk/+/

(Continued)

http://www.dh.gov.uk/en/Publicationsandstatistics/Publications/PublicationsPolicyAndGuidance/
DH_4006585 (accessed October 30, 2020).
- National Institute for Health and Care Excellence (NICE) (2007) *Acutely Ill Patients in Hospital: Recognition of and Response to Acute Illness in Adults in Hospital* (Clinical Guideline 50). London: NICE. Available from www.nice.org.uk/guidance/cg50 (accessed October 30, 2020).

Do you think the evidence presented above, which was published between 2000–2007, has been implemented, or does it still reflect some of the issues in acute care?
There is no template answer to this question as it is based on your reflection.

Advances in therapeutic interventions, diagnostics, and monitoring require progressive thinking about how people are assessed as suitable for Critical Care admission. We need to consider how such advances can affect each individual's recovery with a consideration of the risk versus benefits that these interventions pose.

Critical care is a research-intensive area although nursing research is in its infancy. As evidence is generated, as noted in Chapter 1, practice needs to change to incorporate these new research findings. Having an awareness of the theory that can support changes in practice can support the healthcare practitioner in this process.

THIS TOPIC
IS ALSO
COVERED IN
CHAPTER 1

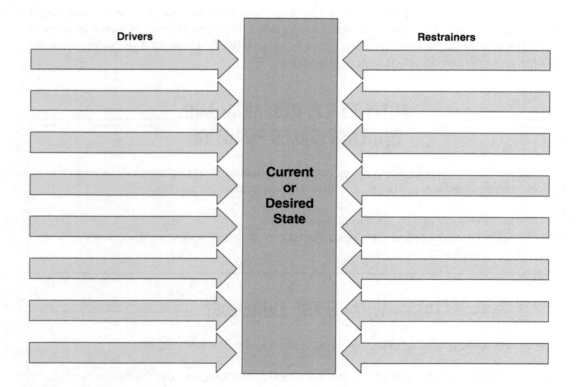

Figure 3.1 Force field analysis

Source: K. Lewin's force field analysis (1951), Figure 9.3 in Burns (2019) 'Developing practice and managing change',p. 229.

ACTIVITY 3.3: THEORY STOP POINT

There are a number of change management theories. One popular theory you may have read about is Lewin's (1951). Before any change in practice is considered, Lewin suggests that the drivers for the change or the barriers should be identified. He refers to this as a force field analysis.

Consider a change of practice you think you would like to implement.

Use Figure 3.1 to consider drivers or barriers.

1.   If you have too many barriers, how could you overcome these?

There is no template answer to this activity, as it is based on your reflection.

To understand more about change management read:

Burns, D. (2019) 'Developing Practice and Managing Change', in D. Burns (ed.), *Foundations of Adult Nursing* (2nd edition). London: Sage. pp. 221-46.

ORGANISATIONAL APPROACHES TO CRITICAL CARE

Critical care units are one part of a much larger institution. Optimal utilisation of critical care beds as part of this larger structure is a complex task of balancing need and availability. Ideally, there would always be a level 2 or level 3 bed available for every admission that requires it so that we may smoothly move patients along the continuum.

To manage the resource, it is necessary to have an overview of the whole organisation, to decide on the most appropriate use of beds. This may mean an elective surgical procedure is cancelled, as the bed is needed for someone acutely deteriorating, who takes priority. These are decisions that senior nurses and doctors are making every day. We will look at these pressures in the context of the most extreme situations, such as a major incident, later in this chapter.

THIS TOPIC IS ALSO COVERED IN CHAPTER 1

To address these pressures, several approaches have been employed at local, regional, and national levels. Locally, specialist teams and individuals fulfil roles of reviewing anyone deteriorating within the ward environment and intervene. This is to prevent further deterioration and possibly the need for a critical care admission or managing the situation whilst waiting for a critical care bed to become available. Similar teams and specialists can support those going to a ward, facilitating an earlier discharge from critical care and preventing re-admissions.

Regional Critical Care networks promote cooperation between hospitals in neighbouring areas. As well as a shared approach to research and education to ensure best practice, beds can be optimised regionally through agencies that record and share bed availability. Regional networks have specialist working groups looking at all aspects of critical care, including a broad view regarding the patients' pathway before and after their critical care admission.

AIMS OF CRITICAL CARE OUTREACH

The general aims of critical care outreach are:

*   To assess the acutely unwell person, advise the personal care team, and stabilise
*   To ensure timely referral and admission to critical care, if appropriate

- To follow up those who transfer out of critical care
- To share knowledge and skills with the team of staff working in the ward environment

Unfortunately, there is no one approach to the provision of critical care outreach services and the level of provision can vary enormously across the UK and internationally. The National Outreach Forum (NOrF, 2012: 4) defines Comprehensive Critical Care Outreach (C3O) as 'A multidisciplinary organisational approach to ensure safe, equitable and quality care for all acutely unwell, critically ill and recovering patients irrespective of location or pathway.'

Nurse-led critical care outreach teams (CCOTs) will have broad experience, skills, and competencies. This is to support the ward staff when caring for a deteriorating person, with the aim of preventing critical care admissions or acknowledging the need for admission and facilitating this quickly. Education through sharing knowledge and skills with ward staff completes the three core functions of such teams.

These teams are staffed by experienced senior critical care nurses with the ability to assess and manage someone who is becoming acutely unwell. They will guide and support ward nurses in caring for the acutely unwell. They provide support with clinical skills, create a management plan, and liaise with all relevant teams to ensure the correct input and support is received.

EDUCATIONAL STRATEGIES

The Resuscitation Council UK (RCUK, 2015) list education as the first link in the 'Chain of Prevention' for cardiac arrest.

One approach would be to employ the service to improve the education of staff working with the acutely ill in Level 1 areas. A criticism of CCOTs has been that they de-skill ward-based nurses. On the contrary, CCC (2000) foresaw a central role of these teams as educational. Equipping staff with the skills to accurately monitor, correctly interpret observations, recognise deterioration, and implement an ABCDE approach to stabilising the patient requires multiple formal and informal approaches.

> [...] ability of a system to achieve [its] goals hinges on [...] continual training (and retraining) of clinical staff (Rothman, 2018).

Some care providers have an escalation model that relies solely on a ward level response with assigned responder roles and responsibilities for interventions when someone becomes acutely unwell. Ongoing education for these staff with no support external to the ward is paramount. In Activity 3.4 you will be looking into your local provision in relation to critical care outreach services.

ACTIVITY 3.4: RESEARCH AND EVIDENCE-BASED PRACTICE

Take some time to explore your local provision in relation to critical care outreach services.

1.   What do you think are the limits of these services and the challenges of their implementation?

OTHER MODELS OF CRITICAL CARE SERVICES

Other approaches implemented to manage the deterioration of someone acutely unwell in a ward setting may be to utilise teams external to the ward areas. This may be a medical emergency team or rapid response team, a multidisciplinary team experienced in emergency medicine or critical care. A medium level response strategy can be a nurse led Critical Care Outreach Team (CCOT), Hospital at Night team, or a specialty trainee (NICE, 2007).

Locally agreed policies will stipulate why and when these teams will be contacted and the remit of the team. This variety and team structure, response, and name have led to difficulty in assessing their effectiveness (Garry 2018). This, along with a lack of robust trials when they were first implemented, has made research in this area limited and **equivocal** (Bedaya 2019). In an era of limited resources, the cost-effectiveness of all services is a moral responsibility for all service providers. Quantitative research in this area will usually focus on the length of stay hospital, cardiac arrest calls, and **mortality**. Data is generally found to lack figures that show overwhelming statistical significance in favour of this approach to service provision (Garry et al., 2018; Rocha et al., 2018; Bedoya et al., 2019). Nevertheless, culturally, anecdotally and qualitative research clearly illustrates the value of their presence (Garry et al., 2018).

Assessment of the acutely unwell person

It is widely acknowledged that the recognition and treatment of an acutely deteriorating person is an ongoing challenge (McQuillan et al., 1999; NCEPOD, 2005, NICE, 2007). Failure to recognise those who are becoming unwell prevents them from receiving the care and management they require. A delay to definitive treatment has been shown as a prognostic indicator of a poor outcome (Fernando, 2019).

A report by The National Confidential Enquiry into Patient Outcome and Death (2005) found alarming data which confirmed that this lack of recognition was a national issue and urgent action was required.

McQuillan et al. (1999) produced a seminal study highlighting the urgency and gravity of the systematic failure to recognise the deteriorating person. The initial challenge is for the deterioration to be acknowledged in a timely way. Early identification of a person who is becoming acutely unwell continued to be an ongoing problem (NPSA, 2007b).

ACTIVITY 3.5: REFLECTIVE PRACTICE

1. Can you think of an occasion when you were looking after someone who became unwell?
2. How did you know they were deteriorating?
3. Who did you tell? What happened next?
4. Were they transferred to a higher level of care?
5. Could the management of the situation have been improved?

There is no template answer to this activity as it is based on your reflection.

As noted earlier, there are several routes a person can take before their admission to critical care. Those admitted via the elective post-operative route have either been booked in for a critical care bed due to the nature of the surgery or their current comorbidity. The mechanism for recognising a person on the ward or within an emergency department that needs expert assessment and input, and possibly an escalation of care, is a more complex task. Activity 3.5 asks you to reflect on a time where you have looked after someone who may be deteriorating.

There are nationally agreed programmes of study that relate to the management of those who are deteriorating. You may want to find out if your undergraduate organisation or employer provides the Acute Illness Management or Acute Life-Threatening Events Recognition and Treatment Course or similar.

A strategy that assists the clinician with timely recognition of deterioration is a physiological track and trigger scoring system or Early Warning Score (EWS). Used alongside observations, the system generates an aggregate score; a locally agreed response strategy will direct action according to the score. Use of such a track and trigger system is widespread throughout the UK and there is a move towards a standardization of the tool throughout all health care facilities and providers to promote continuity (Royal College of Physicians, 2017). Different early warning scores exist and can be related to specific client groups such as maternal or paediatric. Further differences in EWS tools may be related to the preference of the hospital where a locally agreed modified tool is employed. It has been argued that this can lead to an error when clinicians are moving between different care providers or clinical areas using different tools (Downey et al., 2019). Variety can also be seen in how documentation of observations and scores are managed. Paper charts can still be found but are being replaced with electronic systems, which may help to prevent charting and calculation errors. These systems can also remove the subjectivity of the decision to escalate by generating automatic notifications according to present escalation parameters. In Activity 3.6 you will reflect on the use of track and trigger systems.

ACTIVITY 3.6: REFLECTIVE PRACTICE

In light of what you have read so far, consider acute areas where you have worked.

1. What track and trigger tools have you used?
2. What were the different mechanisms you have encountered for raising concerns about someone when they are deteriorating?

A national track and trigger tool has been implemented (NEWS 2) and you can access more information via www.england.nhs.uk/ourwork/clinical-policy/sepsis/nationalearlywarningscore/ (accessed October 30, 2020).

3. Is this different from any track and trigger tools you have previously used?
4. Is it a better tool? What could the benefits or drawbacks of a national tool be?

There is no template answer to this activity as it is based on your reflection.

Alongside the physiological track and trigger system, an objective tool, we also rely upon subjective assessment by staff. Observations and EWS will form part of the assessment but there is a need to ensure that the multi-disciplinary team has the skills and experience to recognise when someone is becoming unwell (NICE, 2007). It is not unusual for a person to be deteriorating with stable observations, and therefore an Early Warning Score, within normal parameters (Fernando et al., 2019). Professional concern should demand a senior review and possibly assessment from critical care teams as appropriate.

The minimum set of observations are:

Respiratory Rate

Heart Rate

Blood pressure

Saturations

Temperature

Level of consciousness

(NICE, 2007)

The clinician performing the observations should be someone trained and capable of doing so correctly with the knowledge of how to respond appropriately. In the following case study about Carol, you will need to consider what the change to her condition is indicating.

ACTIVITY 3.7: CASE STUDY

You have been looking after Carol, 64, for the last 2 days. Carol is being treated for infective **exacerbation** of Chronic Obstructive Pulmonary Disease. Today, whilst Carol's observations are within a normal range, you feel she isn't as well. Carol is drowsy and lethargic with some subtle signs of confusion; her respiratory rate is normal but her breathing looks laboured.

1. What could these changes be a sign/symptom of?
2. How will you escalate your concerns?

ONGOING ASSESSMENT AND MONITORING

NICE (2007a) and NPSA (2007b) demand that for 'high- and medium-score groups', health care professionals should:

- Initiate appropriate interventions
- Assess response
- Formulate a management plan, including location and level of care

The ABCDE approach (also known as the A-E approach)

Following these and other recommendations (NCEPOD, 2005; NICE, 2007) clinicians should employ an:

Airway

Breathing

Circulation

Disability

Exposure

approach (RCUK, 2015).

Using this structured approach addresses and treats life-threatening problems in order of priority (RCUK, 2015). That is, an airway problem must be assessed and treated before moving on to the breathing assessment and interventions, and so on. The clinician needs to re-assess to ensure the impact of each intervention has been beneficial. Throughout the assessment, the clinician must consider if additional help is required and request this in an appropriate and timely way.

Communicating the assessment to colleagues with a clear request for specific support is preferably performed using a structured communication tool. In Activity 3.8 you will look at one of the most commonly used communication tools.

ACTIVITY 3.8: CRITICAL THINKING

The RCUK (2015) suggests the use of the SBAR communication tool.

Situation
Background
Assessment
Recommendation

SBAR is a structured method for communicating critical information that requires immediate attention.
Access more information here: https://improvement.nhs.uk/documents/2162/sbar-communication-tool.pdf (accessed October 31, 2020) or on the RCUK website: www.resus.org.uk/resuscitation-guidelines/in-hospital-resuscitation/ (accessed October 31, 2020).

1. Have you used the SBAR tool in your practice and if so, was it effective?
2. If not, can you see how it may help deliver information?
3. Are there any limitations to the tool?

Appropriate monitoring should be instigated; this may be possible through standard ward equipment. Alternatively, a monitor may be required for greater supervision of the person's condition. This can give a constant display of heart rate and rhythm, oxygen saturation, and respiratory rate and can be set to cycle through regular blood pressure checks. It needs to be considered if there are staff present who are familiar with the equipment, skilled in recognising problems, and whose workload will allow for regular inspection of the monitor. If a person requires this level of monitoring, they should be in a clinical area that can facilitate this.

Additional information as part of the assessment will be gained from taking a history from the person and reviewing notes, medications, results, and Recommended Summary Plan for Emergency Care and Treatment (ReSPECT) forms. They can be found at https://www.resus.org.uk/respect/respect-healthcare-professionals (accessed October 31, 2020). The ReSPECT form is a summary plan that records recommendations to guide clinical decision-making in a future emergency.

In the case below about Julia, you will need to consider what she is at increased risk from, and the potential interventions and monitoring you may need to think of.

ACTIVITY 3.9: CASE STUDY

Julia, 43, is currently receiving chemotherapy for breast cancer. She has been admitted with a three-day history of **diarrhoea** and vomiting and had her last cycle of chemotherapy 6 days ago. Julia is hypotensive and tachycardic.

1. What is Julia at risk of?
2. What interventions and monitoring would you implement?

ESCALATION OR DE-ESCALATION OF CARE

An additional function of the Critical Care Outreach team members is that they start to raise questions regarding escalation or de-escalation of care and resuscitation decisions (Pattison, 2015). Despite best practice recommending early discussion regarding wishes around resuscitation and the need for more intensive interventions, these issues are usually only discussed once the person starts to deteriorate. Pattison (2015) found frequent input from CCOTs involved prompting these considerations and discussions when reviewing a deteriorating person. Garry (2018) highlighted CCOTs acted as advocates and mediators when broaching End of Life Care. In the case study about Andrew, you will need to consider if and how his care should be escalated.

ACTIVITY 3.10: CASE STUDY

You are caring for Andrew, who is 89 years old. He was admitted 6 days ago with heart failure, reduced mobility, poor nutritional intake, and not coping well. Today he has acutely deteriorated and has an elevated EWS due to **hypotension**, tachypnoea, low saturations and has stopped passing urine.

1. What issues do you think should be discussed around the escalation of care for Andrew?

THIS TOPIC IS ALSO COVERED IN CHAPTER 16

The decision about limiting care or deescalating care is not made by the nurse but through a team discussion with the person and after consideration of the family view. The lead consultant then makes the final decision. More guidance and information on this topic can be found in Chapter 16.

ACTIVITY 3.11: CASE STUDY

David, 39, is a type 1 insulin-dependent diabetic with epilepsy. He is in hospital for IV antibiotics due to an infected foot ulcer. David deteriorated this afternoon after a fall and has been reviewed by the CCOT and the critical care medical team and he is scheduled for admission to the critical care unit. He also needs to go for a CT scan of his head.

Currently, David is on 15 lpm oxygen non-rebreathe mask achieving SpO2 94% with a respiratory rate of 9 bpm. His breathing is shallow.

Heart rate is 103 BPM and Blood pressure is 92/52. David is apyrexial.

On the ACVPU scale, David is responding to pain and has had three seizures in the last hour. ACVPU is quick and simple and is particularly helpful when there is a need to make a rapid assessment of a patient's level of consciousness. (For more details see Chapter 11).

1. What preparations are required for this transfer?
2. Consider what equipment is needed.
3. Which staff are needed?
4. What communication needs to take place prior to the transfer?

THIS TOPIC
IS ALSO
COVERED IN
CHAPTER 11

If the decision has been made to de-escalate care, then the outreach team will ensure support is offered for both staff and family. This will normally be the end of their involvement in the person's care although the team will remain a point of contact if required. Sometimes it will be more about supporting the ward team than directly supporting the person or their family.

Transfer of the critically ill

A pre-requisite for admission to a critical care area, aside from the person requiring single or multi-organ support, is that the person will benefit from the support and that the acute condition is reversible.

Transferring the critically ill carries an inherent risk. It exposes the vulnerable person to the possibility of harm from adverse events. Possible causes include equipment failure or human error. We also need to consider that critically ill people are at risk of acute changes in their condition leading to deterioration without being transported (Droogh et al., 2015) and that movement may precipitate this. We must 'anticipate and prepare for all foreseeable adverse events' according to Droogh et al. (2015). Flabouris et al. (2006) found that 91 per cent of adverse incidents during transfers were preventable. The speciality has progressed since this research and local and national guidelines exist along with specialist training to ensure that clinicians are appropriately qualified to transfer someone who is critically ill.

Before moving it should be considered by clinicians if the benefit of the transfer outweighs any likelihood of harm. A transfer may be required to access specialist services, procedures, or interventions such as diagnostic imaging, surgery, or accessing specialist departments. The transfer may need to occur if a critically ill person is moving to a different level of care requiring them to be in a different clinical environment.

Once it is established that the person must be moved, an appropriately qualified and experienced team will prepare the person, equipment, and documentation. As with many situations, clear communication is crucial. Delays between departments must be avoided to prevent unnecessary time in public or less than ideal environments.

The privacy and dignity of the individual being transferred must be protected. Managing possible harms due to pressure area damage, falls, misplacement of lines or other indwelling tubes should be foreseen. Specialist transfer equipment is mandated by regional and national guidelines. This equipment is for the sole use of transfers and is otherwise left charging to ensure full batteries are maintained. A specialist ambulance compatible transfer trolley may be used if transferring the individual on their bed is not suitable. A transfer ventilator may be required so you should be familiar with this piece of equipment. Dedication of specialist equipment for this task has in some way led to a reduction in equipment errors. Further safety initiatives include the use of a checklist (ICS, 2011) during a verbal bedside handover with the allocation of roles and responsibilities for the transfer. Appropriate levels of meticulous planning are required to safely provide this 'mobile' critical care unit (Droogh et al., 2015). Transfer to or from a higher level of care will be an anxious time for the individual. You will need to explain what is going to happen and you may need to answer concerns that will help to allay any fears. In the following case study about David, you need to consider all elements of his transfer.

An additional transfer bag is always taken, which will include a standardised selection of equipment that may be required. You will need to ensure the contents of the bag are regularly checked to guarantee all equipment is present and within expiry dates. You must complete any transferring of notes or personalised documentation in accordance with General Data Protection Regulations. You will need to make special consideration if medications or blood/blood products are being transferred with the critically ill person. You will be supported when learning about all of these checks and procedures.

PREPARATION PRE AND POST-OPERATIVE MANAGEMENT

Recognition that a person who has undergone a surgical procedure is high risk and needs critical care may occur intra- or post-operatively. An urgent critical care bed must then be negotiated. In some cases, the need for a critical care bed may be recognised before the surgery. This may be due to the high-risk nature of the surgery or pre-existing comorbidities. Preparing this cohort for their hospital admission and procedures requires a pre-operative assessment and enrolment in an education programme, which is concerned with optimisation prior to the surgery. These types of initiatives are becoming common practice along with post-operative multi-disciplinary pathways in an effort to reduce preventable surgical mortality and postoperative **pulmonary** complications, and reduce the Length of Stay (Goldhill, 2005). Interventions are 'prescribed' for the post-operative phase and are concerned with respiratory function, oral hygiene, mobility, pain relief, and positioning. Cassidy et al. (2020) has devised the mnemonic 'iCough' which is designed to reduce pulmonary complications following surgery.

Pathways like the iCough protocol are used whether the person is going to a ward or critical care after surgery. For those being admitted to a critical care area after their procedure Berg et al. (2006) suggest information-giving as a method of reducing anxiety, which many people awaiting elective surgery suffer from. Informing the person about the nature of interventions and monitoring they may experience, and in some hospitals offering a visit prior to the surgery, can help dispel fears. As mentioned in Chapter 1, the critical care environment can be overwhelming due to noise, lighting, lack of sleep, and levels of interventions. Some people can suffer from anxiety, **delirium**, sleep disturbance, and **PTSD**-like symptoms after a critical care admission, and this group of people admitted electively may experience these as much as any other group. They should be assessed, and their post Critical Care rehabilitation planned, as with any other admission (NICE, 2007). Rehabilitation after critical care will be expanded upon in Chapter 17.

THIS TOPIC
IS ALSO
COVERED IN
CHAPTER 17

Individuals who are admitted to critical care via one of the unplanned pathways miss out on this level of intervention and support.

THE MAJOR INCIDENT AND CRITICAL CARE

Never are the finite resources of hospitals, and, more specifically for our discussion, critical care facilities, under greater pressures than during a major event. NHS England (2015) defines a major incident as one 'whose impact cannot be handled within routine services arrangements' and where there is a 'serious threat to health'. The NHS England (2015) preparedness, resilience, and response framework describes nine types of Major Event. Forward planning within the NHS and critical care services needs to consider managing these different types of incidents which can affect the provision of services in different ways. A major incident will create a demand surge and capacity pressures, but these may present in differing ways:

- 'Big blast' scenario, such as a bomb blast
- Air crash
- Major RTA (road traffic accident)

These will create an immediate need for greatly increased resources that will then peak and settle over a short period of time. The second scenario type is of a slower onset but the increased capacity needs to be extended over longer periods such as an epidemic or pandemic. Both of these scenarios present their own challenges.

A mass casualty event

With a mass casualty event, the focus will initially be the Emergency Department, triage will be crucial to ensure the individuals with the most need have access to critical care; this will include those not involved in the incident. There will be a need to determine how critical care facilities can be increased by accessing additional staff and utilising additional areas of the hospital with the infrastructure to support critical care admissions such as theatres and recovery. Alternatively, reducing resource usage can be beneficial by cancelling planned procedures, postponing any tests and investigations. To be able to deliver a major event plan, Carter (2014) talks of the need for staff to be educated and trained regarding the plan. A resilient communication and collaboration system needs to be in place between critical care and 'key interface departments [...] locally regionally and nationally'.

A slower onset event

The extended response required of a pandemic or epidemic may be further complicated with staff absence due to sickness. Staff support post-event may take the shape of an acute 'hot' debrief, a 'cold' debrief, or a longer-term therapeutic intervention dependent upon the needs of the workforce.

Critical Care is no longer just a department within a hospital but a clinical need of an individual. This must be provided wherever they are and means that the right people with the right skills go to the person at the right time. The responsibilities of the Critical Care team extend far beyond the walls of the Critical Care Unit and also beyond the days spent on the unit to the entire pathway either side of the critical care admission.

CHAPTER SUMMARY

This chapter has supported your understanding of the following topics:

- The development and provision of critical care services
- The importance of following a structured assessment when with someone who is deteriorating
- The roles and responsibility of critical care outreach
- The pathways of admission to a critical care unit

GO FURTHER

Books

Adam, A.K., Odell, M. and Welch, J. (2009) *Rapid Assessment of the Acutely Ill Patient.* Oxford: Wiley Blackwell.

Clarke, D. and Malecki-Ketchell, A. (2016) *Nursing the Acutely Ill Adult* (2nd edition). London: Palgrave.

Tait, D., James, J., Williams, C. and Barton, D. (2012) *Acute and Critical Care in Adult Nursing* (2nd edition). London: Sage.

- All of these books will give you detailed information on the assessment and management of the acutely unwell person with more of a ward-based context.

Useful websites

www.ics.ac.uk/ (accessed October 30, 2020).

- This is a website run by the ICS, however, the guidelines and standards they publish are accessible for non-members. It does have more of a medical focus but has useful guidelines on the provision of intensive care services.

www.respectprocess.org.uk/ (accessed October 30, 2020).

- This website contains further information about the ReSPECT form, which is a summary plan that records recommendations to guide clinical decision-making in a future emergency.

www.norf.org.uk/ (accessed October 30, 2020).

- This website is for the National Outreach Forum. There are several resources on the site regarding various aspects of care related to outreach services.

Journal articles

Harris, S., Singer, M., Sanderson, C., Grieve, R., Harrison, D., and Rowan, K. (2018) 'Impact on mortality of prompt admission to critical care of deteriorating ward patients', *Intensive Care Medicine*, 55 (5): 606–15.

So, H.M., Yan, W.W., Ying, S. (2018) 'A nurse-led critical care outreach programme to reduce readmission to the intensive care unit: A quasi-experimental study with a historical control group', *Australian Critical Care*. doi.org/10.1016/j.aucc.2018.11.005

Fritz, Z., Slowther, A.M. and Perkins, G. (2017) 'Resuscitation policy should focus on the patient, not the decision', *British Medical Journal*, 356: j813.

REFERENCES

Audit Commission (1999) *Critical to Success: The Place of Efficient and Effective Critical Care Services Within the Acute Hospital*. London: Audit Commission.

Bedoya, A.D., Clement, M.E., Phelan, M., Steorts, R.C., O'Brien, C. and Goldstein. B.A. (2019) 'Minimal impact of implemented Early Warning Score and best practice alert for patient deterioration', *Critical Care Medicine*, 47 (1): 49–55. doi.org/10.1097/CCM.0000000000003439

Berg, A., Fleischer, S., Keller, M. and Neubert, T.R. (2006) 'Preoperative information for intensive care unit patients to reduce anxiety during and after the ICU stay: Protocol of a randomised controlled trial', *BMC Nursing* 5: Article #4. doi.org/10.1186/1472-6955-5-4

Carter, C. (2014) 'Managing a major incident in the critical care unit', *Nursing Standard*, 28 (31): 39–44. doi.org/10.7748/ns2014.04.28.31.39.e8566

Cassidy, M.R., Rosenkranz, P., Macht, R.D., Talutis, S. and McAneny, D. (2020) 'The ICOUGH Multidisciplinary Perioperative Pulmonary Care Program: One decade of experience',. *The Joint Commission Journal on Quality and Patient Safety*, 46: 241–49. https://doi.org/10.1016/j. jcjq.2020.01.005. (accessed January 7, 2021).

Department of Health (2000) *Comprehensive Critical Care: A Review of Adult Critical Care Services*. London: Department of Health. http://webarchive.nationalarchives.gov.uk/20130107105354/ http://www.dh.gov.uk/prod_consum_dh/groups/dh_digitalassets/@dh/@en/documents/ digitalasset/dh_4082872.pdf (accessed October 30, 2020).

Downey, C.L., Tahir, W. Randell. R., Brown, J.M. and Jayne, D.G. (2017) 'Strengths and limitations of early warning scores: A systematic review and narrative synthesis', *International Journal of Nursing Studies*, 76: 106–19. doi.org/10.1016/j.ijnurstu.2017.09.003

Droogh, J.M., Smit, M., Absalom, A.M., Ligtenberg, J.J.M., and Zijlstra, J.G. (2015) 'Transferring the critically ill patient: Are we there yet?', *Critical Care*, 19 (1): Article #62. doi.org/10.1186/s13054-015-0749-4

Fernando, S.M., Fox-Robichaud, A.E., Rochwerg, B., Cardinal, P., Seely, A.J.E., Perry, J.J., [...] and Kyeremanteng, K. (2019) 'Prognostic accuracy of the Hamilton Early Warning Score (HEWS) and the National Early Warning score (NEWS2) among hospitalised patients assessed by a rapid response team', *Critical Care*, 23: Article #60. doi.org/10.1186/s13054-019-2355-3

Flabouris, A., Runciman, W.B. and Levings, B. (2006) 'Incidents during out-of-hospital transportation', *Anaesthesia and Intensive Care*, 34 (2): 228–36.

Garry, L., Rohan, N., O'Connor, T., Patton, D. and Moore, Z. (2018) 'Do nurse led critical care outreach services impact inpatient mortality rates?', *Nursing in Critical Care*, 24 (1): 40–6. doi. org/10.1111/nicc.12391

Goldhill, D.R. (2005) 'Preventing surgical deaths: Critical care and intensive care outreach services in the postoperative period', *British Journal of Anaesthesia*, 95 (1): 88–94. doi.org/10.1093/bja/aeh281

Intensive Care Society (2011) *Guidelines for the Transport of the Critically Ill Adult* (3rd edition). London: Intensive Care Society.

McQuillan, P., Pilkington, S., Allan, A., Taylor, B., Short, A. and Morgan, G. (1998) 'Confidential inquiry into quality of care before admission to intensive care', *British Medical Journal*, 316 (7148): 1853–8.

National Confidential Enquiry into Patient Outcomes and Death (NCEPOD) (2005) *An Acute Problem?* London: NCEPOD. Available from https://www.ncepod.org.uk/2005aap.html (accessed October 31, 2020).

National Health Service (NHS) (2015) *Emergency Preparedness, Resilience and Response Framework*. Redditch: NHS. Available from https://www.england.nhs.uk/ourwork/eprr/ (accessed October 31, 2020).

National Institute for Health and Care Excellence (NICE) (2007) *Acutely Ill Patients in Hospital: Recognition of and Response to Acute Illness in Adults in Hospital* (Clinical Guideline 50). London: NICE. Available from www.nice.org.uk/guidance/cg50 (accessed October 30, 2020).

National Outreach Forum (NOrF) (2012) *Operating Standards and Competencies for Critical Care Outreach Services*. National Outreach Forum. Available from www.norf.org.uk/Resources/Documents/NOrF%20CCCO%20and%20standards/NOrF%20Operational%20Standards%20and%20Competencies%201%20August%202012.pdf (accessed October 30, 2020).

National Patient Safety Agency (NPSA) (2007a) *Safer Care for the Acutely Ill Patient: Learning from Serious Incidents*. London: NPSA. Available from https://webarchive.nationalarchives.gov.uk/20171030124149/http://www.nrls.npsa.nhs.uk/resources/?entryid45=59828&p=15 (accessed October 30, 2020).

National Patient Safety Agency (NPSA) (2007b) *Recognising and Responding Appropriately to Early Signs of Deterioration in Hospitalised Patients*. London: NPSA. Available from https://webarchive.nationalarchives.gov.uk/20171030124453/http://www.nrls.npsa.nhs.uk/resources/?entryid45=59834&p=13 (accessed October 30, 2020).

Pattison. N., O'Gara, G. and Wigmore, T. (2015) 'Negotiating transitions: Involvement of critical care outreach teams in end-of-life decision making', *American Journal of Critical Care Medicine*, 24 (3): 232–40. doi.org/10.4037/ajcc2015715

Resuscitation Council UK (RCUK) (2015) *Advanced Life Support Manual* (7th edition). London: RCUK.

Rocha, H.A.L., de Castro Alcantara, A.C., Rocha, S.G.M.O. and Toscano, C.M. (2018) 'Efetividade do uso de times de resposta rápida para reduzir a ocorrência de parada cardíaca e mortalidade hospitalar: Uma revisão sistemática e metanálise [Effectiveness of rapid response teams in reducing intrahospital cardiac arrests and deaths: A systematic review and meta-analysis]', *Revista Brasileira de Terapia Intensiva*, 30 (3): 366–75. https://pubmed.ncbi.nlm.nih.gov/30328990/ (accessed January 7, 2021)

Royal College of Physicians (RCP) (2017) *National Early Warning Score 2 (NEWS 2): Standardising the Assessment of Acute Illness Severity in the NHS*. London: Royal College of Physicians. Available from https://www.rcplondon.ac.uk/projects/outputs/national-early-warning-score-news-2 (accessed October 30, 2020).

INFECTION PREVENTION AND CONTROL IN THE ADULT CRITICAL CARE UNIT

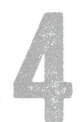

MARK COLE

> " When you start your nurse education, you hear a lot about infection control and vulnerable patients. But it's not until you experience something like critical care that you begin to really appreciate it. The devices, the antibiotics, the other co-morbidities, it really makes you think. What can I do and how can I do it better? "
>
> **Lizzie, 3rd Year Nursing Student**

> " (The Adult Nurse) Initiates and maintains appropriate measure to prevent and control infection according to route of transmission of micro-organism, in order to protect service users, members of the public and other staff.
>
> **(Nursing and Midwifery Council, 2018)** "

LEARNING OUTCOMES

When you have finished studying this chapter you will be able to:

- Describe and apply the cycle of infection
- Appreciate the enhanced risk to patients in critical care environments
- Understand the importance of optimum antibiotic stewardship
- Recognise the role hand hygiene plays as a mediator of cross infection
- Have an awareness of the bundled approach to prevent infection.

INTRODUCTION

HealthCare Associated Infection (HCAI) can be defined as an infection a patient acquires while receiving medical treatment that was not present or incubating at the time of admission (World Health Organisation (WHO), 2011). It is the most common adverse incident experienced by people in hospital and is something that permeates all health care systems regardless of the resources available. In Europe, on any given day, approximately 80,000 individuals have at least one HCAI, entwined with increased **morbidity, mortality**, antibiotic resistance, prolonged lengths of stay and overall social and economic costs. This can result in people experiencing unnecessary levels of fear and anxiety who have been fed a media diet of superbugs, dirty hospitals and flesh-eating bacteria. The Adult Critical Care Unit (ACCU) has the highest prevalence of HCAI. In a recent European study that examined the incidence and distribution of HCAI in ACCU, 8.4% of patients whose stay exceeded two days had either healthcare associated pneumonia, bloodstream infection or a urinary tract infection (European Centre Disease Prevention and Control (ECDPC), 2016).

CHAIN OF INFECTION

The 'chain or circle of infection' is a well-established framework that helps us to understand how disease causing microbes can move between people (Centre for Disease Control (CDC), 2016) (see Figure 4.1). It is called a chain because it is built on the idea that for an infection to occur a series of sequential links, or events, needs to take place. Like any chain however, transmission is only as strong as its weakest part. If, as healthcare professionals, you can target the chain at single or multiple points, through evidence-based **intervention**s, the transmission of HCAI becomes less likely. This chapter will use the chain of infection as a backdrop to discuss the infection risks that are present within the ACCU and how you can use infection prevention and control (IPC) strategies to prevent and control infection. We can begin this by considering the factors in Activity 4.1.

ACTIVITY 4.1: CRITICAL THINKING

Think of patients you have cared for in a critical care setting.

1.   What factors do you think made them more vulnerable to HCAI?

It might help to think of these in terms of the treatments they have received, the co-morbidities they have, plus the resources available to you and the behaviour of your colleagues.
    Write these down and we will return to them later in the chapter.

MICROBES AND THEIR RESERVOIRS

The first two components of the chain, the infectious agent and its reservoir, describe a microbe that has the ability to cause disease and the 'place' where it can live and multiply. Broadly the 'place' could be a person, for example, a health care worker (HCW) a patient or relative. Or it could be the inanimate

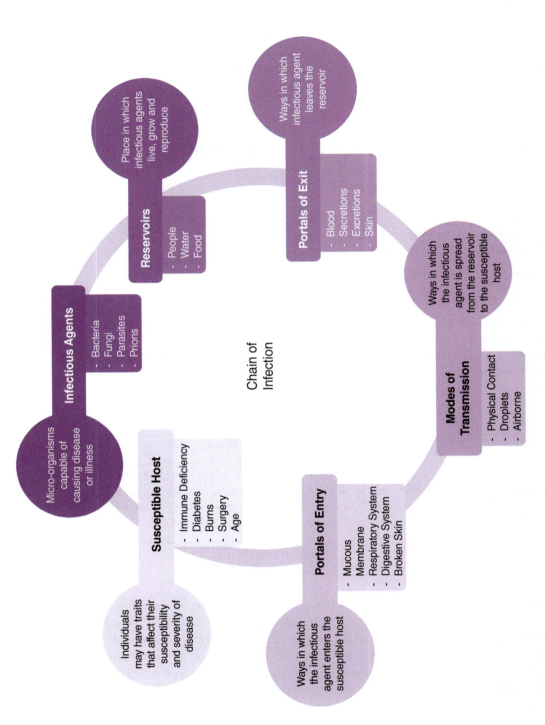

Figure 4.1 The Chain of Infection

environment, a building, its furnishings or the equipment that you use in the delivery of care. The human body is a rich reservoir of bacteria and can be colonised by up to 39 trillion bacterial cells. This is referred to as the human microbiota. In health the human microbiota is restricted to certain body zones where it performs the vital role of microbial antagonism. That is, the more benign, health promoting organisms colonise the body the more they 'crowd out' and remove the space required for more pathogenic material to grow and cause disease.

ACTIVITY 4.2: REFLECTIVE PRACTICE

Think of a patient who has a critical illness.

1. What parts of their body are normally 'sterile', and which are colonised with bacteria?
2. How does their body function to separate the two zones?
3. What treatments might someone receive that compromises this?

However, an individual's microbiota is a dynamic process that is sensitive to environmental factors, to the insertion of devices that promote the formation of abnormal colonisations and to therapeutic agents like antibiotics. Due to the severity of individuals' clinical conditions, the demand for antibiotics in ACCU is high.

WHAT'S THE EVIDENCE?

In a recent nationwide prevalence study in England the number of patients on at least one antibiotic in ACCU was 60.8%. This compared to 34.7% in the general adult sector (Health Protection Agency, 2012). In 2019 antibiotic usage in ACCU was 55.6 defined daily doses (DDDs) compared to an average of 4.28 DDDs in other areas of a hospital (Public Health England, 2020).

The high use of antibiotics in the ACCU is problematic as it creates something called a selective pressure on a person's microbiota. Selective pressure can be thought of as an influence that is exerted by some factor (such as an antibiotic) on natural selection to promote one group of organisms over another. So, in other words, the use of broad-spectrum antibiotics depletes the population of commensal microbes and replaces them with multidrug-resistant or extensively drug-resistant bacteria. The group of microbes implicated in this have been given the acronym ESCAPE. This has been summarised by Johnson and Banks (2017) and we have captured this in Table 4.1.

Table 4.1 Multi drug resistant organisms in the ACCU

	ESCAPE
E	Enterococcus faecium (vancomycin resistance – VRE)
S	Staphylococcus aureus (methicillin resistance – MRSA, vancomycin intermediate resistance – VISA, vancomycin resistance – VRSA). S. pneumoniae (penicillin resistance)
C	Clostridium difficile
A	Acinetobacter baumannii (carbapenem, cephalosporin, aminoglycoside and quinolone resistance)
P	Pseudomonas aeruginosa (carbapenem resistance) This can occur within 48-72 hours of admission and worsens during a patient's stay in the hospital
E	Enterobacteriaceae (which encompasses K. pneumoniae, Enterobacter species and E. coli – 3rd generation cephalosporin and carbapenem resistance)

Source: Johnson, I. and Banks, V. (2017) Antibiotic stewardship in critical care, *BJA Education* 17: 111-16.

The same process of selective pressure can take place in the patient's immediate environment. How far inanimate surfaces form reservoirs of cross infection is a contentious point. But there is an increasing evidence base that suggests they can be a significant source of HCAI.

=== **WHAT'S THE EVIDENCE?** ===

A systematic review by Mitchell et al. (2015) concluded that admission to a room or bed space where a previous occupant was infected or colonised with a specific pathogen increased the risk for subsequent residents.

Authorities in hospital cleaning argue that work specifications should focus on high risk sites. These can be defined as those that are frequently touched, like handles, switches, buttons, knobs and equipment that surrounds the person's bed. The idea here is that the closer you get to the patient the greater confusion on whose responsibility it is to clean and how it should be done (Dancer, 2014). Whether it is the patient's own microbiota or that of the environment, careful **antibiotic stewardship** can reduce the negative impact of selective pressure.

Johnson and Banks (2017 p.112) state that the aim of antibiotic stewardship is to:

administer the right drug at the right time, at the right dose, and for the right duration in order to eradicate infection whilst minimizing collateral damage such as nosocomial infection, drug toxicity, and the emergence of resistance and resultant escalating health care costs.

In an effort to improve antimicrobial prescribing through an organised antimicrobial management programme, Public Health England (2015) recommended a *Start Smart: Then Focus* approach to antibiotic prescriptions. Public Health England prepared a tool kit which is captured by the treatment algorithm in Figure 4.2.

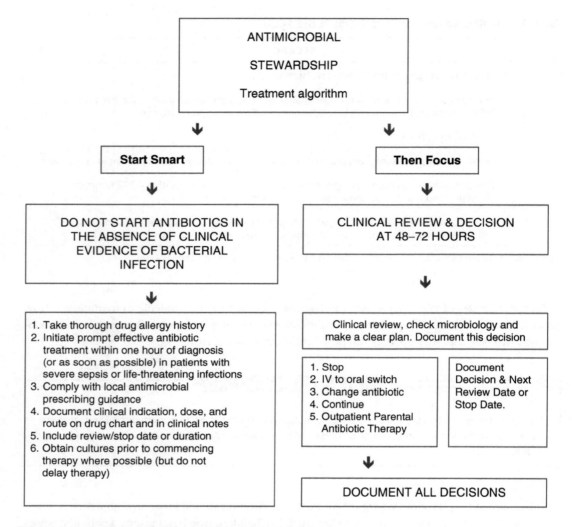

Figure 4.2 Antimicrobial Stewardship Treatment Algorithm

Source: Contains public sector information licensed under the Open Government Licence v3.0. License: http://www.nationalarchives.gov.uk/doc/open-government-licence/version/3/

ACTIVITY 4.3: REFLECTIVE PRACTICE

1. How far does your department follow the principles of Start Smart Then Focus?
2. Do you have local evidence-based guidelines?
3. Are these reviewed regularly?
4. Is prescribing practice audited?
5. Are the results of the audit fed back to prescribers?
6. What more do you think you could do?

There is no template answer to this activity as it is based on your own reflection.

PORTAL OF EXIT - MODE OF TRANSMISSION

Trying to prevent a difficult to treat, multi drug resistant bacteria microbiota in the ACCU are the first two stages of the chain of infection. Judicious antibiotic stewardship programmes and targeted cleaning specifications are both seen as effective preventative strategies. The next links to the chain of infection are the *portal of exit and the mode of transmission*. The portal of exit attends to how the microbe leaves its reservoir and this is traditionally associated with the place where it is normally found. For example, Clostridium difficile exits via the gastrointestinal tract; influenza via the respiratory tract, **Hepatitis** C through breaks in the skin or mucus membranes and the Scabies mite through shedding of the skin.

The mode of transmission has its focus on how the microbe is transmitted to a new host. Loosely, this can be labelled as indirect or direct. Airborne is an example of indirect transmission. Some pathogens will exit the respiratory tract through aerosols, which are very small, lightweight particles that remain suspended in the air for a long time period and can travel lengthy distances. Tuberculosis, Chickenpox and Measles are all examples of microbes that can be transmitted through an airborne route. On occasion you might perform aerosol generating procedures (AGPs). These are procedures where you would put sufficient energy into infectious body fluids to break them up into small enough particles to form aerosols. In this scenario you would need to wear a Fit tested respirator as personal protective equipment (Coia et al., 2013). However, AGPs are not an efficient mechanism to create airborne transmission and close proximity is usually required for cross infection to arise.

In the greater scheme of things airborne transmission is relatively uncommon (Coia et al., 2013). Primarily respiratory pathogens would leave your patient through droplets. This is a form of direct transmission. Droplets are small particles, but they are a lot larger than aerosols. They do not suspend in the air, will often travel less than a metre and fall to the ground within seconds. An example of a droplet infection is influenza. The important point here is that because most patients in ACCU are confined to their beds, direct transmission by some kind of mediator is the most probable cause of cross infection. Logically your contaminated hands, the soiled gloves and aprons you are wearing, or the unclean equipment you are using, are the likely perpetrators. It is important to consider your own safety. Blood and body fluids can be splashed or sprayed during surgical procedures and your eyes, nose and mouth can be vulnerable points of entry. Completing a risk assessment of the task and patient and donning the correct facial protection are important protective measures.

HAND HYGIENE

Hand hygiene, perhaps more than any other topic, has dominated IPC. In their quality standard, NICE wrote:

> Effective hand decontamination, even after wearing gloves, results in significant reductions in the carriage of potential pathogens on the hands and decreases the incidence of preventable healthcare-associated infections, leading in turn to a reduction in morbidity and mortality (NICE, 2014: 17).

Despite its central role the literature is awash with rich descriptions of hand hygiene compliance and how behaviour will often fall short of policy mandates. Typically, these reports come from observational studies, in ACCUs, where care processes can be more predictable and easily observed. Hand hygiene compliance has become an enduring problem and the challenges can be best understood in two areas. The first is when you should decontaminate your hands, the frequency; the second how you should complete the task, your technique.

WHAT'S THE EVIDENCE?

A systematic review by Erasmus et al. (2010) reported that average hand hygiene compliance in ACCUs was 30-40%. It was lower among physicians (32%), than nurses (48%), and lower before patient contact (21%) than following patient contact (47%).

ACTIVITY 4.4: REFLECTIVE PRACTICE

1. Do the figures reported by Erasmus et al. (2010) surprise you?
2. Do wards and departments you have worked on report hand hygiene compliance?
3. Are the figures similar or different to the 30-40% reported in the research literature?
4. If there is a difference, what might explain this?

FREQUENCY

The WHO's five moments for hand hygiene (Figure 4.3) has been widely endorsed throughout the NHS as the times when you should decontaminate your hands. But as indicated by Erasmus et al. (2010) and countless

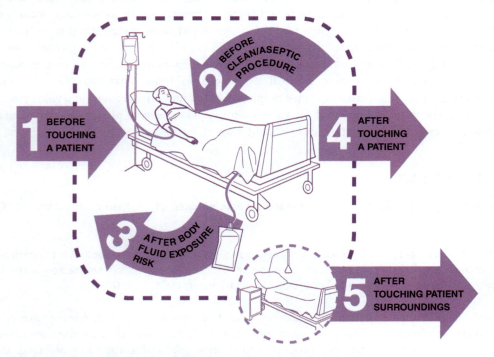

Figure 4.3 World Health Organisations Five Moments of Hand Hygiene

Source: Reproduced by kind permission of the World Health Organization https://www.who.int/campaigns/world-hand-hygiene-day

studies since, compliance with this is often sub-optimum. The reasons for this have become a congested area of research and a large number of organisational and behavioural features have been implicated (WHO, 2009) (see Table 4.2).

Table 4.2 Compliance Factors

Heavy workload	High demand	Lack of role models
Frequent interruptions	Access to facilities	Workplace culture
Distraction	Lack of knowledge	Lack of accountability
Forgetfulness	Sore hands	Scepticism about its value
Other priorities	Wearing gloves	Duration of contact

ACTIVITY 4.5: REFLECTIVE PRACTICE

Think of the list given in Table 4.2. Now think about your own hand hygiene.

1. Which of these factors are the most important to you?
2. How do you think compliance could be improved?

There is no template answer to this activity as it is based on your own reflection.

Something that Erasmus et al. (2010) alluded to and which has been picked up by a number of other authors is that 'the five moments' is not a homogenous model. That is, performance across the five moments varies. For example, compliance is often found to be better after patient contact than before. It is greater if there is contact with body fluids compared to contact with the environment.

ACTIVITY 4.6: CRITICAL THINKING

Think a bit more about the differences in performance across the five moments of hand washing described by Erasmus. What could explain these differences?

Whitby et al. (2007) gave a compelling explanation for why compliance may be better for certain types of contact. He argued that hand hygiene is a habitual practice that is triggered by an emotional feeling of dirtiness, not the removal of transient micro-organisms. In other words, people are programmed from a young age to wash their hands when they feel dirty. As such contact with body fluids makes people feel dirty and it brings out an instinct to wash hands. It is the need for personal protection that drives this behaviour. Contact with a 'clean' environment or social contact, for example taking someone's blood pressure, does not activate the same response. Omissions of hand hygiene are typically seen after these types of clean activities.

Technique

The hand hygiene technique of HCWs has not received the same exposure as their compliance with the five moments of hand hygiene. In part this may be a pragmatic decision based on the view that an opportunity taken is better than no opportunity at all. It may also be due to the practicalities of covertly watching and assessing someone's technique. This is misleading, as a still contaminated hand could become a mediator of cross infection. Skodová et al. (2015) assessed the technique of HCWs using a UV lamp. He found that only 9.5% covered the 5 regions of both hands. The thumbs and fingertips were the most common areas missed. Moreover, staff would frequently wear wrist-watches, bracelets, rings or embellish their hands with long and polished nails that hindered good hand hygiene.

Taking a multimodal approach to compliance is now generally accepted as the most effective method for sustainable hand hygiene improvement (Loveday et al., 2014b). This began with something called the 'Geneva Model', developed by WHO, and implemented as the 'Clean Your Hands Campaign (CYHC)' in England and Wales. The CYHC ran from 2004–2008 across 187 NHS Trusts. It was sponsored by the Department of Health and focussed on the provision of near patient alcohol hand rub (AHR), visual cues in the environment, regular audit and feedback and empowering service users to remind you to clean their hands. The move from washing hands with soap and water to using AHR has possibly become the greatest shift in hand hygiene policy. As stated earlier, the greater the demand for hand hygiene, the more compliance becomes a problem. It has been argued that full compliance using soap and water is not time sustainable (WHO, 2009). AHR on the other hand can be made available at the point of care, is quick to apply and is fast acting. That it is more effective and kinder to hands are other compelling reasons why it compliments, but will not totally replace soap and water. In their evaluation of the CYHC, Stone et al. (2012) reported that the procurement of soap and AHR tripled across 4 years and there were significant reductions in MRSA and C.difficile. You will probably see many aspects of these campaigns still present in clinical practice today. Feel assured they have done much to prevent the burden of HCAI amongst your service users.

ACTIVITY 4.7: CASE STUDY

You, as a student nurse, are working with your practice assessor in an ACCU. You go to use the AHR after completing a patient's clinical observation. Your practice assessor remarks, 'don't use that, you can't beat a bit of soap'.

1. Why do you think she might say that?
2. What impact do you think this standpoint would have on her hand hygiene behaviour?
3. How would you respond?

Gloves and aprons

Over 1.5 billion boxes of disposal gloves are supplied to the NHS each year. These, as well as plastic aprons, are worn by you as a means of interrupting the mode of transmission. Pineles et al.

(2017) swabbed the gloves and aprons of HCWs after completing care in an environment where MRSA was endemic. Across 1,543 interactions, 20% of gloves and 11% of gowns were found to be contaminated with the organism. However, there seems to be a negative correlation between glove use and hand hygiene behaviour: here people use gloves as a substitute for hand hygiene and wear them, as well as plastic aprons, for multiple contacts. The position is clearly complex as gloves and aprons also seem to be worn when they are not indicated. Loveday et al. (2014a) observed 163 glove-use episodes on four wards over 13 hours. Their usage was inappropriate in 42% of cases. The reasons why they were worn when not indicated were personal protection, confusion about when to wear them, social norms and peer pressure and the assumptions that patients preferred it that way. The importance of using gloves and aprons appropriately rests with three arguments. Contaminated apparel if not changed may act as a mediator of cross infection, their unnecessary use is expensive and excessive use of gloves will exacerbate skin problems caused by over-hydration of the skin.

PORTAL OF ENTRY AND SUSCEPTIBLE HOST

Earlier in the chapter you were asked to consider the factors that made individuals in ACCU vulnerable to HCAI. You may have come up with a number of concerns. For ease, in Table 4.3 they have been separated into intrinsic, extrinsic, organisational and behavioural factors.

Table 4.3 Risk Factors for HCAI

Intrinsic	Extrinsic
Age	Invasive devices
Long term conditions	Surgery
Chronic wounds	Antibiotics
Immunosuppression	Corticosteroids
Trauma	
Impaired cognition	

Organisational	Behavioural Factors
Lack of available bed stock	Knowledge and skills
Organisational compliance with regulations	Leadership
Insufficient single rooms	Accountability
Poor access to equipment	Compliance
Length of hospital stay	
Inadequate staffing levels	
Hospital cleanliness	

===== **ACTIVITY 4.8: REFLECTIVE PRACTICE** =====

Consider the list in Table 4.3.

1.   Was it similar to yours?
2.   What do you feel are the major issues in your department?
3.   How easy are these to address?
4.   What can you do to improve matters?

There is no template answer to this activity as it is based on your own reflection.

INVASIVE DEVICES

In this chapter we have considered a range of factors that increase the risk of HCAI in vulnerable critical care populations. However, it is the presence of invasive indwelling devices that breach the skin, or enter a sterile organ, that particularly escalate that level of risk.

Intravascular access devices

The use of intravascular access devices can include peripheral, central venous and arterial catheters. They are an inevitable component of critical care and can be used to administer fluids, blood products, medications, parental nutrition and provide access for **haemodynamic** monitoring. They are also often implicated in a range of local and **systemic** infections. The latest national prevalence survey reported that 64% of bloodstream infections occurred in patients with a vascular access device (Health Protection Agency, 2012). Moreover, bloodstream infections in an ACCU can have a mortality rate of up to 70% (Brooks et al., 2018). The more complex multi-lumen catheters often carry a greater risk, but the cause of infection is similar for all devices and can come in two forms. First, the microorganisms that surround the patient's skin may contaminate the catheter during insertion and migrate along the cutaneous catheter track. Or second, your contaminated hands could transfer microbes to the catheter hub during an episode of care (Loveday et al., 2014b). If you ensure safe maintenance of an intravascular catheter and attend to the insertion site, you will decrease transmission of microorganisms, delay colonisation and reduce the rate of HCAI. The interventions you could employ include initiating maximal sterile barrier precautions for insertion of central lines. Strict ANTTT for the insertion of peripheral lines, antisepsis of the patient's catheter hub and connection port and effective hand hygiene before contact with key parts and sites (Wasserman and Messina, 2018).

Urinary catheters

Many of your patients will have a decreased consciousness level, require close fluid monitoring, may be immobile and have other pathologies. For these reasons the use of short-term indwelling urethral catheters is sometimes unavoidable. The ECDC (2016) found that urinary catheters were used in 81% of ACCU patient-days and 99.3% of UTIs were associated with a catheter. Catheter Associated Urinary Tract Infection (CAUTI) is strongly associated with the choice of catheter, the method of its introduction, its duration and maintenance. The risk of bacteriuria will increase by 5% each day your patient has a catheter. By day 30 bacteria in their urine is almost inevitable. Approximately 24% of these patients will go on to develop a CAUTI, and of these, up to 4% a severe, life-threatening secondary infection such as bacteraemia or **sepsis** (Loveday et al., 2014b). Urinary catheters predispose to infection in similar ways to other foreign bodies. In brief, they allow the passage of bacteria from the person's perineum, their distal urethra or your hands to the sterile bladder. It could occur at the time of insertion or during maintenance and come from contamination of the outer aspect of the catheter, or the inner lumen. Voiding is nature's way of removing transient contamination of the urinary tract, but the retention balloon in a catheter prevents this. Instead unwelcome bacteria that have transgressed into the bladder will multiply in the residual urine (Weston, 2013). By maintaining a sterile, continuously closed urinary drainage system you play a central part in the prevention of CAUTI.

Ventilator associated pneumonia (VAP)

The ECDC epidemiological survey (2016) found that where length of stay exceeded 2 days, 6.3% of patients experienced at least one episode of pneumonia, 97% of these were associated with intubation. The pathogenesis of VAP rests, first with the replacement of normal flora by more virulent and resistant strains in the surrounding anatomic structures, such as the stomach, sinuses, nasopharynx and oropharynx. These strains then collect and pool above and around the inflated cuff and silently and continuously aspirate past the **endotracheal** or tracheostomy tube to the lower respiratory tract (Gunasekera and Gratrix, 2016). The exact mortality attributed to VAP is a contentious point, but it is thought to be associated with increased duration of ventilation, length of stay in ACCU and hospital and a significant increase in healthcare costs. It has been proposed that the prevention of VAP is one of the most cost-effective interventions currently attainable in the ACCU. You can play your part if you halt the repeated micro-**aspiration** and colonisation of the upper airway and GI tract with potentially pathogenic organisms and prevent the contamination of ventilator/respiratory equipment (Wasserman and Messina, 2018).

THIS TOPIC IS ALSO COVERED IN CHAPTER 5

Biofilms

An additional problem that is implicated in most invasive devices is the production of biofilms. As a rule, the surfaces of devices have no inherent defence mechanisms. Bacteria will attach themselves to the device and then secrete a polysaccharide matrix that consists of sugars and proteins. This creates and encases a large colony of bacteria. If you remove a device you might see a slimy coating, this is called a biofilm. The organisms contained within a biofilm have considerable survival advantages as they function as a community and communicate closely with one another. This gains them protection from the action of antibiotic therapy and phagocytosis.

System interventions for reducing the risk of infection

In recent times there has been an abundance of national and international evidence-based guidelines that advise on best care practices to prevent device-related infections. The popular view is that a bundled approach offers the best solution. A care bundle is a set of evidence-based measures that when implemented together have a greater impact, and produce a better outcome, than when implemented in isolation (Resar et al., 2012). As part of the Department of Health's Saving Lives pro-gramme, the care bundle approach was adopted throughout the NHS and a number of 'high impact interventions' (HII) were introduced. Not only did these HII group together the critical elements of a clinical procedure, they also provided a means for organisations to audit compliance.

ACTIVITY 4.9: REFLECTIVE PRACTICE

Take a minute to read through the post-insertion high impact interventions for VAP, peripheral and urinary catheters (Tables 4.4–4.6).

1.   Do you use these in your department?
2.   Reflect on your own strengths and weaknesses and those of your colleagues.
3.   What do you think could be done to improve practice in these areas?

There is no template answer to this activity as it is based on your own reflection.

Table 4.4   Ventilator Associated Pneumonia

1	• Elevation of the head of the bed
	The head of the bed is elevated to 30–45° (unless contraindicated).
2	• **Sedation** level assessment
	Unless the patient is awake and comfortable, sedation is reduced/held for assessment at least daily (unless contraindicated).
3	• Oral hygiene
	The mouth is cleaned with chlorhexidine gluconate (≥1–2% gel or liquid) 6 hourly (as chlorhexidine can be inactivated by toothpaste, a gap of at least 2 hours should be left between its application and tooth brushing).
	Teeth are brushed 12 hourly with standard toothpaste.
4	• Subglottic aspiration
	A tracheal tube (endotracheal or tracheostomy) which has a subglottic secretion drainage port is used if the patient is expected to be intubated for >72 hrs.
	Secretions are aspirated via the subglottic secretion port 1–2 hourly.
5	• Tracheal tube cuff pressure
	Cuff pressure is measured 4 hourly, maintained between 20-30cm H2O (or 2cm H2O above peak inspiratory pressure) and recorded on the ACCU chart.
6	• Stress ulcer **prophylaxis**
	Stress ulcer prophylaxis is prescribed only to high-risk patients according to locally developed guidelines Prophylaxis is reviewed daily.

Source: Adapted from Infection Prevention Society in association with NHS Improvement 2017.

Table 4.5   Peripheral Cannulas

1	Site inspection
	Regular observation for signs of infection, at least daily.
2	Dressing
	An intact, dry, adherent transparent dressing should be present.
3	Cannula access
	Use 2% chlorhexidine gluconate in 70% isopropyl alcohol and allow to dry prior to accessing the cannula for administering fluid or injections.
4	Administration set replacement
	Immediately after administration of blood, blood products.
	All other fluid sets after 72 hours.
5	Routine cannula replacement
	Replace in a new site after 72-96 hours or earlier if indicated clinically.
	If venous access limited, the cannula can remain in situ if there are no signs of infection.

Table 4.6   Urethral Catheters

1	Hand hygiene
	Decontaminate hands before and after each patient contact.
	Use correct hand hygiene procedure.
2	Catheter hygiene
	Clean catheter site regularly as per local policy.
3	Sampling
	Perform aseptically via the catheter port.
4	Drainage bag position
	Above floor but below bladder level to prevent reflux or contamination.
5	Catheter manipulation
	Examination gloves should be worn to manipulate a catheter, and manipulation should be preceded and followed by hand decontamination.
6	Catheter needed?
	Remove as soon as possible.

ACTIVITY 4.10: CASE STUDY

Suzanne is an experienced nurse on the Level 3 critical care unit. She has been asked by the Matron to take on the position of Infection Prevention and Control Link Nurse for the unit. One of her objectives is to relaunch the Saving Lives programme. This has recently stalled but Suzanne is unsure of the reasons why.

What should Suzanne consider to ensure the successful implementation of this project?

In summary, over the last two decades IPC has moved from something of a Cinderella service to a health service of priority. Historically seen as a regrettable consequence of interventionist care, there is now a drive to reduce these to the irreducible minimum. Central to the task is the acceptance that infection control is everybody's business. By looking at IPC through the lens of the cycle of infection this chapter has illustrated how this may work. Where nurses collaborate with cleaners, reservoirs of environmental contamination can be removed. When they work with pharmacists and doctors, good antibiotic stewardship can prevail. The co-ordination of IPC often falls to nurses who are the biggest professional group with the most consistent clinical profile. However, this also means they have the greatest direct patient contact and logically hold considerable risk of being mediators of cross infection. Because of the surfeit of invasive devices people in ACCU have enhanced risk of HCAI. The bundles of care that have been developed through the Saving Lives programme have done much to clarify the critical elements of a particular procedure in vulnerable patients, the key actions required and the means of demonstrating compliance. Every clinician has the potential to significantly reduce the risk of HCAI by adopting these principles and ensuring they perform them every time for every patient.

CHAPTER SUMMARY

This chapter has supported your understanding of:

- The cycle of infection
- Risk and the critically ill patient
- The nurse's role of antibiotic stewardship
- Healthcare worker-mediated cross infection
- The role of bundles in preventing device related infection

GO FURTHER

Books

Damani, N. (2019) *Manual of Infection Prevention and Control* (4th edition). Oxford: Oxford University Press.

- An excellent introductory text that offers a reference point for Infection Prevention and Control Practice.

Van Saene, H.K.F., Silvestri, L., de la Cal, M.A. and Gullo, A. (eds) (2012) *Infection Control in the Intensive Care Unit* (3rd edition). Berlin: Springer.

- This offers a more specialist text on infection control and the intensive care unit for those who want to go further.

Ward, D. (2016) *Microbiology and Infection Prevention and Control*. London: Sage.

- This short, easy to read book gives a good overview of the principles of infection control, linking it to microbial transmission and reproduction.

Articles

European Centre for Disease Prevention and Control (2019) 'Healthcare-associated infection in intensive care units. Annual epidemiological report for 2017', Stockholm: ECDC. Available from https://www.ecdc.europa.eu/en/publications-data/healthcare-associated-infections-intensive-care-units-annual-epidemiological-1 (accessed October 31, 2020).

- This presents the results of a large scale, international study on the incidence, aetiology and causative organisms responsible for HCAI in Intensive Care.

Loveday, H., Wilson, J., Pratt, R. Golsorkhia, M., Tinglea, A. Baka, A., Brownea, J., Prietob, J. and Wilcox, M (2014) 'epic3: National evidence-based guidelines for preventing healthcare-associated infections in NHS hospitals in England', *Journal of Hospital Infection*, 86S1: S1–S70.

- UK evidence-based guidelines on the prevention of HCAI. These are typically used to form policy and guidelines within NHS trusts.

Department of Health (2007) 'High Impact Interventions: Care processes to Prevent Infection'. 4th edition of Saving Lives. NHS Improvement.

- A group of evidence-based care bundles that highlight the critical elements of a procedure or care process. These often form the basis of audit in infection prevention and control.

Useful websites

Royal College of Nursing (2018) www.rcn.org.uk/library/subject-guides/infection-prevention-and-control-subject-guide (accessed October 31, 2020).

- A useful resource that offers a wealth of accessible information on different topics

GOV.UK (2014 [updated 2018]) 'Healthcare associated infections (HCAI): Guidance, data and analysis'. www.gov.uk/government/collections/healthcare-associated-infections-hcai-guidance-data-and-analysis (accessed October 31, 2020).

- This site includes all the latest information produced by Public Health England on the topic of HCAI.

Health Education England (n.d.) 'Antimicrobial Resistance', Health Education England. www.hee.nhs.uk/our-work/antimicrobial-resistance accessed October 31, 2020).

- This site outlines the work that Health Education England are undertaking to promote awareness of **antimicrobial resistance**, and how it is included in the prevention, management and control of infection curricula for human medicine, nursing, pharmacy, dentistry and other professionals.

REFERENCES

Brooks, D., Polubothu P., Young, D., Booth , M.G. and Smith, A. (2018) 'Sepsis caused by bloodstream infection in patients in the intensive care unit: The impact of inactive empiric antimicrobial therapy on outcome', *Journal of Hospital Infection*, 98 (4): 369–74.

Centres for Disease Control and Prevention (2012) Principles of Epidemiology in Public Health Practice, Third Edition. *An Introduction to Applied Epidemiology and Biostatistics*. Lesson 1: Introduction to Epidemiology. Section 10: Chain of Infection. Available from https://www.cdc.gov/csels/dsepd/ss1978/lesson1/index.html (accessed January 7, 2021).

Coia, J., Ritchie, L., Adiseh, A. Makison Booth, C., Bradley, C., Bunyan, D. […] and Zuckerman, M. (2013) 'Guidance on use of respiratory and facial protection equipment', *Journal of Hospital Infection*, 85 (3): 170–82.

Currie, K., Melone L, Steward, S., King, C., Holopainen, A., Clark, A.M. and Reilley, J. (2018) 'Understanding the patient experience of health care–associated infection: A qualitative systematic review', *American Journal of Infection Control*, 46: 936–42.

Dancer, S. (2014) 'Controlling hospital-acquired infection: Focus on the role of the environment and new technologies for decontamination', *Clinical Microbiology Reviews*, 27: 665–90.

Erasmus, V., Daha, T.J., Brug, H., Richardus, J.H., Behrendt, M.D., Vos, M.C. and van Beeck E.F. (2010) 'Systematic review of studies on compliance with hand hygiene guidelines in hospital care', *Infection Control Hospital Epidemiology*, 31 (3): 283–94.

European Centre for Disease Prevention and Control (ECDC) (2019) 'Annual Epidemiological Report: Healthcare-associated infection in intensive care units'. Stockholm: ECDC. Available from https://www.ecdc.europa.eu/en/publications-data/healthcare-associated-infections-intensive-care-units-annual-epidemiological-1 (accessed January 7, 2021).

Gunasekera, P. and Gratrix, A. (2016) 'Ventilator-associated pneumonia', *BJA Education*, 16: 198–202.

Health Protection Agency (2012) *English National Point Prevalence Survey on Healthcare-associated Infections and Antimicrobial Use 211: Preliminary Data*. HPA. Available from https://webarchive.nationalarchives.gov.uk/20140714085429/http://www.hpa.org.uk/Publications/Infectious Diseases/AntimicrobialAndHealthcareAssociatedInfections/1205HCAIEnglishPPSforhcaiandamu 2011prelim/ (accessed October 31, 2020).

Johnson, I. and Banks, V. (2017) 'Antibiotic stewardship in critical care', *BJA Education*, 17: 111–16.

Loveday, H., Lynam, S., Singleton, J. and Wilson, J.A. (2014a) 'Clinical glove use: Healthcare workers' actions and perceptions', *Journal of Hospital Infection*, 86 (2): 110–16.

Loveday, H., Wilson J., Pratt, R., Golsorkhia, M., Tinglea, A. Baka, A., Brownea, J., Prietob, J. and Wilcox, M. (2014b) 'epic3: National evidence-based guidelines for preventing healthcare-associated infections in NHS hospitals in England', *Journal of Hospital Infection*, 86S1: S1–S70.

Mitchell, B., Dancer, S., Anderson, M. and Dehn, E. (2015) 'Risk of organism acquisition from prior room occupants: A systematic review and meta-analysis', *Journal of Hospital Infection*, 91: 211–17.

National Institute for Health and Care Excellence (NICE) (2014) *Infection Prevention and Control* (Quality Standard S61). London: NICE. Available from https://www.nice.org.uk/guidance/qs61 (accessed November 1, 2020).

Pineles, L., Morgan, D. and Lydecker, A. (2017) 'Transmission of methicillin-resistant Staphylococcus aureus to health care worker gowns and gloves during care of residents in Veterans Affairs nursing homes', *American Journal of Infection Control*, 45: 947–53.

Public Health England (2015) *Start Smart: Then Focus: Antimicrobial Stewardship Toolkit for English Hospitals*. London: Public Health England.

Public Health England (2020) *English Surveillance Programme for Antimicrobial Utilisation and Resistance (ESPAUR)*. London: Public Health England.

Resar, R., Griffin, F., Haraden, C. and Nolan, T.W. (2012) *Using Care Bundles to Improve Health Care Quality* (IHI Innovation Series White Paper). Cambridge, MA: Institute for Healthcare Improvement.

Sender R. Fuchs S. Milo R. (2016) 'Revised estimates for the number of human and bacteria cells in the body'. bioRxiv 036103. doi: https://doi.org/10.1101/036103. Now published in *PLOS Biology* doi: 10.1371/journal.pbio.1002533 (accessed January 7, 2021).

Skodová, M., Garcia Urra, F., Gimeno Benítez, A., Jiménez Romano, M.A. Gimeno Ortiz, A. (2015) 'Hand hygiene assessment in the workplace using a UV lamp', *American Journal of Infection Control*, 43 (12): 1360–2.

Stone, P., Fuller, C., Savage, J., Cookson, B., Hayward, A., Cooper, C., […] and Charlett, A. (2012) 'Evaluation of the national Cleanyourhands campaign to reduce *Staphylococcus aureus* bacteraemia and *Clostridium difficile* infection in hospitals in England and Wales by improved hand hygiene: Four year, prospective, ecological, interrupted time series study', *British Medical Journal*, 344: e3005.

Wasserman, S. and Messina, A. (2018) 'Bundles in Infection Prevention Safety', in G. Bearman, M. Doll, S. Mehtar, Z.A. Memish, S. Ponce de León Rosales, V. Rosenthal and M. Stevens (eds) *Guide to Infection Control in Hospital* (6th edition). Brookline, MA: International Society for Infectious Diseases. https://isid.org/wp-content/uploads/2018/02/ISID_InfectionGuide_Chapter16.pdf (accessed November 1, 2020).

Weston, D. (2013) *Fundamentals of Infection Prevention and Control: Theory and Practice*. Oxford: Wiley.

Whitby, M., Pessoa-Silva, C., McLaws, M., Allegranzi, B., Sax, H., Larson, E., Seto, W.H., Donaldson, L. and Pittet, D. (2007) 'Behavioural considerations for hand hygiene practices: The basic building blocks', *Journal of Hospital Infection,* 65: 1–8.

World Health Organisation (WHO) (2009) *Guidelines on Hand Hygiene in Health Care*. Geneva: WHO.

World Health Organisation (WHO) (2010) *Hand Hygiene Self-assessment Framework*. Geneva: WHO.

World Health Organisation (WHO) (2011) *Report on the Burden of Endemic Healthcare Associated Infection: Clean Care is Safe Care*. Geneva: WHO.

CRITICAL CARE RELATED TO THE RESPIRATORY SYSTEM

COLIN STEEN, SAMANTHA FREEMAN AND GREGORY BLEAKLEY

> **"**
> Providing supporting breathing to a patient who is struggling is both challenging and rewarding. It is the fundamental strategy we can use to help support life. It can often be confused as the media call it a 'life support' machine but really it's just support for a single failing organ.
>
> **Jane, Nurse Practitioner, 35 Years' Experience**
> **"**

LEARNING OUTCOMES

When you have finished studying this chapter you will be able to understand:

- The overview of anatomy and physiology
- some types of respiratory failure
- how to care for a person with an artificial airway
- the basics of artificial ventilation
- some of the available **interventions** in the management of respiratory failure

INTRODUCTION

This chapter aims to provide you with an overview of the relevant anatomy and physiology and provides signposting for those who need more in-depth revision. The focus will be on assessment, the nursing interventions relating to the airway, and then breathing, with topics such as the use of artificial airways and adjuncts, tracheostomy management and care. In relation to breathing, topics covered will be the types of respiratory failure, respiratory management including invasive and non-invasive ventilation, oxygen therapy, **prone** positioning and Extra Corporeal Membranous Oxygenation.

OVERVIEW OF THE ANATOMY AND PHYSIOLOGY OF THE RESPIRATORY SYSTEM

Respiration is usually an effortless physiological process characterised by the inspiration and expiration of air. Breathing occurs as an involuntary reflex controlled by the medulla oblongata and pons, which are part of the brain stem (Waugh and Grant, 2018). A normal adult's breathing rate is approximately 12–18 breaths per minute (bpm). However, the respiration rate can increase or decrease as a result of exercise, ill health and/or drug therapy.

Tortora and Derrickson (2016) describe the key anatomical structures of the respiratory system as including the nose, pharynx (throat), larynx (voice box), trachea (windpipe), bronchi and two lungs. Functionally, the respiratory system is divided into two components. First, the upper respiratory tract includes the nares (nostrils), nose, naso-pharynx (nasal cavity) and pharynx. Second, the lower respiratory tract includes the larynx, trachea, bronchi and two lungs (see Figure 5.1).

Crucially, the respiratory system allows gas exchange to occur. This includes the intake (inspiration) of oxygen (O_2) for delivery to body cells and removal of carbon dioxide (CO_2) following cellular activity, helping to regulate blood pH and maintain **homeostasis**. The normal level for blood pH is 7.35–7.45 and acidosis occurs when the pH of the blood falls below 7.35. Respiratory acidosis is usually caused when blood pH falls below 7.35 as a result of CO_2 levels being abnormally high as a consequence of ill health or disease. Conversely, respiratory alkalosis occurs when blood pH rises above 7.45 as a result of breathing too fast and reducing CO_2 levels below normal (Brinkman and Sandeep, 2018).

Inspired air travels down the bronchial tree towards the distal end of the respiratory tree, the terminal bronchioles. The trachea is a tubular passageway for air, which splits into a right main bronchus and is connected to the right lung and a left primary bronchus which is connected to the left lung. The point where the trachea divides is known as the carina. On entering the lung, the bronchi further divide to form smaller bronchi (secondary bronchi), continuing with smaller divisions to form bronchioles. The extensive branching from the trachea resembles an inverted tree (Tortora and Derrickson, 2011).

The terminal bronchioles end in a collection of microscopic air sacs called alveoli. In the alveoli, gas exchange arises, and oxygen rich air is absorbed into the blood steam. Carbon dioxide travels from the blood steam to the alveoli, where it is exhaled. A thin layer of cells called the interstitium is found throughout the body, but in the lungs it is situated between the alveoli and terminal bronchiole. It contains a network of small blood vessels and cells which supports gas exchange (breathing) (Cook et al., 2021).

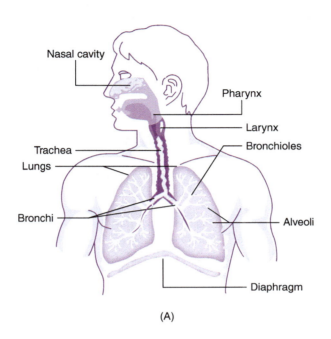

(A)

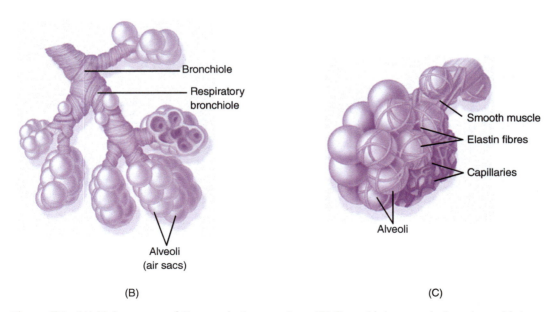

(B)   (C)

Figure 5.1 (A) Main organs of the respiratory system. (B) Bronchioles, respiratory bronchiole and alveoli. (C) Smooth muscle is shown in the walls of the bronchioles

Source: Ashelford et al., *Pathophysiology and Pharmacology in Nursing*, 2nd Edition, Learning Matters.

The lungs are the largest organ of the respiratory system and located in the thorax. Each lung is protected by its own double thin layer of tissue known as the plural membrane. The outer layer, or parietal pleura, lines the inside of the rib cage and the diaphragm while the inner layer, or visceral pleura, covers the lungs. Between the parietal and visceral pleura is a space referred to as the pleural cavity. The membranes of each pleura secrete lubricating fluid into the plural cavity which reduces friction during respiration (Waugh and Grant, 2018).

In some conditions the pleural cavity fills with air (pneumothorax), blood (haemothorax) or pus or chyme (pleural effusion). Air, blood, pus and/or chyme in the pleural cavity are abnormal and their presence can indicate trauma to the lung, infection or **inflammation**.

ACTIVITY 5.1: REFLECTIVE PRACTICE

Consider the roles of key anatomical structure involved in respiration.

1. What are the names and key function?
2. Consider what barriers may occur in the respiratory tree that can impede gaseous exchange.
3. Can you list some of the common causes of air, blood, pus or chyle entering the pleural cavity?

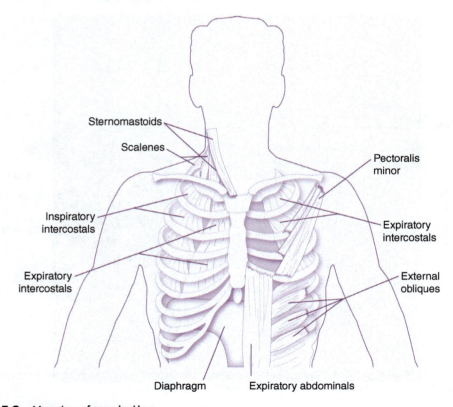

Figure 5.2 **Muscles of respiration**

Source: Cook et al. (2021).

The most significant muscle involved in the physiological process of respiration is the diaphragm. This is a dome shaped muscle and located in a gap between the thoracic cavity above and the abdominal cavity below (see Figure 5.2).

During respiration, the diaphragm contracts and pulls in a downward direction, which encourages greater space in the thoracic cavity (Cohen and Hull, 2015). The movement of the diaphragm results in the inhalation of air (breathing in). Equally, movement of the intercostal muscles creates additional room for inspired air. The intercostal muscles are located between the ribs and can be visualised during laboured or rapid breathing.

RESPIRATORY FAILURE

Respiratory failure is a condition that affects the gas exchange within the lungs. It occurs when either the gas exchange organ (lung) and/or the ventilatory pump (respiratory muscles and the thorax) fail to work properly. Respiratory failure is divided into Type I and Type II. Type I is characterised by low O_2 levels (hypoxaemia) with normal or low CO_2 levels (hypocapnia) and occurs because of damage to lung tissue, which prevents adequate oxygenation of the blood (hypoxaemia). Typical causes of Type I respiratory failure include **pulmonary** oedema, pneumonia, acute lung injury (ALI), acute respiratory distress syndrome (ARDS), idiopathic pulmonary fibrosis, and lung cancer.

Type II respiratory failure involves low O_2 levels, with high CO_2 levels (hypercapnia). This type of respiratory failure or 'ventilatory failure' occurs when alveolar ventilation is insufficient to remove residual carbon dioxide from the blood stream. It is frequently caused by chronic obstructive pulmonary disease (COPD), asthma, and other respiratory muscle weaknesses (e.g. Guillain-Barré syndrome).

Interventions in the management of respiratory failure

Oxygen therapy

When people have abnormally low oxygen levels in their blood, they may require oxygen therapy to be prescribed. Oxygen is classed as a drug and requires a prescription. There are several different kinds of oxygen therapy.

1. Long-term oxygen therapy (LTOT)

This is used to describe the oxygen therapy people receive when they require the use of oxygen to maintain their blood oxygen levels within normal range.

2. Nocturnal oxygen therapy (NOT)

This term is used when oxygen therapy is administered to people who experience a reduction in blood oxygen levels whilst they are asleep.

3. Ambulatory oxygen therapy (AOT)

If, whilst a person is active or involved in physical exertion, their blood oxygen levels fall, then they receive ambulatory oxygen therapy.

4.   Palliative oxygen therapy (POT)

Oxygen therapy may be prescribed to people who experience severe breathlessness that is unresolved by the use of other treatments. See previous section on Type II respiratory failure in this chapter.

People who are acutely unwell may be prescribed oxygen to maintain blood oxygen saturation levels to within normal range. The exception to this is the administration of oxygen to Type II respiratory failure. In these cases, the target SaO_2 for treatment, the therapeutic endpoint, is 88–92%.

There are a number of different devices that are used to deliver oxygen therapy. The non-rebreathing mask or reservoir bag mask (Figure 5.3) delivers oxygen at high concentrations. The precise percentage is unknown but is judged to be in the region of 80%, but this requires oxygen flow rates to be at 15 litres per minute (L/min). The reservoir bag needs to be filled with oxygen prior to positioning the mask on the person and a close fit over the mouth and nose is required.

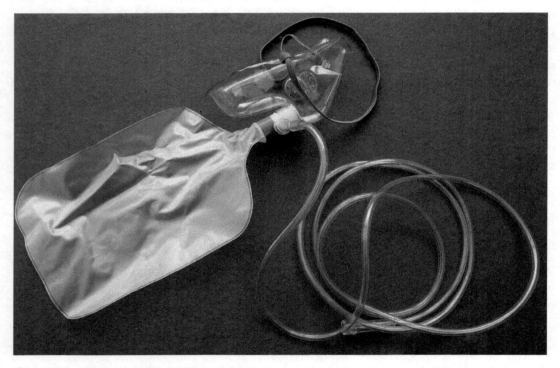

Figure 5.3   Oxygen Mask with Reservoir Bag

© C. Steen.

A simple facemask (Figure 5.4) is intended for short-term use such as following surgery. Oxygen is delivered at 2–10 L/min. The concentration of oxygen inspired is unknown as air is drawn into the mask during breathing, diluting the oxygen concentration.

Nasal cannulae are a method of delivering oxygen nasally. They do not impact on the patient's ability to eat or drink and are generally well tolerated. These are used in situations where a low concentration of oxygen is required. Typically, the oxygen flow rate is between 2–4 L/min. Caution is needed in this method of delivery as high flow rates via nasal cannulae can cause drying of the nasal mucosa.

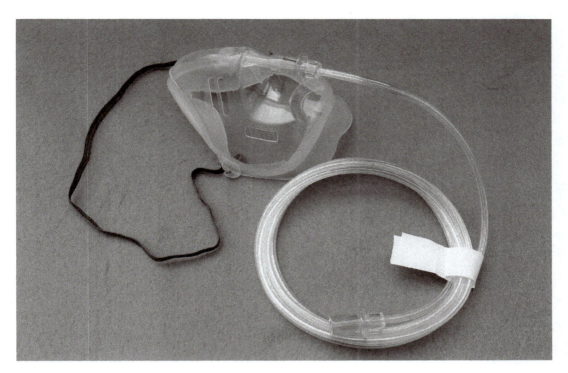

Figure 5.4   Simple Oxygen Mask

© C. Steen.

Fixed performance devices deliver oxygen via a Venturi valve, which gives an accurate and known concentration of oxygen (Figure 5.5). The flow rate varies between manufacturers and is dependent upon the concentration of oxygen required.

When caring for patients receiving oxygen therapy it is important to continue to monitor their oxygen saturation regularly using a pulse oxymeter and for those patients who require oxygen therapy longer than 24 hours, humidification is required to be added to the oxygen delivery system. As oxygen is a dry gas, it can affect the mucosal membranes of the upper respiratory tract as well as trying secretions in the lungs, which can lead to infection.

Patient comfort is paramount and having dried nasal secretions stuck to the inside of the nose is very uncomfortable and painful. I need to understand and ensure that the treatment I apply tries to avoid this.

Jenny, Registered Nurse, 8 Years' Experience in Level 2 Care

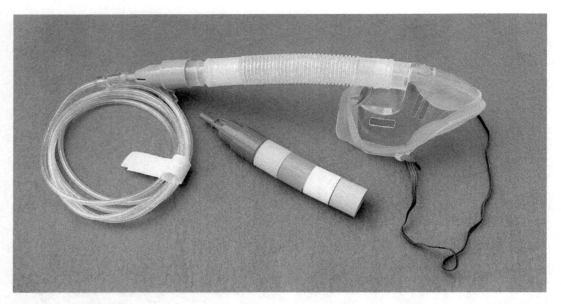

Figure 5.5 Venturi Mask. The adaptors shown are colour-coded to indicate the different oxygen concentrations available

© C. Steen.

WHAT'S THE EVIDENCE?

Read the British Thoracic Society's guidelines (2017):

O'Driscoll, B.R., Howard, L.S., Earis, J. and Mak, V. (2017) 'BTS guideline for oxygen use in adults in healthcare and emergency settings', *Thorax*, 72: i1 – i90. doi.org/10.1136/thoraxjnl-2016-209729

This document describes the national guidelines for the use of oxygen in adults suffering acute illness.

When you're assessing patients in practice, review the measurements of the patients' clinical status and, based on the evidence you have read, consider whether the person requires oxygen or not.

UNDERSTANDING ARTERIAL BLOOD GAS (ABG) ANALYSIS

A common assessment carried out by the team in critical care is arterial blood gases. Normally the sample will be obtained from the invasive arterial pressure monitoring system. The system allows for a small sample of blood to be withdrawn for testing. An appropriately trained member of the team should carry out this procedure. Once you have a sample, the department will have a blood gas analysis machine and you can use this to get a result within a minute or two. There are many parameters such as potassium or haemoglobin levels, which are also obtained on this sample.

As mentioned previously, the normal pH range 7.35 to 7.45 and is affected by changing levels of carbonic acid. This acid is produced as a result of cellular metabolism. It results from metabolic activity that produces CO_2 and water (H_2O) and these two chemicals combine to produce carbonic acid (H_2CO_3). Carbonic acid is unstable in water. Plasma, the liquid portion of blood, contains 92% water, and, as carbonic acid is unstable in water, it splits into hydrogen ions (H^+) and bicarbonate (HCO_3^-). The pH scale measures the amount of H^+ in the blood. Consequently, the higher the H^+ in the blood the more acidic the blood is and the lower the pH level will be. In order to maintain homeostasis, CO_2 is carried to the lungs and excreted, thus reducing the amount of carbonic acid, H^+ and restoring pH to normal levels. This is a rapid response to a change in **metabolic** activity, however there are alternative ways of controlling the pH level that are slower, such as the kidneys excreting H^+ in the urine or retaining HCO_3^-. When someone is unwell, the body will respond by trying to maintain normal homeostasis through these compensatory changes, and it is the role of the nurse and medical teams to detect these mechanisms working in this way. It provides vital information that illness is present and its severity.

The partial pressure of oxygen (PaO_2) dissolved in arterial blood should be >10kPa and the partial pressure of carbon dioxide ($PaCO_2$) dissolved in arterial blood should be between 4.5kPa and 6.1kPa. The bicarbonate (HCO_3^-) reading should be between 22 and 26mmol/l.

Before analysing the blood result, you need to know what level of oxygen the person is receiving. This is because there is a difference between the levels of oxygen we inhale and the PaO_2 dissolved in arterial blood. The difference is normally around 10 kilopascals (kPa). In a person with damage to their lungs, either by infection or illness, this difference will be bigger. The size of the gap between what concentration of oxygen the person inhales and their PaO_2 indicates the degree of damage. This difference is referred to as the Alveolar–arterial (A-a) gradient.

When we start to interpret the ABG we can use five simple questions:

1. Is the patient hypoxic?
2. How does this relate to the inspired O_2?
3. Do they have an acidosis or alkalosis (the pH level)?
4. Is the cause respiratory or metabolic (determined by $PaCO_2$ and HCO_3^-)?
5. Is there any attempt at compensation (determined by $PaCO_2$ and HCO_3^-)?

These last two questions can sometimes be challenging, however using the diagram below may help. If the results are marked on the same side as the pH, then that is the cause of the deterioration, and if the result is on the opposite side, it is the compensatory mechanism trying to correct the pH.

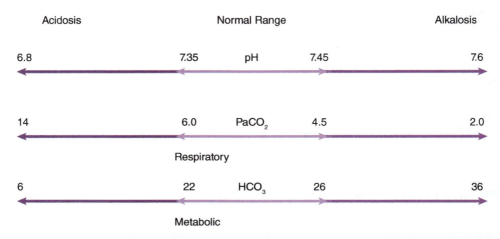

Figure 5.6 Method of determining the outcome of arterial blood gas analysis

Source: Freeman et al. (2019).

"I found this diagram really helpful. I even printed it out and put the questions on the back. Its small so fits in my pocket and is laminated. I use it in placement with real ABGs. It really helped me learn how to read them"

Louise, 3rd Year Student Nurse

ACTIVITY 5.2: CASE STUDY HAROLD

Harold is an 86 year old male who is experiencing a persistent cough and is easily short of breath. He is wheezy during cold weather and is more chesty than usual. He is married to Hilda and lives in a terraced house. He stopped smoking ten years ago and is a retired mill worker. Harold has become more forgetful recently and is developing Alzheimer's disease. On admission to hospital, his respiration rate is 28 breaths per minute and his arterial blood gas (ABG) analysis is pH 7.30; pCO_2 8kPa; pO_2 7.5kPa.

1. What is causing Harold's respiration rate to increase?
2. What type of respiratory failure is Harold likely to be experiencing?

AIRWAY

Caring for somebody who has an artificial airway in place can feel frightening as it poses a number of nursing challenges related to maintaining the safety of the person.

Before establishing artificial ventilation, you will need to secure the airway, and there are a number of ways you can do this. Simple airway protective procedures such as the recovery position and oropharyngeal or nasopharyngeal airways are not suitable for invasive ventilation. Occasionally devices such as laryngeal masks or subglottic masks, which are inserted into the upper airway but remain above the vocal cords, are used in emergency situations. These are more advanced than oropharyngeal/nasopharyngeal airways and can facilitate artificial ventilation. These are preferred as they are easy to insert but are only used until the patient is stabilised and then they are exchanged for more substantial airways such as an endotracheal tube (ET tube) (Figure 5.7) or a tracheostomy tube (Figure 5.8). These are more secure airways and enable prolonged artificial ventilation. To insert an ET tube, the person needs to be anaesthetised and paralysed. The tube is inserted through the oropharynx, which can trigger the gag reflex, therefore continuous background **sedation** is required so the tube can be tolerated.

Caring for a person with an artificial airway

An artificial airway is a medical device that can be inserted into the upper or lower respiratory tract to secure the airway and to facilitate respiration and/or ventilation and the removal of secretions. Firstly, the airway needs to be secure and not easily dislodged or it will cause unnecessary damage to the trachea. Then the nurse needs to ensure the patency of the artificial airway,

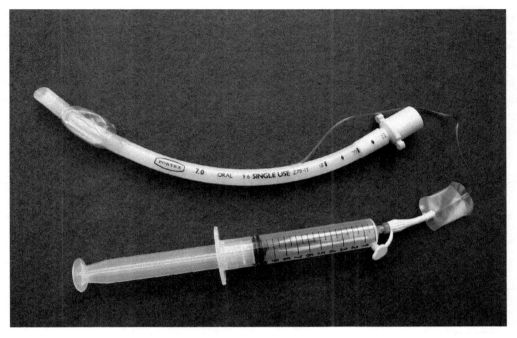

Figure 5.7   Endotracheal tube with syringe attached to inflate cuff

© C. Steen

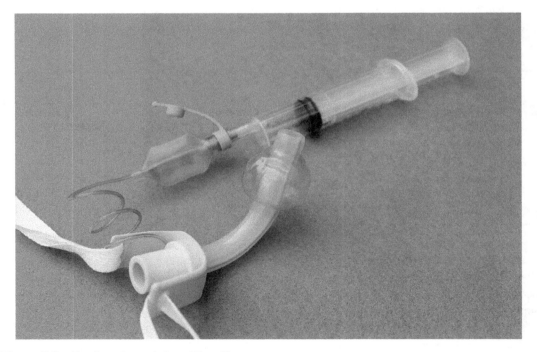

Figure 5.8   Tracheostomy tube with cuff

© C. Steen

prevent **aspiration** of any secretions, or in the case of a tracheostomy, liquids or food, which can result in aspiration pneumonia. This is achieved through endotracheal **suctioning**. You can read further details on this technique later in this chapter in the section on 'Nursing interventions: Endotracheal suctioning'.

Endotracheal tubes (ET) and temporary tracheostomies are the two most common artificial airways you will in see in critical care units. There are other airway adjuncts, such as oropharyngeal or naso-pharyngeal, which you may observe in some units such as accident and emergency and specialist head and neck surgery departments.

ACTIVITY 5.3: REFLECTIVE PRACTICE

Both the insertion of an ET tube or a tracheostomy bypasses the normal physiology of the person's upper airway.

1. Consider what natural defences the insertion of the airway bypasses.
2. Consider how the bypassing of these defences may affect the person.
3. What assessment and management strategies do we need to consider that will assist the person's natural defences?

Endotracheal tube insertion

There will be a number of staff from the multidisciplinary team involved in an airway insertion. The anaesthetist leads the procedure. All equipment will be checked ready before the procedure.

WHAT'S THE EVIDENCE?

All equipment should be checked before, during and after intubation and a full list of all the equipment that may be used can be seen on the Faculty of Intensive Care Medicine website. Read the Faculty of Intensive Care Medicine (2019) detailed guidance and invasive procedure checklist with a specific list for ITU Intubation:

www.ficm.ac.uk/sites/default/files/safety_checklist_-_itu_intubation-final_0.pdf (accessed November 2, 2020).

If the person is awake prior to the procedure, it is likely to be a frightening experience for them and they will require constant reassurance and information about what is happening. The area around the bed space is often noisy and busy and there are a lot of people so try to remain aware of this and offer support to the person and remind the staff of the person's presence.

If not already, you should make access to the head of the bed by removing the headboard of the bed, as this makes positioning the person easier. The person will receive a period of pre-oxygenation and then be laid flat. Should the person be considered high risk of aspiration during the procedure you may hear the anaesthetist ask for someone to apply cricoid pressure (also known as cricothyroid pressure). This is a technique where the anaesthetist's assistant presses on the cricoid cartilage during endotracheal intubation, thus occluding the oesophagus which passes directly behind it. The purpose is to reduce the incidence of aspiration of gastric contents from occurring, however there is some debate as to the effectiveness of this procedure, and some anaesthetists may request this whilst others may not.

WHAT'S THE EVIDENCE?

The **mortality** rate of aspiration pneumonia is very high but preventable. To help prevent this from occurring during intubation cricoid pressure is applied. Listen to this podcast https://theresusroom. co.uk/cricoid-pressure/ and read this paper:

Birenbaum, A., Hajage, D,. Roche, S., Ntouba, A., Eurin, M., Cuvillon, P. [...] and Riou, B. (2019) 'Effect of cricoid pressure compared with a sham procedure in the rapid sequence induction of anesthesia: The IRIS randomized clinical trial.' *JAMA Surgery*, 154 (1): 9-17. doi.org/10.1001/jama surg.2018.3577

The person will need to have **intravenous** (IV) access prior to the procedure to administer the drugs. Monitoring such as electrocardiograph (ECG), heart rate (HR), blood pressure (BP), oxygen saturation (SaO_2), and end tidal carbon dioxide measurement ($EtCO_2$) is used to monitor the condition of the patient during the procedure and to confirm correct positioning of the ET tube.

Once all the team and equipment are ready the person is given a combination of drugs: sedation, analgesia and a paralysing agent. Once the patient is asleep and relaxed, the ET tube is inserted directly into the trachea with the aid of a laryngoscope. Once the tube is inserted, the cuff, which is at the distal end of the ET tube, is inflated and checked for pressure with a manometer. The optimal pressure for a cuff is 20–30cmH$_2$O (Sole et al., 2011). An over-inflated ET tube cuff can cause damage and/or necrosis to the trachea. Conversely, an underinflated ET tube can cause air to leak from the lungs and allow aspiration of gastric content into the trachea. The cuff pressure should be frequently monitored and recorded in the medical/nursing case notes. The person's chest will be observed for equal expansion and auscultation performed to ensure gas is entering both lungs.

The ET tube is then secured in place with a tie and attached to an appropriate ventilator.

Following the procedure, arterial blood gases and a chest X-ray are performed to determine the tube position and to guide the settings of the ventilator. In addition, a nasogastric (NG) tube should be inserted to reduce the possibility of aspiration pneumonia and/or facilitate nutritional intake (Faculty of Intensive Care Medicine, 2019).

The nurse's role following ET tube insertion

The nurse's role is to monitor and maintain the position and patency of the ET tube. The ET tube has markings in centimetres on the outside to indicate how deep the tube is placed in the trachea. The length of the tube should be noted at either the lips or the teeth. This gives you a baseline position and should be recorded in the medical/nursing case notes. To identify whether the tube has moved or dislodged, you should check the position particularly after repositioning the patient. Any suspicion of

ET tube movement or displacement should be treated as an emergency and the airway assessed by an appropriately trained and skilled clinician.

There may be post-intubation complications you need to be aware of, such as:

- Hypoxia
- Trauma to lips, teeth and vocal cords
- Transient cardiac **arrhythmias** due to vagal nerve stimulation
- Hypertension, tachycardia or raised intracranial pressure
- Aspiration
- Missed placement – potential oesophageal intubation
- Infection/pneumonia
- Reduced cough reflex
- Bronchial and tracheal ulceration or stenosis
- Laryngeal oedema (swelling of the larynx)
- Bronchospasm
- Discomfort and anxiety
- Endotracheal tube kinked or damaged
- Damage to the tracheal mucosa

Tracheostomy tube insertion

Typically, a tracheostomy is performed to support weaning from mechanical ventilation. A prolonged period of mechanical ventilation is associated with significant **morbidity** and mortality. Consequently, weaning from ventilation should be initiated at the earliest opportunity and formation of a tracheostomy makes this possible. A tracheostomy is a tube inserted through the anterior wall of the trachea, just below the larynx and cricoid cartilage. The insertion procedure can be either surgical insertion or by percutaneous dilatation. The insertion via percutaneous dilatation is often carried out within the person's bed area rather than in a theatre environment. It involves a very small incision being made in the skin and the anterior wall of the trachea. Then, dilators of increasing width are used and, once sufficiently dilated, a tracheostomy tube is inserted and secured in place.

Either way the procedure is not without risk and insertion will be based on clinical need in conjunction with discussion with the family. The most common problems with tracheostomy tubes are obstruction or displacement of the tube. The Intensive Care Society (2014) published *Standards for the Care of Adult Patients with a Temporary Tracheostomy*. This is open access and provides a detailed breakdown of the procedure. Some of the potential complications are:

- Airway occlusion
- Displaced tubes or blocked tubes
- Air leaks
- Impaired cough
- Surgical emphysema – when gas or air enters the layer under the skin
- Infection-wound/chest
- Haemorrhage
- Tracheal stenosis – narrowing of the windpipe
- Ulceration tissue damage
- Altered body image

The Intensive Care Society (2014) states there are four indications for a temporary tracheostomy to be sited. These are:

- Maintenance of a patent airway
- Protection the airway
- Aid the removal of excessive secretions
- Aid weaning from intermittent, positive pressure ventilation

ACTIVITY 5.4: REFLECTIVE PRACTICE

1. Given the potential risks of the procedure, why do you think it would be in a person's best interest to have a tracheostomy inserted? Write this down in a list.
2. Look at your list. Do your items link to any of the four indications above?

Temporary tracheostomies are commonplace in critical care and you will need to be aware of the additional equipment required, the potential risks and how to manage these. Table 5.1 below outlines the minimum equipment required at the bedside.

Table 5.1 Equipment checklist for temporary tracheostomies

Suction	A suction unit, which should be checked at least daily, with suction tubing attached
	Appropriately sized suction catheters
PPE	Non-powdered, latex-free gloves, aprons, and eye protection
Safety Equipment	Spare tracheostomy tubes of the same type as inserted: one the same size and one a size smaller
	Tracheal dilators
	Re-breathing bag with tubing and a connection to an oxygen supply
	Catheter mount or connection
	Tracheostomy disconnection wedge
	Tracheostomy tube holder and dressing
	Easy access to resuscitation equipment
	10ml syringe (if tube cuffed)
	Artery forceps
	Easy access to resuscitation equipment
	Manometer to measure cuff pressure

Source: Adapted from Intensive Care Society (2014).

There are various types of tracheostomy tube. They either have a cuff, which can be inflated during mechanical ventilation, or not (Myatt, 2015). The purpose of the cuff is the same as that of an ETT (see section on 'Cuff Management' later in this chapter). The other difference is whether the tracheostomy has a removable inner tube. The different types of tube are listed on the National Tracheostomy Safety Project (2013) website.

www.tracheostomy.org.uk/storage/files/Tube%20types.pdf (accessed November 2, 2020).

You should note that there are some differences in resuscitation approaches for individuals who have a temporary tracheostomy. If effective ventilation can be provided with a bag/valve, then continual chest compressions should be carried out along with ventilation at approximately 10 breaths/minute (Resuscitation Council UK, 2015).

ACTIVITY 5.5: REFLECTIVE PRACTICE

1. Consider which members of the multidisciplinary team are required to establish artificial ventilation.
2. Consider why it is necessary to have a dedicated department, i.e. intensive care, to look after these patients.

Nursing assessment

It does not matter which of the two artificial airways the person you are caring for has, fundamentally the assessment will be the same. Working in ACCU, you will notice that there are comprehensive respiratory assessments carried out at the start of a shift, after any significant change in the person's condition, or following repositioning. The person's chest will be auscultated, and the staff will be observing for bilateral air entry, which is equal in all lobes, and abnormal air noises that may be a result of moisture, secretions or airway changes.

Nursing interventions

Endotracheal suctioning

Suctioning is one of the most common procedures performed to help maintain patency of the endotracheal tube or tracheostomy. There are many things you need to consider before, during and after endotracheal suctioning. ET tube suction is an uncomfortable and distressing experience. It can lower the person's oxygen saturation and their heart rate and therefore should only be carried out following a clinical assessment. NICE has provided this document outlining the full procedure: http://rc.rcjournal.com/content/respcare/55/6/758.full.pdf.

When performing endotracheal suctioning via tracheostomy, if the person can cough loose sections into the end of the tube then shallow suctioning can be sufficient (Myatt, 2015). However, for those sedated and ventilated with thick sections this may not be effective and deeper bronchial suction may be required.

This should be carried out by an appropriately trained practitioner as it can lead to complications such as hypoxia, mucosal trauma, cardiac arrhythmias, and raised intracranial pressure, and increases the risk of infection (Dougherty and Lister, 2008). This is a sterile procedure and the person may require pre-oxygenation administration beforehand. Guidance from the National Tracheostomy Safety project (NTSP) (2013) states that the suction catheter is advanced until resistance felt, this is at the carina, and is then withdrawn slightly before the application of suction. The procedure should not last more than ten seconds (NTSP, 2013). Suctioning can be painful and distressing so adequate pain relief and reassurance should be given (Freeman, 2011).

There are different types of suction systems in use. They are termed 'closed' and 'open' suction systems and which you should use is dependent on local policy. The size of the suction catheter should be equal to or less than half the inner diameter of the ET tube or tracheostomy tube. This is to allow air into the lungs during suctioning and prevent alveolar collapse and atelectasis, and reduce the risk of hypoxia and cardiovascular instability.

ACTIVITY 5.6: RESEARCH AND EVIDENCE-BASED PRACTICE

Carry out some research and further reading on the benefits and disadvantages of open and closed suction systems.

Following your reading of the evidence base, review your local policy to determine how it compares to your findings.

There is no template answer to this activity as it is based on your own reflection.

Humidification

The insertion of an artificial airway disrupts the normal humidification of the airway. Dry sections can lead to blockage of the tube with thick, difficult to expectorate sputum. All oxygen administered to those with an artificial airway should be humidified. The type and level of humidification will be affected by the way in which the person is ventilated and their clinical picture. The NTSP (2013) offers suggestions to help decision making as to the type and level of humidification required with the humidification ladder, which is in Table 5.2.

Table 5.2 Requirements for types of humidification

Method of humidification	Presenting symptoms
Heated water bath (active humidification)	Ventilated patient with thick secretions Self-ventilating patient (on oxygen) with thick secretions
HME for breathing circuit	Ventilated patient with minimal secretions (replace every 24 hrs) Monitor effectiveness (less likely to be effective if required for more than 5 days)
Cold water bath	Self-ventilating patient (on oxygen)
HME: (Buchanan bib, Swedish nose)	Self-ventilating patients (no oxygen)
Add saline nebulisers or mucolytics and ensure adequate hydration if secretions are not improving	

Source: National Tracheostomy Safety Project (2013).

Management of tracheostomy inner cannula

Many tracheostomy tubes are manufactured with an inner cannula. One of the advantages of an inner cannula is it can provide immediate relief of life-threatening airway obstruction in the event of blockage of a tracheostomy tube (Intensive Care Society, 2014). The National Tracheostomy Safety Project (NTSP) (2013) recommends the inner cannula is removed and cleaned at least once per eight-hour shift, however NCEPOD (2014) suggested this should be every four hours. Consequently, you may see some clinical variation in the frequency of cleaning and you should learn which is applicable in your ACCU. The inner cannula can be cleaned with sterile gauze or cannula brushes. The soaking of the inner cannula is not recommended as it has been shown to increase the risk of exposure to pathogens (Intensive Care Society Standards, 2014; NCEPOD, 2014).

Stoma care and tracheostomy tube securement

The stoma, like any wound, requires appropriate care. The application of a sterile dressing absorbs secretions from the stoma and reduces the risk of pressure damage caused by the tracheotomy (Mallet et al., 2013). Regular checking for any signs of wound breakdown is important and as this is a surgical wound it requires aseptic cleaning with 0.9% sodium chloride at least once every 24 hours (Intensive Care Society, 2014). To prevent the accidental removal of the tracheostomy during dressing changes, two staff are required to carry out the procedure (Freeman, 2011). The tracheostomy tube is secured around the person's neck with either a commercial tracheostomy holder or tracheostomy tapes (Myatt, 2015). These tapes need to be secure but not too tight to cause any damage to the skin, and in severe cases compromise venous return. It is recommended that once tied you should be able to insert one or two fingers between the tape and the person's neck (Mallet et al., 2013).

Cuff management

The cuff creates a sealed airway in both an ETT and a tracheostomy. Underinflation of the cuff leads to ineffective ventilation, leakage of gastric contents into the lungs and risks the airway being dislodged. Overinflation can lead to damage and complications within the trachea. Further information can be found in the 'What's the evidence' box below.

WHAT'S THE EVIDENCE?

Read the detail guidance on cuff management provided by the National Tracheostomy Safety project (2013)

http://www.tracheostomy.org.uk/storage/files/Cuff%20management.pdf (accessed November 3, 2020)

Mouth care

As the normal flow of air had been disrupted, oral secretions are reduced (Myatt, 2015). Meticulous mouth care is vital to maintain the comfort and hygiene of the person. It may also reduce the risk of ventilator-associated pneumonia (Hellyer et al., 2016). The concentration of chlorhexidine may also influence the effectiveness of the oral hygiene (Andrews and Steen, 2013). There is some discussion and controversy regarding the use of chlorhexidine in the prevention of pneumonia, please see 'What's the evidence' box for further guidance.

WHAT'S THE EVIDENCE?

It is recommended by NTSP, 2013 that chlorhexidine mouthwash is used in between twice daily teeth brushing. Research the current evidence about the benefits and risks of using chlorhexidine mouthwash.

1. Read the detailed guidance on the use of chlorhexidine provided by the National Tracheostomy Safety Project (2013): http://www.tracheostomy.org.uk/storage/files/Cuff%20management.pdf
2. Also, read this Cochrane review:

Hua, F., Xie, H., Worthington, H.V., Furness, S., Zhang, Q. and Li, C. (2016) 'Oral hygiene care for critically ill patients to prevent ventilator-associated pneumonia', *Cochrane Database of Systematic Reviews*, 10: Article #CD008367. doi.org/10.1002/14651858.CD008367.pub3
   There is also a podcast of this review, which can be heard here: www.cochrane.org/pod-casts/10.1002/14651858.CD008367.pub3

Nutrition and hydration and swallowing

A person with an artificial airway inserted is likely to have a nasogastric tube. Adequate nutrition and hydration are vitally import in the critically ill. The presence of a tracheostomy increases the risk of the person developing dysphagia or swallowing difficulties. It is vital that **speech and language therapists** are involved in the person's care to assess the person's swallow and gag reflex to minimise any complications.

THIS TOPIC IS ALSO COVERED IN CHAPTER 10

COMMUNICATION

In any clinical setting communication is a vital component in supporting person-centred care, and this is no different in critical care. Communication will be covered in more detail in Chapter 10.

It is important to acknowledge this here, as this is the most likely point where the person loses their ability to verbalise their wishes. Critical care survivors, even when the person was unconscious or sedated, may often recall communication at the bedside. The conscious and subconscious recall of the noises and conversations at the bedside and can have an adverse impact on long-term psychological outcomes. You need to aware of the techniques and technology available for those intubated to engage in communication, including the use of spelling boards, icon charts, and electronic aids.

THIS TOPIC IS ALSO COVERED IN CHAPTER 10

It is vital that the person is able to convey their thoughts, feelings and concerns to us by using alternative means when they cannot vocalise.

Sarah, 28 years' experience working in level 3 critical care department

VENTILATION

There are many different strategies and methods of ventilating people, but the two main and basic methods will be presented here. These are invasive and non-invasive ventilation. As to which is used depends on the type and severity of the underlying pathology. The terminology and delivery of ventilation can vary according to the manufacturer of the equipment used.

Non-invasive ventilation

Non-invasive positive pressure ventilation (NIPPV) is a method of enhancing gas exchange in the lungs. It is typically delivered via a tight-fitting face or nasal mask. This is offered to avoid the need for invasive ventilation and the associated increased risks. It is also used to help with weaning from invasive ventilation (see the section on weaning from ventilation later in this chapter). An advanced method of NIPPV is bi-level ventilation.

NIPPV differs from invasive ventilation in that the stimulus to breathe comes from the patient. Once the machine recognises this effort, it blows gas into the lungs under positive pressure. This pressure is sustained at a pre-set level until the machine senses that the patient starts the expiration phase and then it ceases to blow. The clinician determines the amount of assistance provided during the inspiration phase. For those patients who are very tired or struggling to breathe then the pressure is set higher than for those who are recovering or only require a low level of support.

A positive pressure can be retained within the respiratory circuit at the end of expiration to splint the lungs open. This pressure is termed continuous positive airway pressure or CPAP. When CPAP is used, it helps to recruit redundant alveoli and improves gaseous exchange in the lungs. It also helps to reduce the work of breathing in as the lungs are already partially inflated, meaning the patient doesn't have to work so hard to inflate their lungs with each inspiration. For those patients who have to work hard to maintain effective breathing CPAP helps in reducing this workload.

As CPAP and PEEP, which relates to invasive mechanical ventilation and is discussed below, increase intrathoracic pressure, the effect on the cardiovascular system can have advantages and disadvantages. There is evidence that CPAP can assist in patients suffering from acute myocardial infarction, however it can reduce cardiac output in patients who have heart failure.

Invasive mechanical ventilation (MV)

Invasive mechanical ventilation (MV) requires inserting an endotracheal tube through the mouth and into the trachea. The end of the tube should rest 2-3cm above the carina. The carina is the bifurcation of the trachea into the left and right main bronchi. The purpose of MV is to take over the process of breathing, thus reducing the workload associated with breathing, reducing **fatigue** and the associated oxygen consumption. The indications for implementing MV are loss of consciousness and loss of the ability of the individual to protect their own airway, respiratory distress and failure and to improve gaseous exchange in the lungs. To provide MV the person is sedated and paralysed to establish the airway and to facilitate compliance with ventilation. This process can have an adverse effect on the blood pressure and associated oxygen delivery to tissues, resulting in tissue hypoxia. Depending on the condition of the person and their compliance with MV, sedation and paralysis may continue until such a time that their lung function and haemodymanic state has recovered and is stable.

The type of ventilation required will determine the equipment used. With invasive ventilation an artificial ventilator is attached to either the endotracheal tube or tracheostomy. Gas, a mixture of air and oxygen at a pre-prescribed concentration, is forcibly blown through the tube, inflating the lungs. This positive pressure ventilation differs from the normal method of breathing where the chest cavity expands, resulting a reduction in intrathoracic pressure to less than atmospheric pressure and air is sucked into the lungs. Using invasive ventilation requires forcibly blowing air into the lungs and can cause a variety of problems.

ACTIVITY 5.7: CRITICAL THINKING

1. How does positive pressure ventilation adversely affect the lungs?
2. What issues can you think of that can arise from the use of sedation and paralysing agents to facilitate positive pressure ventilation?

The main problems with forcing air into the lungs are barotrauma (trauma caused to the lungs by the force, which can result in pneumothorax), inflammation, selective ventilation of areas of the lung that are more flaccid, and under-ventilation of areas of the lung that are redundant. These redundant areas of the lungs can result in infection. The forces involved can induce bronchospasm similar to that seen in asthma where gas becomes trapped in the lungs.

Invasive ventilation needs to be very careful managed and closely observed by the multidisciplinary team. Doctors specialising in intensive care medicine working with intensive care nurses are required to manage the ventilation and interpret the biological findings that are frequently monitored and need to adjust the ventilation accordingly.

Nurses are required to manage the ventilation, oral hygiene to prevent lung and oral infection, and to ensure the airway remains secrete and patent. Frequent endotracheal suctioning is required to ensure the tube remains patent.

Physiotherapists are required to help maintain optimal lung function and gas exchange in the lungs. Radiographers perform regular chest X-rays so the condition of the lungs can be observed.

THIS TOPIC IS ALSO COVERED IN CHAPTER 6

The ventilator is a machine that has a number of different modes of ventilation that can be used to reduce trauma to the lungs and attempt to improve the optimal gas exchange. The ventilator is designed to force gas into the lungs at a set respiratory rate (breaths per minute). Forcing gas into the lungs under positive pressure can have negative effects on cardiac output.

In adults there are two differing forms of MV, volume and pressure control ventilation. Volume ventilation is where a set volume and set respiratory rate are provided. For example, 14 breaths per minute of 70mls of gas for each breath, resulting in a minute volume of 980mls/min (9.8l/min). The hazard of this type of ventilation is that the inhaled gas goes to the area of least resistance, resulting in atelectasis in other areas; and these selected areas of the lung are exposed to excessively high pressures, resulting in barotrauma. The alternative to volume ventilation is pressure-controlled ventilation. This is where the pressure at which the gas is forced into the lungs is controlled, the rate of ventilation is set, and the volume varies. Where the lungs are stiff and hard as seen in acute lung injury, infection and oedema, higher pressures may be needed, but when the lungs are flaccid and clear the pressure required to obtain the same volume is less. Controlling pressure this way means clinicians can control the extent of the barotrauma more effectively. Manipulating the inspiratory and expiratory time along with pressure control ventilation means more areas of redundant lung can be recruited for gas exchange. In order to maintain the effectiveness of the recruited areas of the lung additional pressure can be applied within the circuit to prevent the lungs from collapsing completely at the end of each breath. This additional pressure is called 'positive end expiratory pressure' or 'PEEP'. This means that at the end of expiration the lungs are 'splinted' open by the presence of this pressure, alveoli can be recruited, drainage of sections is facilitated, and gaseous exchange is more efficient. The concern when applying PEEP in ventilation is the unnatural state of retaining a positive pressure within the lungs, which can contribute to barotrauma and increase afterload.

If it is likely that direct access to the lungs will be required for a prolonged period, then a tracheostomy may be considered.

ACTIVITY 5.8: CASE STUDY

Sandra, 72 years old, is admitted to hospital following a bout of flu. She is diagnosed with community acquired pneumonia. Her condition is deteriorating, and she is exhausted. Her pattern of breathing is very laboured, and the healthcare professional team review her condition and the decision is to admit her to the intensive care unit, intubate and ventilate.

1. What type of respiratory failure does Sandra have?
2. How would you persuade Sandra to consent to this treatment plan?
3. What resources do you need to prepare prior to Sandra's admission to your ACCU?
4. Which members of the multidisciplinary team are required to support Sandra?

Prone positioning

In ACCU a strategy to help improve blood oxygen levels in people who, despite high levels of ventilation, continue to have poor gas exchange in the lungs, is to turn the person to lie on their front in the prone position. This is a widely practised procedure that is poorly supported by the research evidence. There is anecdotal evidence that it improves oxygenation in some specific groups of patients but any improvement in mortality requires more robust research. Nursing people in the prone position is problematic due to the reduced access to the front of the person. There is an increased risk in the airway being dislodged and IV access being accidentally removed. It is not possible to reposition the person for pressure area relief resulting in pressure sores, including facial sores, which, along with facial oedema, can be distressing for the relatives. Often the absorption of nasogastric feed is disrupted resulting in malnutrition.

THIS TOPIC IS ALSO COVERED IN CHAPTER 9

WHAT'S THE EVIDENCE?

Read the Cochrane review on prone positioning. This paper is a systematic review of the evidence related to prone positioning.

Bloomfield, R., Noble, D.W. and Sudlow, A. (2018) 'Prone position for acute respiratory failure in adults', *Cochrane Database of Systematic Reviews*, 11: article# CD008095. doi.org/10.1002/14651858. CD008095.pub2

Extra corporeal membranous oxygenation (ECMO)

If you are looking after a very severely ill person you may hear an alternative to positive pressure ventilation being discussed. This is extra corporeal membranous oxygenation (ECMO), which is an advanced form of supporting the failing lungs and heart. It is a highly specialised treatment and only performed in selected intensive care units in the UK. There are two types of ECMO, venovenous to support failed lungs and venoarterial to support both lungs and heart.

Working on the same principles of a **cardiopulmonary bypass** machine that is used in cardiac surgery, venovenous ECMO is used in people who have a reversible, i.e. potentially curable, lung condition such as ARDS, chest trauma or severe infection. It requires the insertion of two large bore cannulas into two large veins such as the groin or neck. Deoxygenated blood is drawn from one vein, passed through an oxygenator where carbon dioxide is removed and the blood oxygenated. It is then returned to the person through the second vein.

Venoarterial ECMO works in the same way but the main difference is that the oxygenated blood is returned to the arterial system. This method is typically used in the management of either lung or cardiac failure.

WHAT'S THE EVIDENCE?

These two papers give national guidance on the selection and administration of ECMO in adults.

Read the NICE guidance (IPG391) on ECMO and severe acute respiratory failure in adults www.nice.org.uk/guidance/ipg391 (accessed November 3, 2020)

and

NICE guidance (IPG482) in ECMO use for acute heart failure in adults. www.nice.org.uk/guidance/ipg482 (accessed November 3, 2020)

As the blood is drawn from the body into an external circulatory system, passed through an artificial oxygenator and then returned to the patient, the main complication that can arise is the development of thrombi. Consequently, people on ECMO are also receiving IV anticoagulation, the dose of which is constantly monitored and adjusted accordingly. Other hazards are a leak in the circulation resulting in major blood loss and the risk of air embolism is high and needs careful monitoring and management. The care of these patients is complicated and requires the nurse to be very knowledgeable and skilled in the discipline. In very unstable patients two nurses may be deployed to look after the one patient.

As the lungs are rendered mostly useless during the process, artificial ventilation may not be required and, although unusual, in some stable patients, the patient can be awake and extubated whilst receiving this treatment.

In people with lung failure, withdrawal of the treatment is dependent on the recovery of the lungs, which can be judged by X-ray analysis, improvement in the compliance of the lungs and the improvement in gas exchange gained through the lung function. Withdrawal of ECMO from people who need it for lung and cardiac support is more difficult as an assessment of the recovery of both lung and cardiac function is required (NICE, 2011).

Discontinuation of mechanical ventilation

THIS TOPIC IS ALSO COVERED IN CHAPTER 11

Ventilatory support should ideally follow a **continuum**, beginning with the initial support for respiration and hopefully ending with the ability to sustain independent spontaneous breathing (Haas and Loik, 2012). For some people the process is quick, a few hours, while other people require more time, which can be as long as several weeks. The discontinuation of mechanical ventilatory support is known as 'weaning' (Blackwood et al., 2011). Weaning should be considered as early as possible, as early liberation from mechanical ventilation has many positive effects. Once the patient is assessed as ready to commence weaning, sedation is reduced (Blackwood et al., 2011).

Weaning can be an immediate move from full ventilatory support to breathing without assistance from the ventilator or a gradual reduction in the amount of ventilator support. The process of ventilatory weaning can be categorised as simple, difficult, or prolonged (Cederwall et al., 2018). Those who experience a difficult or prolonged weaning process spend longer on the mechanical ventilator and in critical care. This increased length of stay is linked to a number of negative outcomes including **depression**, agitation and **delirium** as well as increasing the risk of hospital-acquired infection, **sepsis** and lung damage. The weaning process should ideally be structured, and the plan clearly communicated to the person, their family and the wider clinical team. Within the evidence-base and the critical care communities there is uncertainty about the best approach to weaning. Weaning protocols have been developed which promote different methods such as a physician-driven approach, a nurse-led strategy or a protocol-driven team approach to weaning (Smyrnios et al., 2002). The evidence supports a variety of methods which work in different ways to support a person's unique needs.

WHAT'S THE EVIDENCE?

The ideal strategies to promote timely and successful weaning from mechanical ventilation remain a research and quality improvement priority (Rose, 2015). With no consensus on the approach, reading the following articles will help you understand the different issues:

https://warwick.ac.uk/fac/sci/med/research/ctu/trials/critical/breathe (accessed November 3, 2020)

https://erj.ersjournals.com/content/29/5/1033.long (accessed November 3, 2020)

www.crd.york.ac.uk/crdweb/ShowRecord.asp?LinkFrom=OAI&ID=12001008306 (accessed November 3, 2020)

When you are working in a critical care unit, ask if you can read the weaning protocol and try to find out what evidence supports its use.

Extubation

Extubation is the term used to describe the removal of the ETT and is a hopefully final step in the person's liberation from the ventilator. After assessment it should be clear that the person no longer requires ventilation, and can maintain their airway with a good cough effort. Once this is established, the process of removing the ETT can begin.

ACTIVITY 5.9: RESEARCH AND EVIDENCE-BASED PRACTICE

1.   Look at the local practice policy on how to remove the ETT.

There is no template answer to this activity as it differs depending on location.

Post extubation risks

Following extubation, vigilant observation is required. Despite someone being deemed to be ready to be extubated, approximately 15% of people will need re-intubating (Thille et al., 2016).

Other common risk factors you need to be aware of are:

- Pharyngeal or Laryngeal obstruction due to trauma, increased swelling and oedema
- Laryngospasm
- Bleeding
- Reduced cough and increased secretions
- Latent effect of previously given medication causing drowsiness, reducing conscious level and subsequent risk to their ability to maintain their airway

DECANNULATION

As the person starts their recovery and becomes independent of any respiratory support their artificial airway can be removed. The term 'decannulation' refers to the removal of the person's tracheostomy tube and is a significant event in the person's recovery. Again, there are a number of different ways in which the person can be weaned from their tracheostomy and the process will be guided by the clinical condition of the individual. The person will be assessed to see if removal of the tracheostomy is appropriate and will probably undergo a period of time with the tracheostomy in place but with the cuff deflated. Nursing assessment of any changes to the respiratory status is vital. The tracheostomy will not be as secure with the cuff deflated and greater care is needed when assisting with movement. With the cuff deflated the person may be able to vocalise, although if this is not the case, you should reassure them that their voice will return following decannulation.

Once all the criteria are met, then the team can carry out the procedure. As a nurse you will need to constantly inform and reassure the person during the procedure, as they will experience discomfort. They may also experience the sensation of shortness of breath as the tracheostomy comes out.

If not already, the cuff is deflated using a 10ml syringe. Suction will be needed via the tracheostomy tube to remove any secretions that may have been on top of the cuff and have now tricked into the trachea. It might be advisable to clean the stoma at this point. The tapes will be cut and removed; the tracheostomy will need to be temporarily supported by hand. The tracheostomy is then removed and the stoma covered with a sterile dressing.

ACTIVITY 5.10: THEORY STOP POINT

Consider the procedure outlined above and list the equipment you think you would need to decannulate a person.

1. What assessment would you carry out before and after this procedure?

WHAT'S THE EVIDENCE?

Take a look at the St George's NHS Trust resources on tracheostomy weaning – www.stgeorges.nhs.uk/gps-and-clinicians/clinical-resources/tracheostomy-guidelines/weaning/ (accessed November 3, 2020)

CHAPTER SUMMARY

This chapter has supported your understanding of the following topics:

- The anatomy and physiology of the respiratory system
- The types of respiratory failure
- The administration of oxygen therapy
- How to read arterial blood gas analysis
- The different types of artificial airways including tracheostomy and endotracheal tubes and the nursing assessment and management.
- Artificial respiration and ventilation
- The use of prone positioning in intensive care
- The process of ECMO
- The ways in which mechanical ventilation is removed

GO FURTHER

Books

The Intensive Care Foundation (2015) *Handbook of Mechanical Ventilation: A User's Guide*. London: Intensive Care Society. Available from https://www.ics.ac.uk/ICS/handbooks.aspx (accessed November 3, 2020).

- The Intensive Care Society, a multidisciplinary organisation that focuses its work on research and pioneering developments in UK critical care, publishes this guide.

Bersten, A.D. and Handy, A.M. (2018) *Oh's Intensive Care Manual* (8th edition). London: Elsevier.

- This book is one of the key texts used by all members of the multidisciplinary team working in the discipline of intensive care.

Albarran, J.W. and Richardson, A. (eds) (2013) *Critical Care Manual of Clinical Procedures and Competencies*. Oxford: Wiley-Blackwell.

- This book is a manual that is aimed at all healthcare practitioners from beginners to experts. It encompasses evidence-based guidelines in all aspects of critical care practices.

Journal articles

National Confidential Enquiry into Patient Outcome and Death (NCEPOD) (2014) *On the Right Trach? A Review of the Care Received by Patients who Underwent a Tracheostomy*. NCEPOD, London. Available from https://www.ncepod.org.uk/2014tc.html (accessed November 3, 2020).

National Tracheostomy Safety Project (2013) *NTSP Manual 2013*. http://www.tracheostomy.org.uk/storage/files/Comprehensive%20Tracheostomy%20Care.pdf (accessed November 3, 2020).

- These two publications, NCEPOD and NTSP, related to tracheostomy care are required reading for those who may care for a person who has a tracheostomy. These texts report the causes of avoidable complications associated with tracheostomy care and provides guidance for future practice to prevent these complications and enhance care.

Boles, J.-M., Bion, J., Connors, M., Herridge, M., Marsh, B., Melot, C. [...] and Welte, T. (2007) 'Weaning from mechanical ventilation', *European Respiratory Journal*, 29: 1033–56. doi.org/10.1183/09031936.00010206

- This paper provides guidance on strategies for weaning from ventilation.

Useful websites

Intensive Care Society (2020) *ICS Standards and Guidelines*. www.ics.ac.uk/ICS/GuidelinesStandards/ICS/GuidelinesAndStandards/StandardsAndGuidelines.aspx (accessed November 3, 2020).

- This website has up-to-date clinical guidelines and professional standards for the multiprofessional body working in intensive care.

European Federation of Critical Care Nursing Associations (2020) 'Ventilation'. www.efccna.org/clinical-practice/info-clinical-practice?id=178 (accessed November 3, 2020).

- This website has guidelines for nurses across the European Union on artificial ventilation in critical care.

British Medical Journal Best Practice (2020) Acute Respiratory Distress Syndrome (ARDS). https://bestpractice.bmj.com/topics/en-gb/374 (accessed November 3, 2020).

- This website gives an overview of acute respiratory distress syndrome that is the major condition that requires artificial ventilation in critical care.

REFERENCES

AARC Clinical Practice Guidelines (2010) 'Endotracheal Suctioning of Mechanically Ventilated Patients With Artificial Airways 2010', *Respiratory Care*, 55 (6): 758–64.

Andrews, T. and Steen, C. (2013) 'A review of oral preventative strategies to reduce ventilator-associated pneumonia', *Nurs Crit Care*, 18 (3): 116–22. doi.org/10.1111/nicc.12002

Ashelford, S., Raynsford, J., & Taylor, V. (2019). *Pathophysiology and Pharmacology in Nursing*. (Second ed.) Sage Learning Matters.

Blackwood, B., Alderdice, F., Burns, K., Cardwell, C., Lavery, G. and O'Halloran, P. (2011) 'Use of weaning protocols for reducing duration of mechanical ventilation in critically ill adult patients: Cochrane systematic review and meta-analysis', *BMJ*, 342: c7237.

Brinkman, J.E. and Sandeep, S. (2018) 'Respiratory Alkalosis'. Available from www.ncbi.nlm.nih.gov/books/NBK482117/ (accessed November 2, 2020).

Cederwall, C.J., Olausson, S., Rose, L., Naredi, S. and Ringdal, M. (2018) 'Person-centred care during prolonged weaning from mechanical ventilation, nurses' views: An interview study', *Intensive and Critical Care Nursing*, 46: 32–7. doi.org/10.1016/j.iccn.2017.11.004

Cohen, B.J., and Hull, K.L. (2015) *The Human Body in Health and Disease* (13th edition). London: Wolters Kluwer.

Cook, N., Shepherd, A. and Boore, J. (2021) *Essentials of Anatomy and Physiology for Nursing Practice* (2nd edition). London: Sage.

Dougherty, L. and Lister, S. (2008) *The Royal Marsden Hospital Manual of Clinical Nursing Procedures* (7th edition). Oxford: Blackwell Publishing.

European Resuscitation Council (2001) *Advanced Life Support Manual* (4th edition). Antwerp: University of Antwerp/European Resuscitation Council.

Faculty of Intensive Care Medicine (2019) 'Invasive procedure safety checklist: NG tube insertion'. Available from https://www.ficm.ac.uk/sites/default/files/safety_checklist_-_ng_tube_insertion_-_final.pdf (accessed November 2, 2020).

Freeman, S. (2011) 'Standards for the care of adult patients with a temporary tracheostomy', *Nursing Standard*, 26 (2): 49–56. doi.org/10.7748/ns2011.09.26.2.49.c8706

Freeman, S., Steen, C. and Bleakley G. (2019) 'Caring for the Critically Ill Adult', in D. Burns (ed) *Foundations of Adult Nursing*. London: Sage. pp. 404–32.

Haas, C.F. and Loik, P.S. (2012) 'Ventilator discontinuation protocols', *Respiratory Care*, 57 (10): 1649–62. Available from http://rc.rcjournal.com/content/57/10/1649 (accessed November 3, 2020).

Intensive Care Society (ICS) (2014) *Standards for the Care of Adult Patients with a Temporary Tracheostomy*. London: The Intensive Care Society. Available from https://www.ics.ac.uk/ICS/ICS/GuidelinesAndStandards/ICSGuidelines.aspx as 'ICS Tracheostomy Standards (2014)' (accessed November 2, 2020).

Mallett, J., Albarran, J.W., Richardson, A. (eds) (2013) *Critical Care Manual of Clinical Procedures and Competencies*. Oxford: Wiley Blackwell.

Myatt, R. (2015) 'Nursing care of patients with a temporary tracheostomy', *Nursing Standard*, 29 (26): 42–9.

National Confidential Enquiry into Patient Outcome and Death (NCEPOD) (2014) *On the Right Trach? A Review of the Care Received by Patients who Underwent a Tracheostomy*. London: NCEPOD. Available from https://www.ncepod.org.uk/2014tc.html (accessed November 3, 2020).

National Tracheostomy Safety Project (NTSP) (2013) *NTSP Manual 2013*. Available from http://www.tracheostomy.org.uk/storage/files/Comprehensive%20Tracheostomy%20Care.pdf (accessed November 3, 2020).

NICE (2011) *Extracorporeal Membrane Oxygenation for Severe Acute Respiratory Failure in Adults* (Interventional Procedures Guidance 391). London: NICE. Available from www.nice.org.uk/guidance/ipg391 (accessed November 3, 2020).

Resuscitation Council UK (RCUK) (2015) 'Resuscitation Guidelines', https://www.resus.org.uk/library/2015-resuscitation-guidelines (accessed November 2, 2020).

Rose, L. (2015) 'Strategies for weaning from mechanical ventilation: A state of the art review', *Intensive and Critical Care Nursing*, 31 (4): 189–95.

Smyrnios, N.A., Connolly, A., Wilson, M.M., Curley, F.J., French, C.T., Heard, S.O., Stephen, O. and Irwin, A. (2002) 'Effects of a multifaceted, multidisciplinary, hospital-wide quality improvement program on weaning from mechanical ventilation', *Critical Care Medicine*, 30: 1224–30

Sole, M.L., Xiaogang, S., Talbert, S., Penoyer, D.A., Kalite, S., Jimenez, E., Ludy, J.E. and Bennett, M. (2011) 'Evaluation of an intervention to maintain endotracheal tube cuff pressure within therapeutic range,' *American Journal of Critical Care*, 20 (2): 109–18.

Thille, A.W., Boissier, F., Ben-Ghezala, H., Razazi, K., Mekontso-Dessap, A., Brun-Buisson, C. and Brochard, L. (2016) 'Easily identified at-risk patients for extubation failure may benefit from noninvasive ventilation: A prospective before-after study', *Critical Care*, 20 (1): 1–8.

Tortora, G.J., and Derrickson, B. (2016) *Principles of Anatomy and Physiology*, Volume 2 (15th edition). Singapore: Wiley and Sons.

Waugh, A., and Grant, A., (2018) *Anatomy and Physiology* (13th edition). London: Elsevier.

CRITICAL CARE RELATED TO THE CARDIAC SYSTEM

6

COLIN STEEN

> When I started in critical care, I hadn't really appreciated that there were two circulatory systems and that they were dependent on each other. Each one is just as important as the other and it is fascinating to see how my interventions and treatments produce instant changes which can improve the person's status.
>
> **Charlie, 2 years, critical care experience**

LEARNING OUTCOMES

When you have finished studying this chapter you will be able to understand:

- The anatomy and physiology of the cardiovascular system
- The factors that influence blood flow around the body
- The left and right heart are affected by different things but are dependent upon each other
- Different treatments available for heart failure
- A brief overview of blood and blood products

INTRODUCTION

This chapter will examine the structure and function of the circulatory system and how these influence the oxygen delivery to tissue. You will also learn how the treatments and **interventions** used in intensive care unit can affect the function of the heart and circulatory system, sometimes with detrimental effects and sometimes with beneficial effects.

In critical care there is effective and accurate cardiovascular monitoring which as a minimum normally consists of cardiovascular monitoring tools such as:

- Continuous electrocardiogram monitors, normally via a three-lead system
- Arterial blood pressure recording
- Central venous pressure measurement
- Cardiac output measurement (several tools are available)
- Fluid balance assessment
- Central temperature recording

Figure 6.1 illustrates the common monitoring wave forms you will see. These monitoring tools are there to assist the assessment and management of the critically ill person in our care. In addition to the monitors we must not forget to also undertake a cardiovascular focused assessment of the person's skin, face, neck, and peripheries.

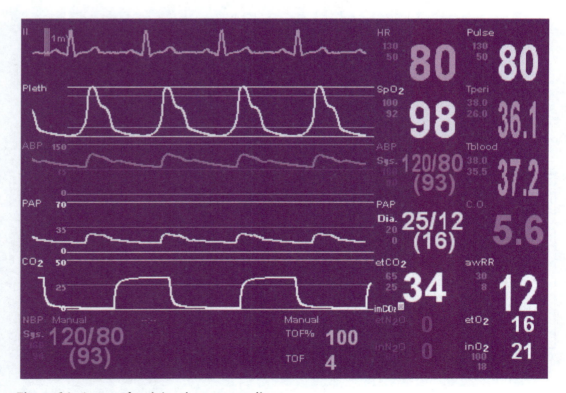

Figure 6.1   Image of an intensive care monitor

ANATOMY

Before we cover critical illness related to the cardiac system it is important that you understand some of the simple gross anatomy and physiology of the heart and blood vessels. If you feel this is an area where you need further support and development, then it is recommended that you access and read an anatomy and physiology book such as Cook et al. (2021).

One of the major processes that keep you alive is the delivery of oxygen and nutrients to all the cells of your body to enable **aerobic** metabolism and the removal of waste products. Every cell receiving an adequate supply of blood should achieve this and the delivery of this blood is enabled by the heart pumping efficiently and the circulation working to provide a blood flow to all areas. If a cell or area of the body does not receive an adequate supply of blood, oxygen and nutrients then normal **metabolic** activity cannot occur and the cell either uses alternative sources that results in anaerobic activity and the production of toxins, or the cell does not function properly. As each cell is part of an organ, then the organ does not function properly: it cannot contribute to the functioning of the body maintaining **homeostasis**, resulting in illness and disease.

THE HEART

The heart sits in the thoracic cavity and is protected by the sternum and rib cage. It is about the size of each individual's closed fist. It requires 4 key components in order for it to function properly, the muscle of the heart, the myocardium, an electrical system, valves to ensure blood flows in one direction. It should also have a blood supply to the myocardium providing it with oxygen and nutrients to be able to function efficiently.

1. The **muscle** of the heart is comprised of three layers, the epicardium (the outside layer); the myocardium (the muscle layer that contracts); the endocardium (the inner layer). Sitting around the heart is another layer, the pericardium. This is a fluid filled sac in which the heart sits. It provides protection and lubrication to allow for smooth functioning of the expansion and contraction of the heart.

    Just as with any other muscle, the heart muscle requires its own blood supply. This is provided through a system of coronary arteries, which branch out and cover the surface of the heart. It is these arteries that, when they become blocked, cause a myocardial infarction (heart attack) or when partially blocked, angina (chest pain).

2. The heart comprises 4 **chambers**, 2 smaller, the left and right atria and 2 larger, the left and right ventricles. Between each chamber and at the outflow from the 2 ventricles is a valve, i.e. 4 valves in total. These valves are vitally important as they ensure that the blood flows in the right direction. If a valve becomes stenotic (stiff) or incompetent (loose) then blood is either unable to flow adequately (stenotic) or can flow in the wrong direction (incompetent), resulting in heart failure and congestion.

3. In order to make the heart muscle contract to pump the blood around the body, the muscle requires an **electrical system** to 'shock' the muscle and make it squeeze the blood out of

the chamber. It has an internal device called a 'pacemaker', which is located in the upper right atrium. This determines when the electrical impulse should commence. It is a finely tuned process and must be working in a very specific way so that the muscle of the heart contracts efficiently. If there is any blockage in the 'electrical wiring' of the heart then the heart will not contract efficiently and this will affect the amount of blood that is ejected from the heart and therefore the oxygen delivery to the cells of the body. This electrical system can be recorded using an ECG machine. The electrical impulse is generated by the cells of the cardiac muscle shifting electrolytes in and out of the cells through the cell membrane. These electrolytes carry a charge, typically a positive charge and this change in electrical charge of the cell creates an electrical impulse that stimulates the muscle. The electrolytes that typically affect the electrical system are potassium (K^+), calcium (Ca^{2+}), magnesium (Mg^{2+}) and, to a lesser extent, sodium (Na^+). All of these electrolytes are positively charged and control frequency and rhythm of the heart which influences the amount of blood that is ejected from the heart per minute. Only under very specific circumstances would you take over control of the person's heart rate, for example when the person's electrical system is not working, and an artificial pacemaker is needed. However, in order to ensure the body's own electrical system is working properly, it is vitally important that you ensure the person's electrolytes are correct by measuring the levels in the blood each day, or more frequently as required. If any abnormality is detected then corrective measures are needed.

ELECTROCARDIOGRAPH (ECG)

The ECG is the method that is used to record the electrical activity of the heart. It can be used in different ways. For example, a basic ECG is when you attach 3 electrodes to the chest wall. This then provides you with a simple recording of an ECG from one perspective (see Figure 6.2, which is an image of a 3 lead ECG). It is the most common system of recording the heart's rhythm. However, it is also possible to record the electrical activity of the heart in different views. If 5 leads are attached to the chest, this typically provides a view of the conduction of electricity through the ventricles. If 10 electrodes are attached to the person, 6 on the chest and one on each of the 4 limbs, this provides a complete 3 dimensional view of the conduction through all chambers of the heart giving 12 different views of the electrical conduction called a 12 lead ECG (see Figure 6.3, which is an image of a 12 lead ECG). The reason why the different views are required is so that it is possible to determine whether there is any damage to the myocardium in one specific area of the heart, which may account for a reduction in cardiac output and efficiency. It may also indicate where there may be a blockage of a specific coronary vessel, which would help the medical team determine where they need to focus their treatment.

It takes a lot of knowledge and many years of practice to accurately read a 12 lead ECG. To begin with you should learn to read the common **arrhythmias** that can be seen in a 3 lead ECG.

ACTIVITY 6.1: THEORY STOP POINT

Review this website on how to read a 3 lead ECG and common arrhythmias that can be detected using 3 leads.

https://patient.info/doctor/ecg-identification-of-arrhythmias (accessed November 4, 2020)

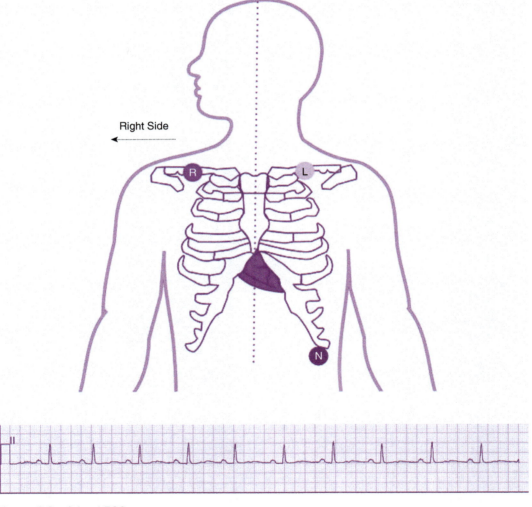

Figure 6.2   3 lead ECG

Source: Adapted from Kumar 2020. Medical Education Resources by LITFL is licensed under a Creative Commons Attribution-NonCommercial-ShareAlike 4.0 International License. Based on a work at https://litfl.com/normal-sinus-rhythm-ecg-library/

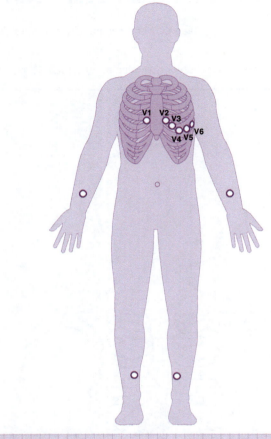

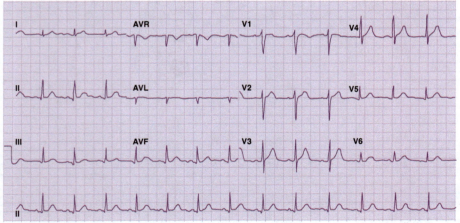

Figure 6.3 12 lead ECG

CARDIAC ARREST AND RESUSCITATION IN INTENSIVE CARE

Despite people in intensive care being the sickest in the hospital the incidence of cardiac arrest occurring in intensive care is significantly lower than people in hospital wards (Armstrong et al., 2019). A potential reason for this is the enhanced monitoring that is undertaken in intensive care which means that any homeostatic imbalances that may have led to a cardiac arrest are detected early and corrected.

Should someone suffer a cardiac arrest, it is handled very differently from a ward. To begin with the cardiac arrest team is not routinely called as there are senior medical staff resident in the department who are very skilled in managing the critically ill. People who do suffer a cardiac arrest are often already intubated and ventilated so the airway and breathing are already protected, which just leaves chest compressions. Owing to the severe illness the person is suffering, resuscitation can often be complicated and not follow the normal process, as the staff already have access to a lot of information regarding the person's blood chemistry.

THE CIRCULATION

The circulation is a closed system of pipes that flows around all the cells of the body conveying blood pumped by the heart. There are 2 circulatory systems, each containing 2 types of vessels. The first and main one is the **systemic** system. This arises from the left ventricle, the main pumping chamber of the heart in the major artery called the aorta. This oxygenated blood passes through the arteries and arterioles to the smaller capillaries where the exchange of oxygen, nutrients and waste products occurs at cellular level. The blood then passes into the veins, which returns the blood to the right atrium of the heart. This is the end of the first circulatory system.

The second system is the **pulmonary** circulation and differs from the arterial system in that deoxygenated blood is carried in the arterial system and oxygenated blood is carried by the venous system. The deoxygenated blood is pumped from the right ventricle through the pulmonary artery to the lungs where gas exchange takes place. It returns to the left atrium of the heart through the pulmonary veins as oxygenated blood. In Table 6.1 there is a summary of the difference between arteries and veins.

Table 6.1 Difference between arteries and veins

Systemic		Pulmonary	
Artery	Vein	Artery	Vein
Carries oxygenated blood away from the heart	Carries deoxygenated blood towards the heart	Carries deoxygenated blood away from the heart	Carries oxygenated blood towards the heart
Are found deeper in the body	Are found closer to the skin	Are found deep inside the thoracic cavity	Are found deep inside the thoracic cavity
Has a narrow lumen	Has a wide lumen	Has a wider lumen	Has a wide lumen

(Continued)

Table 6.1 (Continued)

Systemic		Pulmonary	
The walls are elastic and have a thicker muscle layer which can distend under the pressure of the ventricle pumping	Less elastic and has a thinner layer of muscle	Thick elastic walls to accommodate the pressure from the right ventricle	Thinner walls
Blood flows under the pressure of the left ventricle pumping	The blood flows passively, pushed by the blood flow from behind.	Blood flows under the pressure of the right ventricle pumping	Blood flows under the pressure of the right ventricle pumping
No valves	Contain valves throughout to ensure there's no back flow	No valves	No valves as the pressure from the right ventricle is sufficient to drive the blood through to the left atria.

PHYSIOLOGY

The monitoring of a person's **haemodynamic** status involves measuring, calculating and analysing how the heart is functioning and how the vasculature is influencing the blood flow through the body and the oxygen delivery to tissues. The assessment of the functioning of the heart starts with cardiac output.

CARE OF INVASIVE LINES

People that are admitted to critical care will have a number of invasive lines inserted into veins and arteries. These are in addition to the usual peripheral lines you will have seen used in other clinical areas. The 'lines' are used for the invasive monitoring of haemodynamic parameters (heart rate/blood pressure/cardiac output) and/or administration of fluid and medicine. There are a wide variety of invasive lines used in critical care including:

- Arterial lines
- Central Venous Catheter lines
- Vascaths (to support haemodialysis)
- Pulmonary artery catheters (inserted into a large vein and floated in the pulmonary artery, used to obtain haemodynamic measurements)
- Hickmann lines (inserted into veins and used for the long-term administration of chemotherapy, medicines and/or nutrition)

The more common types of invasive lines are central venous catheters (CVC) and arterial lines. Central lines are typically inserted into large veins like the internal jugular vein, subclavian vein or femoral vein. Certain medicines used in critical care like noradrenaline are not recommended for peripheral use and require administering via a CVC. Additionally, the CVC can be used to administer fluid and nutrition during the period of critical illness. An arterial line is inserted into an artery and provides direct and continual haemodynamic monitoring. Arterial lines are also used to gain samples of blood for arterial blood gas (ABG) for analysis, removing the need to puncture the skin repeatedly, which is painful.

Any invasive line that is inserted into blood vessels carries risk. These risks include dislodgment, extravasation, haemorrhage, infection, and phlebitis. The insertion site offers an opportunity for bacteria to enter the person's blood stream. Therefore, meticulous nursing care is needed to minimise the risk associated with invasive lines.

First, inadequate fixation of the invasive line can lead to dislodgement or cause trauma to surrounding tissue. Central and arterial lines are usually secured with skin sutures. Typically, a transparent dressing is used over the insertion site, so that the nurse is able to check the insertion site for swelling, haemorrhage and infection. These dressings are changed regularly, and you must consult your local hospital policy for further guidance. It is important to document the anatomical site, date and time of the dressing change in the person's clinical notes. If the nurse suspects swelling, bleeding or infection at the site of the invasive line, this must be escalated immediately to a senior clinician for further assessment. Be cautious and always seek guidance. You must never stop an **intravenous** infusion without checking first. Certain medicines, like adrenaline and noradrenaline, can cause cardiovascular collapse if stopped suddenly. The nurse must always decontaminate hands and observe the aseptic non-touch technique (ANTT) when changing invasive line dressings. Central venous catheter related infections that can result in septic shock are significantly high in critical care areas (Bion et. al., 2012) (for a discussion on infection control, see Chapter 4).

THIS TOPIC IS ALSO COVERED IN CHAPTER **4**

WHAT'S THE EVIDENCE?

The following evidence source will help you understand some of the important aspects of invasive line care:

NICE (2016) www.nice.org.uk/guidance/mtg34/resources/policy-for-the-insertion-and-care-of-central-venous-access-devices-cvad-in-hospital-royal-marsden-nhs-ft-pdf-4481503169 (accessed November 4, 2020).

HAEMODYNAMIC MONITORING

Cardiac output

Assuming the structure of the heart is intact then the cardiac output is determined by the contractility of the heart muscle and the heart rate. It can be shown in the simple formula

Cardiac Output (C) = Stroke Volume (SV) x Heart Rate (HR)

(Stroke volume is the amount of blood volume that is ejected from the ventricle with each heartbeat.)

(Cardiac output is the amount of blood ejected from the heart in 1 minute. The Heart Rate is the number of beats per minute.)

Preload

The contractility is dependent on the elasticity of the heart. The Frank-Starling law describes the relationship between fluid loading and contractility and cardiac output. A depiction of this can be seen in Figure 6.4.

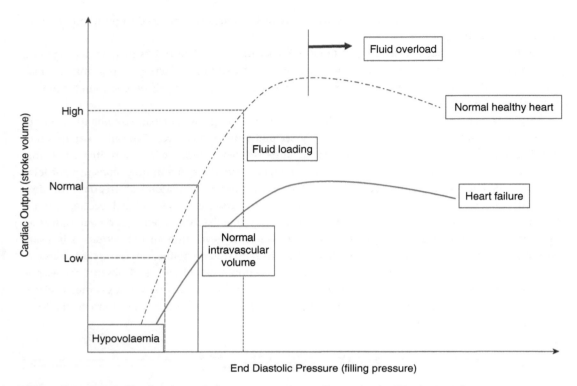

Figure 6.4 Frank-Starling Law of changes seen in cardiac output with changes in venous return/hydration

This law shows as the volume of blood stretches the fibres of the heart, they recoil with sufficient force to eject blood out of the heart and around the body. The stretch of the heart is dependent on the volume of blood, also known as the hydration status of the person. This is why it is very important for you to keep accurate fluid balance records of all people under your care. The more fluid you give a person, the more you make the fibres stretch and therefore the greater the force of the contraction. This is termed the 'preload'. It can be measured through an intravenous line that is inserted into a main vein such as the subclavian or internal jugular. The tip of the line rests near or inside the right atrium and it can measure the pressure in the venous system. This is called the Central Venous Pressure (CVP) and indicates the preload of the heart. The normal CVP is around 2 – 8 cmH$_2$O.

However, there comes a point when the fibres become too far stretched and they become flaccid and do not recoil with the same degree of force, this is called fluid overload. Fortunately, by reducing the amount of fluid in the circulation the force of the recoil improves. This can be achieved by giving a drug, such as a **diuretic**.

ACTIVITY 6.2: REFLECTIVE PRACTICE

It is easy to forget the more 'basic' approaches to assessment when in such a highly technical area, but these assessments offer additional information that adds to a more complete overall assessment. Consider and reflect on the assessments you have undertaken in non-critical care areas.

1. What you think we mean by cardiovascular-focused assessment of the person's skin, face, neck, and peripheries?
2. What abnormalities are we assessing for?

ACTIVITY 6.3: CASE STUDY

You and the staff nurse you are working with, Laura, are waiting for a new admission who is being transferred to critical care from theatre. Over the phone, Laura has received a brief handover and lets you know that you will be caring for Gerry, who is 65 years old. He is being admitted to the department ventilated post elective surgery. He has had a Whipple's procedure or pancreaticoduo-denectomy to remove a pancreatic tumour. The surgeon said they will visit in an hour or so and speak to Gerry's partner. There were some complications, so Gerry was not woken in recovery but brought to critical care. He is to remain sedated and ventilated with a view to wean from mechanical ventila-tion following the surgeon's review.

The team arrives with Gerry and he is transferred onto the critical care monitoring and swapped from the transfer ventilator to the department's ventilator by the anaesthetist.

Gerry's monitor shows:

- Heart rate is 120 beats per minute in sinus rhythm
- Arterial blood pressure is 88/52 mm Hg (**mean arterial pressure**, 64 mm Hg)
- Central venous pressure is 6 mm Hg

He has a 1 litre bag of Hartmann's solution attached but clamped closed during transfer and the transferring nurse says he has 2 units of packed red blood cells in the fridge.

1. What is your first concern and what do you think may be happening to Gerry?
2. Are there any additional assessments you can make?
3. Who do you need to involve in Gerry's care at the moment and what do you think the plan of interventions could be?

WHAT'S THE EVIDENCE?

If left untreated, hypovolemia can result in the **ischaemic** injury of vital organs, leading to multi-system organ failure, and therefore quick effective action is required.

Read the following guidance about:

- resuscitation for **hypovolemic** shock

  https://patient.info/doctor/resuscitation-in-hypovolaemic-shock (accessed November 4, 2020)

- assessment of hypovolaemia in the critically ill

  https://pubmed.ncbi.nlm.nih.gov/29182211/ (accessed November 4, 2020)

(Continued)

- guideline outlined by NICE which relates to fluid therapy

  www.nice.org.uk/guidance/cg174/resources/intravenous-fluid-therapy-in-adults-in-hospital-algorithm-poster-set-191627821 (accessed November 4, 2020)

Afterload

The amount of blood that is ejected from the heart is also dependent on the resistance against which the ventricles have to pump. This is determined by the tension in the arterial circulation. If there is **vasoconstriction**, i.e. the lumen of the blood vessels is reduced (as seen in most types of shock), then the resistance is high and the ventricles have to work harder to overcome this resistance and eject blood from the heart. If there is vasodilation, i.e. the lumen of the vessels is wide, then the resistance is low and the heart has to work less hard to overcome this resistance to eject blood from the heart.

Measurement

The cardiac output and the **afterload** can be measured in a variety of ways. The Pulmonary Artery (PA) catheter used to be gold standard but this was an invasive technique and came with some risks of complications. Therefore, you will see more contemporary ways of monitoring cardiac output, some invasive and some non-invasive. The method will depend on the unit on which you work, but they will all offer the same information. The process is to gather information on blood flow and from this various calculations can be done to determine how much oxygen is delivered to the cells of the person's body and how much of this oxygen the cells consume, which helps to determine whether the oxygen level in the blood is adequate and whether the blood flow to the cells is adequate in order to maintain homeostasis. The different calculations and variables measured can be seen in Table 6.2.

Table 6.2 Haemodynamic variables that can be calculated in intensive care (Vincent, 2014)

Variable to be measured	Formula
Determination of Cardiac Output (CO) per minute.	Cardiac Output = Heart Rate × Stroke Volume
	$CO = HR \times SV$
	Normal = 5 litre/min
Calculation of the oxygen delivery to the tissues (DO_2)	DO_2 = Cardiac Index × PaO_2
	$DO_2 = CI \times PaO_2 \times 10$
	Normal = 500–600 O_2/min/m²
Oxygen consumption (VO_2)	$VO_2 = (PaO_2 - PvO_2) \times x \ CI \times 10$
This is the amount of oxygen that the cells consume. It is a more accurate measurement of cellular activity. Again the higher the number, the more metabolic activity.	Normal = 120-170ml/min/m²

Variable to be measured	Formula
Oxygen extraction ratio (OER). This is the amount of oxygen that is removed from the arterial blood by the cells of the body. The higher the figure, the more metabolic activity is occurring. This can indicate ill health.	Oxygen Extraction Ratio = (Partial Pressure of arterial oxygen – partial pressure of venous oxygen [taken from a central line]) divided by partial pressure of arterial oxygen $$OER = \frac{PaO_2 - PvO_2}{PaO_2}$$ Normal = 22–30%

You will notice the use of CI in the formulae above. When measuring variables such as these, it is important to take the size of the person into account. A smaller person would require and consume a smaller amount of oxygen and correspondingly they would have a smaller cardiac output than a larger person. So a calculation is used to determine the body surface area of the person in metres^2 (see below). In order to do this calculation the height and weight of the person is required. This is why it is very important when you admit a person to hospital that as part of the admission process you measure and record an accurate height and weight.

Formula to calculate body surface area.

$$(BSA = \frac{\sqrt{Weight(kg) \times Height(cm)}}{3600})$$

Arterial pressure (blood pressure)

As mentioned earlier, it is common to record people's blood pressure using an arterial line. The arterial line is rigid and not flexible. It is also not designed to have fluids administered through it. However, it is usually attached to a saline 0.9% infusion that is under pressure through a pressure bag, this is to prevent the person's blood moving up into the infusion set. The pressure bag needs to be at a pressure higher than the systolic pressure to prevent this. This is then attached to a device called a transducer, which in turn attached to the arterial cannula. The transducer has 2 functions. The first is to permit the infusion of the saline at 2–3mls/h, just enough to prevent the line from blocking. The second, and main function, is to convert, or transduce, the physical pressure from the artery into an electronic impulse that is then translated onto a monitor. The pressure trace can then record the systolic and diastolic pressures (see Figure 6.5). Using this trace you can see a beat-to-beat waveform depicting the arterial blood pressure.

However, you can further analyse the waveform and determine other things from its shape and amplitude. For example, if the waveform's amplitude varies in time with the respiration, this is termed respiratory swing, or if the waveform looks like a spike, this can often indicate hypovolaemia or cardiac insufficiency (see Figure 6.6). If the waveform is rounded with little difference between the systolic and diastolic pressures this may indicate that the heart is struggling to pump efficiently.

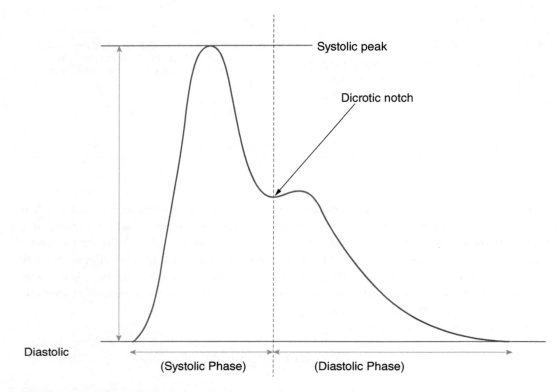

Figure 6.5 An example of an annotated arterial waveform

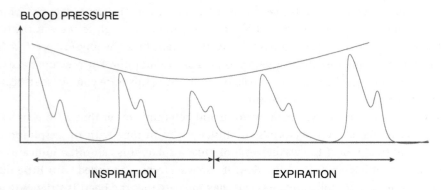

Figure 6.6 Another example of an arterial waveform showing respiratory swing

=== **WHAT'S THE EVIDENCE?** ===

This article provides more in-depth analysis of the reading of an arterial line trace and the errors that can occur in the waveform affecting the measurement.

Saugel, B., Kouz, K., Meidert, A., Schulte-Uentrup, L. and Romagnoli, S. (2020) 'How to measure blood pressure using an arterial catheter: A systematic 5-step approach', *Critical Care*, 24 (1), Article #172. doi.org/10.1186/s13054-020-02859-w

DRUGS USED IN INTENSIVE CARE TO SUPPORT THE HEART AND CIRCULATION

There are a number of key drugs that are used in managing someone's blood pressure and blood flow when in intensive care. Each drug works on a different part of heart and vasculature and the type of drug used depends on the problem faced by the person.

There are specific receptors in the body that, when stimulated or blocked by drugs, affect that part of the body. Typically, these receptors are called alpha 1 (α_1), beta 1 (β_1), beta 2 (β_2) and Dopaminergic although there are many others. Their effect is seen in Table 6.3.

Table 6.3 Receptors found in the body and how they affect blood pressure

Receptor Type	Where found	Effect on that part of the body
Alpha 1 (α_1)	Peripheral vasculature Renal circulation Coronary vasculature	Vasoconstriction
Beta 1 (β_1)	Heart	Increases the contractility of the heart (i.e. the stroke volume) Increases the heart rate
Beta 2 (β_2)	Lungs Peripheral and coronary circulation	Bronchodilation Vasodilation
Dopaminergic	Mesenteric circulation Renal circulation Coronary arteries	Vasodilation

When determining which type of drug to use or which dose you should increase or decrease depends on what you are going to try and achieve to maintain homeostasis. You need to decide whether you are trying to improve cardiac output or change the vascular tone, i.e. vasoconstriction or vasodilation. The initial management of the cardiac output is dependent on the person's Starling curve and a decision is needed as to whether they are at the top of the curve or whether more fluid is required. Once this decision is made, then medication should be considered. There are 4 main drugs used in controlling blood pressure in intensive care; their uses can be seen in Table 6.4.

Table. 6.4 Drugs used in controlling blood pressure in intensive care

Drug	Local of action	Effects	Indication
Dopamine	Dopaminergic receptors	Positive **inotrope**	Dose dependent
		Renal and mesenteric vascular dilation	Improvement of renal and mesenteric blood flow
		Increases vascular resistance (vasoconstriction) elsewhere	At higher doses vasoconstriction and **tachycardia**
Dobutamine	β_1 and β_2	Positive inotrope	Reduced cardiac output/ cardiogenic shock often following acute myocardial ischaemia
		Decreases vascular resistance	
		Increases cardiac output	
Epinepherine (adrenaline)	α_1 β_1 and β_2	Positive inotrope	Increase in cardiac output
		Vasoconstriction	Mainly vasoconstriction
		Increases cardiac output	
		Decreases vascular resistance	
		Increases vascular resistance	
		(this drug has a dual effect and the dose and use in combination with other drugs needs careful titration)	
Nor-epinepherine (noradrenaline)	α_1 β_1 and β_2	Mainly vasoconstriction	Mainly vasoconstriction
		Positive inotrope	

ACTIVITY 6.4: REFLECTIVE PRACTICE

Now that you are informed about the importance of Frank-Starling's Law and fluid management, consider how a person with a low blood pressure might be managed.

1. What would be your first treatment strategy?
2. What would be the ongoing treatment if the first strategy is not effective enough and doesn't restore the blood pressure to normal levels?

CARDIOGENIC SHOCK

Cardiogenic shock occurs when one of the systems that makes the heart pump efficiently fails. For example, if there is damage to the heart muscle, the myocardium, then the muscle of the heart is incapable of pumping efficiently. If there is a failure in the valve, then the blood flow through the heart is affected and the cardiac output will fall. If there is damage to the electrical system of the heart, then the trigger to make the muscle contract fails and the cardiac output is reduced which can result in an enlarged heart and a flatter Starling curve. To treat cardiogenic shock, you need to determine the causes, so if there is a problem with the heart muscle then we need to restore the blood flow to the muscle or reduce the workload of the muscle. If the problem is with valves, then usually surgery is required to repair or replace the valve. If there is a problem with the electrical system then again the cause needs to be determined and treated appropriately, for example ensuring that the blood electrolytes are normal, whether there has been damage to the electrical system that may require a pacemaker, or whether the heart has become distended damaging the conduction process which would require management of the heart muscle. There main drugs used in managing heart failure and cardiogenic shock can be seen in Table 6.5.

WHAT'S THE EVIDENCE?

This guidance from the National Institute for Health and Care Excellence (NICE) (NH106) covers the diagnosis and management of adults with chronic heart failure.

www.nice.org.uk/guidance/ng106/evidence/full-guideline-pdf-6538850029 (accessed November 4, 2020)

Table 6.5 Drugs used to treat heart failure

Drugs used to treat heart failure	Mode of action
ACE inhibitors	ACE inhibitors induce vasodilation resulting in a reduction in afterload, easing the workload of the heart and allowing it to pump more effectively. They also reduce the blood pressure.
Angiotensin receptor blockers (ARBs)	These are used when the side effects of ACE inhibitors are not tolerated by the person. Their action on the body is similar to ACE inhibitors.
Beta blockers	When used in heart failure, Beta blockers slow down the heart rate, allowing the heart the time to fill properly and create a more effective output with each beat.
Mineralocorticoid receptor antagonists (the most common one is Spironolactone)	Often used in combination with the drugs above to reduce blood pressure, these diuretics promote water loss through urination. They encourage a decrease in the reabsorption of sodium in the kidney whilst preserving potassium levels, which are required to maintain a regular heart beat.
Other diuretics	Other diuretics allow for water loss through urination but are less discriminate than Mineralocorticoid receptor antagonists in the electrolytes that are lost.

Diuretics are designed to reduce blood volume. The effect of this is two-fold. Firstly, is reduces the afterload of the heart, reducing the force against which the ventricle has to pump. Second, by reducing the water content of blood volume, an osmotic potential is established that draws in water from extravascular spaces. This is beneficial in people who have oedema, especially of the legs.

Ivabradine	Similar but safer drug than beta blockers but needs to be used with caution when the person has other symptoms or co-morbidities.
Hydralazine	A vasodilator similar to ACE inhibitors but is used when ACE inhibitors or ARBs are not tolerated. Can be used with other vasodilators such as nitrates.

(Continued)

Table 6.5 (Continued)

Drugs used to treat heart failure	Mode of action
Nitrates	Reduce the vascular tone, increasing vasodilation and reducing the afterload of the heart increasing the cardiac output. Can also be used in those who have chest pain as a vasodilator of the coronary vessels, increasing blood flow to the myocardium and reducing pain whilst also reducing the afterload of the heart.
Digoxin	Used in the treatment of atrial arrhythmias such **as atrial fibrillation.** It slows and steadies the heart beat allowing the heart to beat more strongly and with a better rhythm.

DVT PROPHYLAXIS

Venous thromboembolisms (VTE) such as pulmonary **embolism** (PE) and deep venous **thrombosis** (DVT), are a common and severe complication of critical illness. The reason is that the critically unwell person is immobile, and the use of **sedation** and **vasopressors** increases their risk (Minet et al., 2015). Other risk factors are **sepsis**, and vascular injury from indwelling central venous catheters or other invasive interventions (Miri et al., 2017). Therefore, thromboprophylaxis is needed, usually by administering low molecular weight heparin except when **prophylaxis** is contraindicated. The use of prophylactic thromboprophylaxis is normally until the person is awake and mobile. As nurses, we play a vital role in the detection of early DVT as we conduct frequent assessments. To help you remember some key points when assessing the critically ill person in your care O'Brien et. al. (2018) developed the mnemonic STOP*DVTs*:

- S—*S*welling and *S*hortness of breath
- T—Skin on the affected limb that is hot or cold to *T*ouch – The presence of *T*achycardia
- O—*O*peration (Has the person undergone a total hip or knee replacement?)
- P—*P*ain (Has the person got increased pain in the affected limb?)
- D—*D*iscoloration (Is the skin on the affected limb discoloured?)
- V—*V*eins/*V*aricoses (Does the person have swollen/distended varicose veins in the affected limb?)
- T—*T*ime (How many days post-surgery)
- S—*S*till/*S*edentary (The person is less mobile than expected)

It's also important for you to check the limbs where there are invasive lines.

VENTRICULAR ASSIST DEVICES

In specialist critical care units, ventricular assist devices (VAD) can be used to reduce the workload of the heart, or in some cases take over the pumping of blood around the body completely. Depending on the type, these either require the person to have a very large catheter, which has a large balloon on the end, inserted into their femoral artery or a device implanted into either the chest or abdomen, a VAD. The first device has a balloon at the end of the catheter which inflates and deflates in time with the heart to help displace the blood from the descending aorta around the body. Whilst it increases the perfusion of the tissues, it also reduces the afterload of the left ventricle that results in a more efficient working of the heart.

The alternative VAD can be used as a bridge to a heart transplant. The insertion of these requires surgery as they sit inside the thorax and are plumbed directly into the heart. Using **vortex** flow, they draw the blood from the heart and pump it around the body, effectively acting as the heart. The control and power comes from a device that sits outside the body and is attached to the device inside the body by cabling. This is a temporary device whilst a person waits for organ donation. However as technology develops, these devices are increasingly being used for longer periods and may in the future be used as an alternative to transplants.

ACTIVITY 6.5: THEORY STOP POINT

Review this website that focuses on ventricular assist devices.

www.bhf.org.uk/informationsupport/heart-matters-magazine/medical/lvads (accessed November 4, 2020)

1. Watch this video and consider what challenges a person living with a ventricular assist device faces in your opinion

www.bhf.org.uk/informationsupport/heart-matters-magazine/my-story/living-with-an-artificial-heart (accessed November 4, 2020)

ACTIVITY 6.6: CASE STUDY

Brenda is 72 years old. She is active and does regular exercise. She reports feeling excessively tired over the last week. She has some discomfort in the form of indigestion and some pain in her upper back. She has some osteoarthritis for which she takes paracetamol as required. She is tachycardiac with a low blood pressure and sounds of fluid in her lungs. She is admitted to intensive care for non-invasive ventilation and possible insertion of ventricular assist device.

Read this article before answering this question:

- www.ahajournals.org/doi/10.1161/JAHA.119.014733 (accessed November 4, 2020)

1. What might be causing Brenda's symptoms?

Before answering the next question, please review the 2 documents from NICE:

- www.nice.org.uk/guidance/qs68/resources/acute-coronary-syndromes-in-adults-pdf-2098794360517 (accessed November 4, 2020)
- www.nice.org.uk/guidance/cg187/resources/acute-heart-failure-diagnosis-and-management-pdf-35109817738693 (accessed November 4, 2020)

2. What investigations might be requested?

BLOOD AND BLOOD PRODUCTS

This chapter talks about the heart and circulation and part of this is blood. Although blood and blood products could sit within a number of other topics it will be briefly mentioned here. Table 6.6 lists the blood groups.

Table 6.6   The ABO blood type system

Blood Group	
A	A antigens on the red blood cells with anti-B antibodies in the plasma
B	B antigens on the red blood cells with anti-A antibodies in the plasma
O	No antigens, but both anti-A and anti-B antibodies in the plasma
AB	Both A and B antigens, but no antibodies

THE RHESUS SYSTEM

The red blood cells of your blood sometimes have another **antigen** which is the Rhesus antigen (RhD). If you have this then you are positive (+) and if you don't then you are negative (-). Approximately 85% of the UK population is positive and the other 15% are negative.

This means that there are 8 main types of blood group:

A+ and A-

B+ and B-

O+ and O-

AB+ and AB-.

When cross matching blood other factors are taken into account by the haematologist, but broadly speaking these 2 main classifications are the main determiners as to the type of blood you have.

Blood Products

When a blood donor donates blood, they donate whole blood. The whole blood is then slit up into various solutions (see Table 6.7). For example, the most typical type of blood transfusion is red blood cells, or 'packed cells' and this is used for those who are anaemic.

ACTIVITY 6.7: THEORY STOP POINT

Review the NICE guidance (NG24) on blood transfusions.

www.nice.org.uk/guidance/ng24 (accessed November 4, 2020).

Table 6.7 Types of blood products

Packed Red Blood Cells	Used for people with a low haemoglobin level
Platelets	Used in people who have a low platelet count which can cause bleeding
Albumin	Used to increase the levels of albumin in the blood and replace a loss of blood volume. The Albumin helps to regulate the oncotic pressure of the blood drawing in extravascular fluid as necessary
Cryoprecipitate	Contains specific elements of fresh frozen plasma
Fresh frozen plasma	Contains all the clotting factors and is used in people who are bleeding or are at risk of bleeding.

CHAPTER SUMMARY

This chapter has supported your understanding of:

- The anatomy and physiology of the cardiovascular system
- How there are different factors that influence the blood flow around the body
- The factors that influence the blood flow around the body have also been discussed along with the different treatments for heart failure
- The use of ventricular assist devices
- The ABO system of blood transfusion and other blood products that are used in healthcare practice

GO FURTHER

Books

Davies, A. and Scott, A. (2015) *Starting to Read ECGs: The Basics* (4th edition). London: Springer.

- This book is a comprehensive text on how to perform, record and interpret a normal ECG. It also includes the effects of cardiac conditions on an ECG.

Peate, I. and Muralitharan, N. (2017) *Fundamentals of Anatomy and Physiology for Nursing and Healthcare Students* (2nd edition). Chichester: Wiley.

- This text is an overview of the structure and function of the human body.

Aaronson, P.I., Connolly, M.J. and Ward, J.P.T. (2012) *The Cardiovascular System at a Glance*. Hoboken, NJ: Wiley-Blackwell.

- This a guide to understanding the heart and circulation.

Journal articles

van Oosterhout, R.E.M., de Boar, A.R., Maas, A.H.E.M., Rutten, F.H., Bots, M.A. and Peters, S.A.E. (2020) 'Sex differences in symptom presentation in acute coronary syndromes: A systematic review and meta-analysis', *Journal of the American Heart Association*, 9 (9). doi.org/10.1161/JAHA.119.014733

- This is an article assessing the extent of sex differences in symptom presentation with confirmed ACS.

National Institute for Health and Care Excellence (NICE) (2014) *Acute Coronary Syndromes in Adults* (Quality Standard 68). Available from www.nice.org.uk/guidance/qs68 (accessed November 4, 2020)

- The above link takes you to the quality standards regarding diagnosing and managing acute coronary syndromes in adults.

Pena-Hernandez, C. and Nugent, K. (2019) 'One approach to circulation and blood flow in the critical care unit', *World Journal of Critical Care Medicine*, 8 (4): 36–48.

- A guide to clinical information relevant when assessing the critically ill with failing circulation.

Useful websites

www.bhf.org.uk (accessed November 4, 2020)

- The British Heart Foundation's 'For Professionals' section of the website has a variety of sources of information for both you and those in your care.

www.bhf.org.uk/informationsupport/heart-matters-magazine/medical/lvads (accessed November 4, 2020)

- The British Heart Foundation website also contains information on ventricular assist devices.

www.oxfordmedicaleducation.com/intensive-care/cardiovascular-support-on-icu/ (accessed November 4, 2020)

- This website provides additional details on cardiovascular support that is provided in intensive care units.

REFERENCES

Armstrong, R.A., Kane, C., Oglesby. F., Barnard, K., Soar, J. and Thomas, M. (2019) 'The incidence of cardiac arrest in the intensive care unit: A systematic review', *Journal of the Intensive Care Society*. doi.org/10.1177/1751143718774713

Cook, N., Shepherd, A. and Boore, J. (2021) *Essentials of Anatomy and Physiology for Nursing Practice*. London: Sage.

Furst, J. (2017) 'Recording a 12 lead ECG/EKG'. Available from https://www.firstaidforfree.com/recording-a-12-lead-ecgekg/

Kumar, A. (2020) 'Three(3), Five(5), Ten(10) Lead ECG Cable/Electrode Placement'. Available from https://www.biometriccables.in/blogs/blog/three3-five5-ten10-lead-ecg-cable-electrode-placement

Minet, C., Potton, L., Bonadona, A., Hamidfar-Roy, R., Somohano, C.A., Maxime Lugosi, M. [...] and Timsit, J.F. (2015) 'Venous thromboembolism in the ICU: Main characteristics, diagnosis, and thromboprophylaxis', *Critical Care*, *19*: Article #287. doi.org/10.1186/s13054-015-1003-9

Miri, M., Goharani, R., and Sistanizad, M. (2017). 'Deep vein thrombosis among Intensive Care Unit patients: An epidemiologic study', *Emergency (Tehran, Iran)*, 5 (1): e13.

Morton, P.G. and Fontaine, D.K. (2017) *Critical Care Nursing: A Holistic Approach*. Philadelphia, PA: Lippincott Williams and Wilkins.

Naish J., Syndercombe Court, D. (2018) *Medical Science* (3rd edition). London: Elsevier.

O'Brien, A., Redley, B., Wood, B., Botti, M. and Hutchinson, A.F. (2018) 'STOP*DVTs*: Development and testing of a clinical assessment tool to guide a nursing assessment of postoperative patients for Deep Vein Thrombosis', *Journal of Clinical Nursing*, 27 (9–10): 1803–11. https://doi.org/10.1111/jocn.14329

Vincent, J.L. (2014) 'Arterial, Central Venous and Pulmonary Artery Catheters', in Joseph E. Parrillo and R. P. Dellinger (eds) *Critical Care Medicine Principles of Diagnosis and Management in the Adult*. (4th edition). Philadelphia, PA: Elsevier/Saunders.

CRITICAL CARE RELATED TO SYSTEMIC INFLAMMATORY RESPONSE

7

COLIN STEEN

> " I have seen far too many patients suffer and die as a consequence of sepsis. Some of these may have been prevented had the screening and intervention been more rigorous. I have read with increasing interest the evidence supporting the use of sepsis screening tools and treatment plans in areas outside of critical care. I only hope that they are implemented fully to help prevent unnecessary admissions to critical care.
>
> **Erin, Senior Sister, 35 Years Critical Care Experience** "

LEARNING OUTCOMES

When you have finished studying this chapter you will be able to understand:

- The definition of **sepsis**
- A brief overview of what sepsis is and how it occurs
- The warning signs that sepsis is developing
- How you should manage sepsis in line with detailed guidelines
- That sepsis is everyone's responsibility
- The care bundles that are required to ensure the person is getting the right treatment.

INTRODUCTION

Sepsis is a concern for all healthcare staff. It requires everyone to be extra vigilant owing to the very poor outcomes that can arise if treatment is not started in a timely fashion.

This chapter gives an overview of the pathophysiology of sepsis, the importance of early detection in the development of sepsis and its management. It also briefly looks at sepsis and its relationship with coronavirus (Covid-19) according to the evidence that is available at the time of writing. It is a certainty that during your career as a nurse or healthcare professional you will encounter someone who develops sepsis. As you will see, the consequences of sepsis are dire with a very high **mortality** rate or long term/permanent damage to those who suffer from severe sepsis. It is therefore your role to detect the symptoms of sepsis early and ensure that the appropriate action is undertaken immediately to prevent the cascade of events that can lead to death. You must recognise that any patient can develop sepsis arising from many causes and that deterioration can be dramatic, however there are some people who are at greater risk than others and they will require closer monitoring.

Sepsis has a number of terms that can be confusing. You may see the media use the term 'blood poisoning' or colleagues say, 'severe sepsis'. Two terms used are a *sepsis* and *septic shock*. The definitions for these terms are:

Sepsis is a life-threatening organ dysfunction caused by dysregulated host response to infection.

Septic shock is a subset of sepsis with circulatory and cellular/**metabolic** dysfunction associated with higher risk of mortality.

(Singer et al., 2016)

PATHOPHYSIOLOGY OF SEPSIS

Sepsis occurs when the **inflammatory response** is triggered, this could happen for multiple reasons. The first change that occurs in inflammation is vasodilation. This is a normal healthy response and is designed to deliver improved blood flow to the area of damage or infection. This improved blood flow enhances the delivery of proteins, white cells to fight infection, clotting products and improved oxygenation. This is all designed to provide the area of damage or infection with materials for growth and repair of tissue, cells that can fight invading organisms and a heightened oxygen supply to facilitate this increase in metabolic activity. The **coagulation** process is activated but localised, which prevents blood flowing downstream from the site of injury or infection and therefore limits the spread of the invading organism around the body. The blocking of the microcirculation by clots is temporary and once the site of damage has been repaired, the clot is naturally dissolved and blood flows through the circulation again.

Sepsis occurs when the system becomes overwhelmed or dysregulated, which results in the vasodilation occurring systemically rather than just locally. In Chapter 6, you will have seen that blood pressure is partially controlled by the vascular tone, i.e. **vasoconstriction** and **vasodilation**.

Therefore, when there is a **systemic** dilation there is a profound drop in blood pressure, reduction in blood flow, pooling off blood in the peripheral circulation, reduced oxygen supply to tissue, a reduction in venous return to the heart all resulting in tissue hypoxia and **ischaemia** and ultimately cell death. The earlier that this can be detected and the earliest an **intervention** can be implemented, the less damage occurs to tissues.

THIS TOPIC
IS ALSO
COVERED IN
CHAPTER 6

ACTIVITY 7.1: THEORY STOP POINT

Review your knowledge about the control of blood pressure in relation to cardiac output, especially stroke volume, and vascular tone. Consider what conditions may apply to create a drop in cardiac output and blood pressure. Then, consider why sepsis may be overlooked when monitoring patients.

The videos below from the UK Sepsis trust may help you understand how easy it is not to consider sepsis as a possible diagnosis:

https://youtu.be/JYfUPs9pcNE

https://youtu.be/4o45YrYoosI

Epidemiology

As the inflammatory process is occurring all the time in people, and the body is constantly fighting off bacteria and viruses, it is impossible to predict when sepsis is going to occur. Therefore, it is vitally important to be extra observant of people who may be at risk of infections. These are the very young, the older generations, those with immune system compromise through disease or treatment, pregnant women, those without a spleen, inpatients, those with liver failure/cirrhosis or renal disease, or those with indwelling intravascular devices, especially those in intensive care units (WHO, 2019). In England, there was an annual increase of sepsis cases of 11.5% from 2010–11, with 52,000 deaths anticipated in the UK in 2019 (Daniels et al., 2019).

Common causes of sepsis

NICE (2016) identifies those who are most at risk of developing sepsis. As the most common cause of sepsis is infection, it is predictable that those who are at most risk of acquiring an infection and those who are least able to fight it are the most vulnerable. For example, those in the higher age group (<75 years), the very young (<1 year) and those who are frail are more vulnerable to infections. Those who have impaired immune systems, either through disease such as diabetes, or AIDS, or conditions such as splenectomy, or malnutrition are unable to fight any prospective infection. There is also a group of people who have their immune systems depressed intentionally as part of a treatment, such as chemotherapy or radiotherapy.

Screening and detection

So how do you prevent sepsis from occurring? It often falls to the nurse who is responsible for monitoring the routine observations of their patients. Using tools such as the NEWS2 (RCP, 2017) will help to identify changes in the person's physiological state. As soon as there is a suspicion that someone may have an infection, every healthcare professional should ask whether the person may have sepsis. Note, the person does not necessarily have to have a high temperature to have sepsis, in some people the temperature does not change in the initial stages. Part of your role is to routinely measure the person's heart rate, respiratory rate, blood pressure, level of consciousness and oxygen saturation.

It is vitally important that any patient showing signs of deterioration should be considered for sepsis but also, you must also listen to the patient and/or relatives in how they describe the person. If they say that they feel unwell, which is a change in their normal condition, then sepsis must be considered.

The UK Sepsis Trust advocates detecting 'Red Flags' in determining whether sepsis is occurring. These red flags can be seen below. The National Institute for Clinical Excellence breaks down the criteria into high, moderate and low risk and this can be seen in Figure 7.1.

Sepsis red flags

Responds only to voice or pain/unresponsive

Acute confusional state

Systolic BP ≤ 90mmHg (or drop >40 from normal)

Heart rate >130 per minute

Respiratory rate ≥25 per minute

Needs oxygen to keep SpO2 ≥92%

Non-blanching rash, mottled skin/ashen/cyanotic

Not passed urine in last 18 hours / Urine output <0.5 ml/kg/hour

Lactate ≥2mmol/L

Recent chemotherapy

Source: Adapted from UK Sepsis Trust (2019) Sepsis Red Flags URL: https://sepsistrust.org/wp-content/uploads/2018/06/ED-adult-NICE-Final-1107.pdf (accessed November 4, 2020).

ACTIVITY 7.2: CASE STUDY

Massum is a 70 year old lady who has type 2 diabetes and a diabetic leg ulcer that needs weekly dressing by the community nurse. She is clinically defined as obese. As her registered nurse, you visit her for her weekly dressing to find her a little breathless but she explains that she's just been up and down stairs just prior to your visit. Whilst chatting to her during the dressing you find that she is a little vague in recalling the events of the past couple of days.

Things to consider:

1. What are Massum's risk factors for sepsis?
2. What might alert you to investigate Massum's condition in more detail?
3. What observations would you take?
4. Who would you contact for further support or advice?
5. What strategy or method might you use whilst communicating with other healthcare professionals?

Category	High risk criteria	Moderate to high risk criteria	Low risk criteria
History	Objective evidence of new altered mental state	History from patient: friend or relative of new onset of altered behaviour or mental state History of acute deterioration of functional ability Impaired immune system (illness or drugs including oral steroids) Trauma, surgery or invasive procedures in the last 6 weeks	Normal behaviour
Respiratory	Raised respiratory rate: 25 breaths per minute or more New need for oxygen (40% FiO_2; or more) to maintain saturation more than 92% (or more than 88% in known chronic obstructive pulmonary disease)	Raised respiratory rate: 21–24 breaths per minute	No high risk or moderate to high risk criteria met
Blood pressure	Systolic blood pressure 90 mmHg or less or systolic blood pressure more than 40 mmHg below normal	Systolic blood pressure 91–100 mmHg	No high risk or moderate to high risk criteria met
Circulation and hydration	Raised heart rate: more than 130 beats per minute Not passed urine in previous 18 hours. For catheterised patients, passed less than 0.5 ml/kg of urine per hour	Raised heart rate: 91–130 beats per minute (for pregnant women 100–130 beats per minute) or new onset arrhythmia Not passed urine in the past 12–18 hours For catheterised patients, passed 1.5–1 ml/kg of urine per hour	No high risk or moderate to high risk criteria met
Temperature		Tympanic temperature less than 36°C	
Skin	Mottled or ashen appearance Cyanosis of skin lips or tongue Non–blanching rash of skin	Signs of potential infection: including redness, swelling or discharge at surgical site or breakdown of wound	No non–blanching rash

Figure 7.1 **Risk stratification tool for adults, children and young people aged 12 years and over with suspected sepsis**

Source: © NICE (2017) *Sepsis: Recognition, diagnosis and early management*, available from www.nice.org.uk/guidance/ng51. Reproduced under the Open Content License.

The Society of Critical Care Medicine and European Society of Intensive Care Medicine (2019) have produced guidelines on how to manage sepsis. They recommend that within 1 hour of you suspecting sepsis that a lactate level is measured. This indicates the extent of tissue ischaemia occurring within the body. The second recommendation is to obtain blood cultures and then administer broad spectrum antibiotics. The evidence for the early administration of antibiotics indicates that there is a significantly improved chance of survival if blood cultures are taken and broad spectrum antibiotics are administered within 1 hour of the detection of sepsis (NICE, 2017).

The UK Sepsis Trust (2018) and NICE (2017) advocate the use of the 'Sepsis 6' in the management of a patient with suspected sepsis. There are 6 actions that should be taken and completed within 1 hour of the suspicion of sepsis (see Table 7.1). The UK Sepsis Trust (https://sepsistrust.org/) has a lot of information and supporting guidelines and education for the general public and healthcare professionals.

Table 7.1 Sepsis 6

	Action (Complete all within 1 hour)	Rationale
1.	Ensure senior clinical (ST3+, or equivalent senior nurse) attends	Sepsis is a complex condition. Experience is essential to deliver the right care and confirm diagnosis.
2.	Administer oxygen Start if saturations less than 92%. Aim for saturations of 94-98%. If at risk of hypercarbia use target range of 88-92%	There's a critical imbalance between oxygen supply & demand in sepsis. Correcting low saturations helps to reduce tissue hypoxia.
3.	Obtain IV access, take bloods Include cultures, glucose, lactate, FBC, U&Es, CRP, Clotting. Consider lumbar puncture/ other samples as indicated	Lab. tests help stratify risk & identify causative pathogen allowing more targeted antibiotic therapy.
4.	Give antibiotics Maximum dose broad spectrum therapy. According to Trust protocol. Consider allergies prior to administration (*Antibiotic stewardship – seek advice of senior clinician regarding suitability of antibiotics as antibiotics not needed in all cases) Consider antivirals.	To control the source of infection, reducing the stimulus to the immune system.
5.	Give IV fluids Give fluid bolus of 500ml if 16+. (Give fluid bolus of 20 ml/kg if age <16). Repeat if clinically indicated. Use lactate to help guide further fluid therapy.	**Hypovolaemia** (absolute & relative) contributes to shock in sepsis; restoring volume can help correct perfusion.
6.	Monitor Use NEWS2. Measure urine output – may require catheter. Repeat lactate at least hourly if initial lactate elevated or clinical condition changes.	Sepsis is a dynamic state. Urine output and lactate can help guide fluid therapy and determine need for ITU referral.

Source: Adapted from Daniels et al., 2019.

ACTIVITY 7.3: CASE STUDY

Billy is under your care in the high dependency Level 2 area of critical care. He is 78 years old and he was admitted following a fall at home where he hit his head, cannot recall the event and has broken his arm. Whilst you are doing his routine observations one afternoon you detect that his NEWS score is 7. His observations are as follows:

Respiratory rate – 24
Oxygen saturation on room air – 93%
Systolic blood pressure – 145
Heart rate – 95
Conscious level – confused
Temperature – 37.8°C

Consider:

1. Do you think this is sepsis? If so, why?
2. Do you think this is not sepsis? If so, why?
3. Based on your considerations, what would you do next?

In situations such as this, the body's normal response would be to shut down peripheral circulation (vasoconstriction) and shunt blood to the vital organs, however in sepsis the normal inflammatory response is to cause vasodilation. Remember, sepsis is an 'out of control' inflammatory response and so the vasodilation becomes systemic, affecting the circulation throughout the body rather than in the location of the cause. This systemic vasodilation results in a reduction in blood flow and therefore blood pressure. Therefore, in sepsis, the recommendation where there is **hypotension** or when there is a lactate measurement of >4mmol/L is to begin a rapid administration of **intravenous** crystalloid at 30mls/kg body weight in an attempt to return the blood pressure and lactate levels to within normal ranges.

As a nurse, it is your role to carefully record the clinical observations of every patient and to monitor whether there is a chance that sepsis may be developing. As soon as you detect this you should act quickly and assertively. You can refer the person urgently to relevant medical teams but also, if you are skilled and trained, you can start to take blood for lactate measurement and for blood cultures. You could also insert an intravenous cannula and be prepared for a prescription of rapid fluid resuscitation. As part of your initial assessment of the person, you should be able to record their weight which will determine the amount of fluid resuscitation required. If you are not able to perform these tasks, having all this prepared and at hand for the first capable person when they arrive will improve the speed at which the patient receives the appropriate treatment and improve their chance of recovery.

ACTIVITY 7.4: RESEARCH AND EVIDENCE-BASED PRACTICE

The personal impact on people who suffer from sepsis is not limited to their recovery period. Sepsis results in life-long debility which can impact on the individual's quality of life and longevity.

This video is particularly impactful as it tells the story of people who have suffered from sepsis and the long term consequences. It is particularly impactful as it is from healthcare professionals who

(Continued)

have a heightened awareness of their sepsis symptoms. www.youtube.com/watch?v=aq2Jj-QNo_U (accessed November 4, 2020).

1. Consider the enduring influence the death of a class mate on Peter the anaesthetist's mental health, Jill's delay in recovery and the physical and mental impact on Jaco.
2. Review the symptoms the victims recall and consider how many people, including yourself, may have had these symptoms that can cause sepsis and death. Also review the rapid timeframe of the progression of the condition.

Care in Critical Care

THIS TOPIC
IS ALSO
COVERED IN
CHAPTER 5

Those with severe sepsis that cannot be managed on a ward are admitted to critical care for ongoing support of failing organs. Also, a number of people already in critical care due to other factors can develop sepsis during their stay. This arises because many of the normal defence mechanisms are compromised whilst critically ill. For example, the skin is broken and an **invasive device**, i.e. a central venous cannula, is inserted directly into the central circulation, a perfect conduit for bacteria. People requiring mechanical ventilation have an **endotracheal tube** inserted bypassing the buccal and pharyngeal areas where bacteria can be filtered. The tube also compromises the **cilia** that line the respiratory tree which help to remove debris and bacteria into the back of the throat where they are either swallowed or expectorated. The tube itself can act as a conduit for the bacteria to enter the lungs. Any device that breaches the natural anatomical defences can be a cause of infection and sepsis.

Once someone is in critical care, typically they receive artificial ventilation, which involves **sedation**, an endotracheal tube and a ventilator.

As part of the sedation/ventilation process the blood pressure tends to drop below normal levels and the person often requires infusions of drugs and fluid to maintain normal blood flow.

THIS TOPIC
IS ALSO
COVERED IN
CHAPTER 6

These drugs typically are **vasopressors** to control the profound vasodilation that is seen in the inflammatory process of sepsis and occasionally drugs to improve cardiac function to increase the cardiac output to improve blood flow.

As a consequence of the overwhelming inflammatory response and the side effects of some of the medications, along with the psychological impact of a critical care stay, many can suffer long term ill health such as post-traumatic stress disorder, memory loss, **polyneuropathy** and **myopathy**. There may be long term kidney dysfunction and compromise in lung function, all arising from the damage caused by the inflammatory process and the side effects of the treatment.

ACTIVITY 7.5: REFLECTIVE PRACTICE

Review the contents of Chapters 5 and 6 and consider how they work together to help sustain a person who has sepsis. Think about how oxygen is normally delivered to tissue and how this is changed and interrupted in sepsis.

1. Think about how your monitoring is important, what observations you should continually be making and what early signs you might see in a patient in intensive care that may be developing sepsis. Think of this in terms of:

   a. Reflection in action
   b. Reflection on action

Schön's (1991) model of reflection may help you with this process.

Reflection in action (at the time it is happening)

- The experience itself
- Thinking about what's happening
- Deciding how to act
- Act

Reflection on action (after the event)

- Reflect on the event
- Think about what you might do differently
- What new information or knowledge have you gained that will enhance your practice in the future

COVID-19

In 2019 a novel virus emerged that the world had never seen before. Part of the coronavirus family, it is highly infectious and can spread very quickly, overwhelming healthcare provision and resulting in an increase in death rates. In the early days of the pandemic the only preventative approach was to prevent or reduce the extent of cross infections. Countries throughout the world adopted a 'stay at home' policy which meant that people would not be able to mix and mingle and this, along with 'social distancing', meant that the incidence of the spread of the virus was reduced.

A virus in itself is incapable of replication or spread and relies on a host, i.e. a person, to allow it to grow and spread itself around. Once a host is colonised the Covid-19 virus accesses the DNA of cells through the ACE2 receptor on the cell walls of the host. This ACE receptor is designed to accept angiotensin, which is a hormone that contributes to the control of blood pressure. The virus is particularly prevalent in the cells of the lungs and once there it triggers an extreme immune response by the host resulting in pneumonia, lung inflammation and sepsis. In some people the immune response becomes overwhelming and this results in **septic shock** and multi organ failure.

Because of the inflammatory response in the lungs, acute respiratory distress occurs which in some people requires oxygen therapy and in extreme cases ventilation.

At the time of writing scientists around the world are producing **vaccines** for the virus and until then the only way to prevent it spreading is prevent cross infection between people by social distancing, i.e. remaining more than 2 metres away from those not in your household/carer bubble, the wearing of masks in public and vigilant hand hygiene when in contact with hard surfaces.

THIS TOPIC IS ALSO COVERED IN CHAPTER 5

The greater the ventilation of a space the less concentrated the Covid particles and therefore the less likelihood of transmission. There are research trials commencing seeking a treatment for those who are more severely affected by the virus but these are still at an early stage.

The epidemiological evidence is also being gathered and there is no definitive evidence as yet, however anecdotally it seems the older you are the more likely you are to suffer a more severe response to the virus and if you have co-morbidities, such as cardiovascular disease, diabetes or a condition that causes immunosuppression, the higher the morbidity and mortality will be.

WHAT'S THE EVIDENCE?

If you'd like to keep up to date on various issues associated with Covid-19 then the Medscape website is comprehensive. www.medscape.com/resource/coronavirus (accessed November 4, 2020).

CHAPTER SUMMARY

This chapter has supported your understanding of:

- Defining sepsis
- An overview of how sepsis is caused and why it is such an important issue
- Provided an insight into how you should detect and monitor the progression of sepsis in the people in your care
- People who are at high, moderate and low risk of sepsis
- Guidelines, which are clear in what you should do to prevent the progression of the condition and the importance of being vigilant
- The guidelines for early and aggressive intervention. The chapter stressed that it is your responsibility to ensure these are completed within the timeframe recommended.

GO FURTHER

Books

Daniels, R. and Nutbeam, T. (eds) (2019) *The Sepsis Manual* (5th edition). Birmingham: United Kingdom Sepsis Trust. Available from https://sepsistrust.org/wp-content/uploads/2020/01/5th-Edition-manual-080120.pdf (accessed November 4, 2020).

- This manual includes information on the Sepsis Six pathway.

Adam, S., Osborne, S. and Welch, J. (eds) (2017) *Critical Care Nursing: Science and Practice* (3rd edition). Oxford: Oxford University Press.

- This book covers all essential aspects of critical care nursing.

Bersten, A.D. and Handy, J. (2018) *Oh's Intensive Care Manual* (8th edition). London: Elsevier.

- Again, this book covers all aspects of intensive care in detail, for use in daily practice.

Journal articles

Alhazzani W., Møller, M.H., Arabi, Y.M., Loeb, M., Gong, M.N.,Fan, E. [...] and Rhodes, A. (2020) 'Surviving Sepsis Campaign: Guidelines on the management of critically ill adults with Coronavirus Disease 2019 (COVID-19)', *Intensive Care Medicine*, 46: 854–87.

- This article reviews the best evidence available in the management of sepsis and COVID-19. It provides expert opinion proposing 4 best practice statements and 9 strong recommendations and 35 weak recommendations based on the strength of the current evidence [March 2020].

Singer, M., Deutschman, C.S., Seymour, C.W., Shankar-Hari, M., Annane, D., Bauer, M. [...] Angus, D.C. (2016) 'The Third International Consensus Definitions for Sepsis and Septic Shock (Sepsis-3)', *JAMA*, 315 (8): 801–10. doi.org/10.1001/jama.2016.0287

- This article defines and clarifies the latest definition of sepsis and septic shock.

Useful websites

National Institute for Health and Care Excellence (NICE) (2017) *Sepsis: Recognition, Diagnosis and Early Management* (NICE Guideline 51). Available from www.nice.org.uk/guidance/ng51 (accessed November 4, 2020).

- This website is the NICE guidance on the diagnosis and early management of sepsis.

The UK Sepsis Trust. https://sepsistrust.org/ (accessed November 4, 2020).

- This website has a vast amount of up to date information, evidence and guidance for both the general public and healthcare practitioners.

The Global Sepsis Alliance website. www.global-sepsis-alliance.org/covid19 (accessed November 4, 2020).

- This page in the Global Sepsis Alliance website has questions and answers specifically related to the COVID-19 virus and how it relates to sepsis.

REFERENCES

Daniels, R., Nutbeam, T., Sangan, V., Annakin, S., Matthews, L. and Jones, O. (2019) *The Sepsis Manual* (5th edition). Birmingham: United Kingdom Sepsis Trust. Available from https://sepsistrust.org/professional-resources/education-resources/ (accessed November 4, 2020).

National Institute for Health and Care Excellence (NICE) (2017) *Sepsis: Recognition, Diagnosis and Early Management* (NICE Guideline 51). London: NICE. Available from www.nice.org.uk/guidance/ng51 (accessed November 4, 2020).

Royal College of Physicians (RCP) (2017) *National Early Warning Score 2 (NEWS 2): Standardising the Assessment of Acute Illness Severity in the NHS*. London: Royal College of Physicians. Available from https://www.rcplondon.ac.uk/projects/outputs/national-early-warning-score-news-2 (accessed November 4, 2020).

Schön, D. (1983) *The Reflective Practitioner*. London: Temple Smith.

Singer, M., Deutschman, C.S., Seymour C.W., Shankar-Hari, M., Annane, D., Bauer, M. […] Angus, D.C. (2016) 'The Third International Consensus Definitions for Sepsis and Septic Shock (Sepsis-3)', *JAMA, 315* (8): 801–10. doi.org/10.1001/jama.2016.0287

The UK Sepsis Trust (2018) 'ED/AMU Sepsis Screening & Action Tool'. *The UK Sepsis Trust.* https://sepsistrust.org/wp-content/uploads/2018/06/ED-adult-NICE-Final-1107.pdf (accessed November 4, 2020).

World Health Organisation (2019) *Sepsis*. Geneva: WHO. www.who.int/news-room/fact-sheets/detail/sepsis (accessed November 4, 2020).

CRITICAL CARE RELATED TO THE PATHOPHYSIOLOGY AND MANAGEMENT OF RENAL AND LIVER DISORDERS

GREGORY BLEAKLEY AND SAMANTHA FREEMAN

8

> " I hadn't realised that this was a whole sub-speciality within critical care. There is so much to learn about the liver and kidney, it's fascinating.
>
> **Johnathan, 2nd Year Student Nurse** "

LEARNING OUTCOMES

When you have finished studying this chapter you will be able to understand:

- The overview of the anatomy and physiology of the kidney and liver
- The assessment of some common renal and liver disorders that can occur in critical illness

INTRODUCTION

In this chapter we will be exploring the evidence-based care surrounding the more commonly experienced presentations of renal failure, hepatic physiology and pathology, as well as some of the management strategies used to support renal failure such as renal replacement therapies. You need to be aware that you may be placed within one of the many speciality critical units, which will have more in depth or bespoke treatment for those who are critically ill due to lack of renal or liver function. This chapter will give you an overview for those in general critical care departments and, if you are in a specialty unit, the chapter can act as springboard to more comprehensive reading. We will first cover nursing issues related to renal failure progressing to nursing care of those experiencing liver failure.

STRUCTURE AND FUNCTION OF THE RENAL SYSTEM

The renal system is composed of two kidneys, two ureters, the bladder and the urethra, as shown in Figure 8.1.

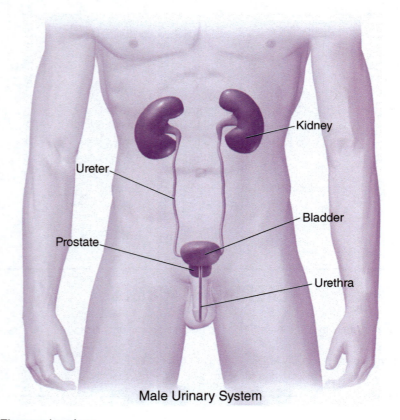

Male Urinary System

Figure 8.1 The renal system

Source: Wikipedia, URL: https://en.wikipedia.org/wiki/Urinary_system#/media/File:Urinary_System_(Male).png (accessed November 5, 2020).
Reproduced under CC BY-SA 4.0

Working together, these anatomical structures process approximately 1700 L of blood and convert approximately 1.5 L of waste products into urine in a twenty-four-hour period (Porth, 2015). Urine flows from the kidneys to the bladder through tubes called ureters. The bladder stores urine until a desire to urinate is reached and urine passes from the bladder through the urethra. The main function of the renal system is to remove waste products from the body. In addition, the kidneys are crucial organs for maintaining homeostatic mechanisms that prevent dehydration and electrolyte imbalance. There are approximately 1 million nephrons in each kidney. Nephrons are the functional part of the kidneys which contain a glomerulus and a tubule (see Figure 8.2). The glomerulus filters waste products from the blood that passes through and the tubule returns essential substances to the system circulation. Essentially, the glomerulus is a network of tiny capillaries located within the Bowman's capsule (Pollak et al., 2014). Blood enters this structure through an afferent arteriole and leaves by an efferent arteriole. A series of renal tubules commence after the Bowman's capsule and are composed of several elements. These include the proximal convoluted tubule (reabsorbs water and other essential substances back to the blood), the Loop of Henle (further reabsorption of critical electrolytes to the blood) and distal convoluted tubule (chiefly responsible for the regulation of sodium and potassium).

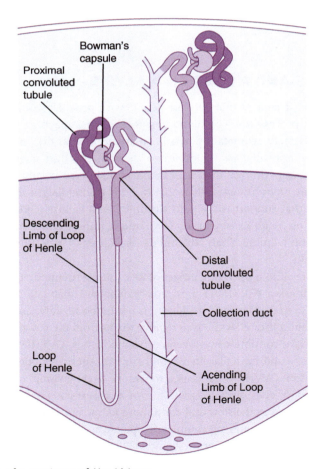

Figure 8.2 Figure of a nephron of the kidney

Source: Wikimedia Commons, URL: https://commons.wikimedia.org/wiki/File:Kidney_Nephron.png (accessed November 5, 2020). Reproduced under CC BY 3.0.

=== **ACTIVITY 8.1: CRITICAL THINKING** ===

High levels of potassium (hyperkalaemia) in the body is dangerous.

1. What might be the effects on the body if the renal system is impaired and unable to regulate potassium levels?

=== **WHAT'S THE EVIDENCE?** ===

A fall in urine output to less than 0.5 ml/kg/hour for more than 6 hours in adults is often associated with an acute kidney injury (AKI). The NICE guidelines (NG 148) (2019) are an excellent evidence-based resource to help you prevent, detect and manage acute kidney injury.

   Access this guidance using the following link: www.nice.org.uk/guidance/ng148 (accessed November 5, 2020).

RENAL SERVICES AND MODES OF DIALYSIS

Renal services are specialist centres that support people with pre-dialysis, dialysis and transplant care. Haemodialysis is a process whereby blood passes through a machine to remove toxins and fluid. Haemodialysis treatment requires the person to attend a renal dialysis unit 3 – 4 times per week. An alternative mode of dialysis is performed through the thin membrane that lines the abdominal cavity known as peritoneal dialysis. Peritoneal dialysis is usually performed each night within the person's home environment (NICE, 2014). Both haemodialysis and peritoneal dialysis are modes of treatment that support those with Chronic Renal Failure (CRF). Alternatively, some critically ill people develop Acute Kidney Injury (AKI) and require renal replacement therapy (RRT) within the critical care unit. Interestingly, this mode of dialysis is very different from those that require dialysis due to CRF.

   In critical care, there are various operating modes of RRT using a haemofilter machine. Continuous venovenous haemodiafiltration (CVVHDF) uses replacement and dialysate (Ede and Dale, 2016). Dialysate, often referred to as dialysis fluid / solution, is a solution of water and electrolytes (sodium and bicarbonate). The main role of dialysate is to remove toxins from the blood stream through a process of diffusion. In contrast, continuous venovenous haemodialysis (CVVHD) removes fluid mainly by diffusion using dialysate and no replacement fluid is used. Another mode of RRT is continuous venovenous haemofiltration (CVVH) which is used to remove larger volumes of fluid mainly via convection. Collectively, these modes of dialysis are known as continuous renal replacement therapy (CRRT). CRRT can be described as the slow and continuous extracorporeal purification of blood (Ede and Dale, 2016). Haemofilter machines are complex to operate and require enhanced nursing knowledge and training. If the critically unwell person requires CRRT, it is usual to insert a vascath. A vascath is a flexible sterile tube that is inserted into a large vein in the neck (internal jugular vein) or groin (femoral vein). Some critical care units refer to the vascath as a dialysis-type central venous catheter.

Vascaths are inserted to treat kidney failure and are designed to remove and return large volumes of blood through the haemofilter machine. Inserting a vascath is a relatively straightforward clinical procedure, but not without risk. Complications can include bruising, bleeding, pneumothorax, tube occlusion, infection and thrombus (Dougherty et al., 2015).

ACTIVITY 8.2: CASE STUDY

Terry is 67 and was admitted to the Emergency Department following an acute onset of confusion and reduction in urine output. He has now been moved to the High Dependency Unit (HDU) due to the sudden deterioration of his renal function under your care.

Terry's renal function is poor, and he will have to start on renal replacement therapy. The first step will be to insert a vascath into a large central vein so that renal replacement therapy can commence.

1. What are the normal serum ranges for the key urea and electrolytes?
2. How much urine would you expect Terry to produce per day?
3. What is a vascath?

PYELONEPHRITIS

A kidney infection (pyelonephritis) is typically characterised by bacteria travelling from the bladder into one or both kidneys. Specifically, pyelonephritis relates to **inflammation** of the renal pelvis (Peate and Wild, 2018). It is more serious than cystitis (inflammation/infection of the bladder) which often makes urination problematic and painful. A kidney infection can develop rapidly over a few hours or days and common symptoms include (Dougherty et al., 2015):

- Pain in the abdomen, lower back or around the genital area
- Pyrexia (temperature may rise above 39°C)
- Rigor, shivering or chills
- Feeling lethargic/general malaise
- Haematuria
- Cloudy or foul-smelling urine
- Nausea

Pyelonephritis is caused by a bacterial infection, most commonly Escherichia Coli (E-Coli). Predisposing risk factors include previous urinary tract infection (UTI) which are more common in women (NICE 2012), sexual intercourse, diabetes and structural problems of the urinary tract (enlarged prostate/kidney stones). Essentially, bowel organisms enter the urinary tract and migrate upwards towards the kidneys. Sometimes organisms enter the kidneys and cause infection from the **systemic** circulation, but this is infrequent. Complications of repeated kidney infection include **sepsis**, kidney failure or kidney abscesses (pus in the kidneys).

WHAT'S THE EVIDENCE?

Current clinical guidelines regarding the management of acute pyelonephritis in adults include (NICE, 2018) https://www.nice.org.uk/guidance/ng111/ :

- Think! Could this be sepsis?
- Being aware the infection can occur in one or both kidneys
- Offer an antibiotic that is mindful of the severity of the symptoms, the risk of developing complications, previous urine culture and previous antibiotic use
- Obtain urine cultures (when available) and review choice of antibiotic
- Refer and seek specialist advice if the person is unable to take oral fluids, significantly dehydrated, pregnant or at higher risk of developing complications (for example, people with diabetes or immunosuppression).

CHRONIC KIDNEY DISEASE (CKD)

Chronic Kidney Disease (CKD) is a long-term condition where the kidneys cease to function normally. The damage to the kidneys can occur over months, even years, and does not often cause symptoms until it reaches an advanced stage. Internationally, CKD is a global health concern which is harmful to health but treatable if detected early (Arici, 2014). CKD is diagnosed from urinalysis and the estimated glomerular filtration rate (eGFR) calculated from serum creatinine. eGFR is calculated by laboratory blood testing (biochemistry) and is often reported alongside the serum creatinine result. Normal eGFR is greater than 90 ml/min and deviation from this value requires causative exploration.

CKD is often aligned to older people and people from south Asian origin. Detection of CKD is enhanced with proactive measurement of blood pressure, serum creatinine, and urinalysis in select populations at risk of developing CKD. The vast majority of CKD cases (up to 80%) are secondary to diabetes or **hypertension** (Arici, 2014; Kerr, 2012). Furthermore, obesity is linked to early onset and acceleration of CKD. Staging of CKD is used to evaluate the severity of disease process on renal function. The eGFR result is reported as a stage from 1 to 5 (DH, 2012):

- **Stage 1:** a normal eGFR > 90ml/min but other tests may indicate signs of kidney damage
- **Stage 2:** a slightly reduced eGFR 60–89ml/min, with other signs of kidney damage
- **Stage 3a:** an eGFR of 45–59ml/min
- **Stage 3b:** an eGFR of 30–44ml/min
- **Stage 4:** an eGFR of 15–29ml/min
- **Stage 5:** an eGFR below 15ml/min, meaning the kidneys have almost lost their function

(Kerr, 2012: 8)

ACTIVITY 8.3: REFLECTIVE PRACTICE

Investigate the stages of chronic kidney disease as advised by Kerr (2012).

1. Reflect back on a person you have cared for and consider their stage of renal disease based on eGFR results.

POLYCYSTIC KIDNEY DISEASE (PKD)

Polycystic kidney disease is a genetic disorder and characterised by many fluid-filled cysts that grown on the kidneys (see Figure 8.3). Unlike simple cysts, PKD produces a more widespread collection of cysts that can alter the structure and function of the kidney (Cowley and Bissler, 2018). Typically, the cysts are non-cancerous cysts that vary in size but can grow very large. PKD can cause other cysts to develop in the body and cause serious health problems, including hypertension and CKD.

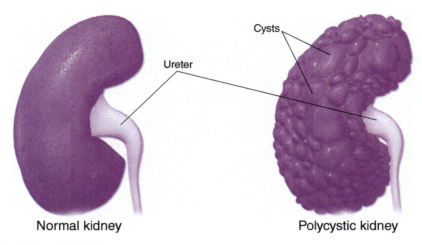

Normal kidney   Polycystic kidney

Figure 8.3 Polycystic kidney disease

Source: Wikimedia Commons, URL: https://commons.wikimedia.org/wiki/File:Polycystic_Kidney.png (accessed November 5, 2020). Reproduced under CC BY-SA 4.0.

ACUTE KIDNEY INJURY (AKI)

Acute kidney injury is a frequent complication of those who are hospitalised, especially those in critical care units. Common causes of AKI include **hypovolaemia** (from dehydration/blood loss/**diarrhoea**), myocardial infarction (cardiogenic shock), major surgery, burn injuries, profound allergic reaction or nephron-toxic effect of drug use (Waikar et al., 2018). A leading cause of AKI is Acute Tubular Necrosis (ATN), a serious condition that involves the death of tubular epithelial cells that form part of the renal tubules in the kidneys. Critical illness is known to be a causative factor in development of AKI but pre-existing CKD, left ventricular dysfunction, liver disease and proteinuria increase susceptibility. Complete recovery from AKI is much less frequent than previously expected, and 'CKD post AKI has now been recognised as a major public health problem' (Waikar et al., 2018: 6–7).

AKI is marked by the sudden loss of renal function with a rise in serum creatinine. Normal serum creatinine level is 55–105μmol/L and elevated creatinine levels are usually indicative of poor kidney function (Dougherty et al., 2015). It is mostly caused by hypo-perfusion of the kidneys due to low circulating volumes of blood or fluid (pre-renal) (Waikar et al., 2018). Intrinsic or intra-renal causes of AKI include ATN, uncontrolled hypertension, infection (pyelonephritis) or drug-induced nephritis. Post-renal failure is caused by any condition which inhibits the flow of urine from the kidneys. This could include an enlarged prostate, tumour, congenital malformation, renal stones or an acquired obstruction from a urinary catheter (O'Callaghan, 2009).

RHABDOMYOLYSIS

Rhabdomyolysis is a serious condition that can have profound effects on renal function as a result of muscle injury. The muscle injury occurs primarily as a result of crush injury, strenuous exercise, infection, a prolonged period of immobility or impaired blood flow to limbs (Stewart et al., 2016). Byproducts of muscle tissue breakdown following injury include a protein called myoglobin. The damaged tissue releases myoglobin into the blood stream and the kidneys attempt to filter out the molecule. Essentially, trapped myoglobin causes AKI and other profound complications including disseminated intravascular coagulopathy (DIC) and compromised circulation to injured limbs (Petejova and Martinek, 2014). Rhabdomyolysis can lead to cardiac **arrhythmias**, hypotension and shock due to **metabolic** changes and systemic fluid shift. Petejova and Martinek (2014) suggest that between 13 and 50% of people with rhabdomyolysis will develop an AKI.

STRUCTURE AND FUNCTION OF THE LIVER

The liver is regarded as one of the **accessory organs** of the gastrointestinal (GI) tract (Porth, 2015). The liver secretes bile which is stored in a collecting pouch known as the gallbladder. Primarily, bile is involved in the digestion of fats in the small intestine. Bile, sometimes called gall, is a dark green to yellowish brown fluid (Cohen and Hull, 2015). Another important role of the liver is the **detoxification** of chemicals and metabolisation of drugs.

Interestingly, the liver is the largest solid organ and the largest gland in the human body. It is located in the upper right portion of the abdomen, beneath the diaphragm and above the stomach (see Figure 8.4).

The liver is divided into two main lobes, the right and left. Each lobe of the liver is further subdivided into many lobules by a network of blood vessels and fibrous strands. These fibrous strands encapsulate the liver in a protective fibro-elastic sheath called the Glisson's capsule (Tortora and Derrickson, 2013).

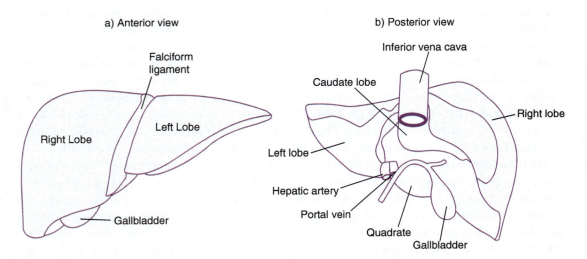

Figure 8.4 Anterior (a) and posterior (b) view of the liver

Source: Cook et al. (2021).

Unlike other organs, the liver has two major blood vessels. The portal vein carries nutrient rich blood into the liver from the digestive system. The hepatic artery transports oxygen rich blood into the liver from the heart. Physiologically, the liver is an active organ and produces bile, metabolises drugs, synthesizes plasma proteins and blood clotting factors, stores vitamins and minerals, and regulates blood glucose levels through storage of glycogen (Porth, 2015; Cohen and Hull, 2015). Many of these vital functions are disrupted by the presence of liver disease.

Alcohol-related liver disease (ARLD) refers to the damage caused by excessive alcohol intake. Unfortunately, ARLD rarely causes any symptoms until the liver has been profoundly damaged. These late symptoms include feeling sick, unplanned weight loss, yellowing of the eyes and skin (jaundice), swelling to the ankles and stomach, confusion and haematemesis (vomiting blood) or passing blood in the stools. Consequently, liver damage is often detected during tests for other conditions. There are three main stages of ARLD: alcoholic fatty liver disease, alcoholic hepatitis and cirrhosis (Sargent, 2009).

HEPATITIS

Hepatitis is known as the swelling or inflammation of the liver. The common cause of hepatitis is from a viral infection. However, hepatitis can occur from non-viral related causes and is divided into 3 types: toxic hepatitis which is caused by chemical or drug ingestion, alcoholic hepatitis which is caused by drinking too much alcohol, and autoimmune hepatitis whereby the immune system attacks the liver cells. There a several classifications of viral hepatitis including types A, B, C, D and E (WHO, 2019). All these types can cause acute hepatitis, but types B and C can cause chronic hepatitis. Different viruses are responsible for each type of virally transmitted hepatitis.

Hepatitis A

Hepatitis A is caused by the Hepatitis A virus. Specifically, Hepatitis A is classified in the hepatovirus genus of the Picornaviridae family (NICE, 2019). The virus is normally transmitted by eating/drinking food contaminated with the faeces of a person infected with the virus. Hepatitis A is common in countries with poor sanitation. The virus replicates in the live cells (hepatocytes), modifying cellular function and causing inflammation of liver cells. The virus is excreted in **bile** from the gallbladder and expelled in the faeces of infected people. Recovery from the virus observes a good prognosis and is typically self-limiting. Nevertheless, the UK does experience community wide outbreaks and point of source outbreaks (related to contaminated food). Furthermore, small outbreaks of the virus can occur in unvaccinated children/adults who have close contact with someone with Hepatitis A, men who have sex with men or people with risky sexual behaviours and **intravenous** drug users (sharing of nonsterile drug paraphernalia) (NICE, 2019).

Hepatitis B

Hepatitis B is caused by the Hepatitis B virus (HBV). It remains a global health challenge and is a significant cause of **mortality** worldwide (Ahmad, 2020). People from endemic areas of Asia and Africa, or intravenous drug users and those with high-risk sexual behaviours are at an increased risk of HBV infection. Normally the HBV is transmitted via percutaneous or mucosal routes, but it is also a sexually transmitted infection. Most adults infected with the HBV recover fully and return to normal health within a few months. However, people who acquire the virus as children can develop long term infection. Long term HBV infection can cause damage to liver cells (cirrhosis) or liver cancer. The UK has a targeted HBV **vaccination** programme for those people in high risk groups including healthcare workers, intravenous drug users, men who have sex with men, infants born to mothers with the virus and those travelling to parts of the world where the virus is endemic. Interestingly, from the 1st August 2017, all UK born babies are given 3 doses of hepatitis B-containing vaccine as part of the NHS routine vaccination schedule (NHS, 2018b). Healthcare workers should apply caution whilst caring for people infected with the HBV due to the risk of accidental needle stick injury (WHO, 2019).

ACTIVITY 8.4: CRITICAL THINKING

Providing nursing care for those with infectious diseases requires careful planning and attention to detail.

1. What personal protective equipment (PPE) would you use for each episode of care and which policies should you follow?

Hepatitis C

Unfortunately, Hepatitis C does not display any noticeable symptoms until the liver has been profoundly damaged. This means that people can carry the virus without realising it. The Hepatitis C virus (HCV) is usually transmitted through blood to blood contact. Therefore, in a similar way to the HBV, HCV is spread through intravenous drug users sharing contaminated needles, infants born to mothers with the virus and through unprotected sex. In severe cases, the HCV can cause damage to hepatocytes which causes cirrhosis and liver cancer. Cirrhosis is the scarring of liver tissue caused by long-term liver damage.

ACTIVITY 8.5: RESEARCH AND EVIDENCE-BASED PRACTICE

There are five main types of the hepatitis virus, referred to as A, B, C, D and E. Types A to C are discussed above.

1. Access the World Health Organisation Fact Sheets for Hepatitis online and explore how types D and E are geographically distributed and transmitted.

www.who.int/features/qa/76/en/ (accessed November 5, 2020)

OBSTRUCTIVE CAUSES OF LIVER FAILURE

Sometimes the flow of bile from the gallbladder is obstructed by **gallstones** in the biliary ducts. Gallstones are often caused by having too much **cholesterol** in the bile. Inflammation of the gallbladder is known as cholecystitis and is characterised by severe pain and fever. Untreated gallstones can lead to severe complications which include jaundice (yellowing of the skin), cholecystitis (inflammation/infection of the gallbladder), sepsis and pancreatic inflammation. Gallstones are often diagnosed using ultrasound, abdominal computerised tomography (CT) scan, endoscopic retrograde cholangiopancreatography (ERCP) (a camera to explore the bile and pancreatic ducts) and liver function blood tests for **bilirubin** level.

HEPATORENAL SYNDROME

Hepatorenal syndrome (HRS) is the development of renal failure which is observed typically in people with underlying liver disease, often caused by cirrhosis. People with HRS are critically unwell and it is almost always fatal unless liver transplantation can be performed rapidly. Usual symptoms of HRS include confusion, vomiting, jaundice, **delirium**, decreased urine output and swollen abdomen. Long term complications for those with HCS include organ damage and fluid overload due to poorly functioning kidneys.

Portal hypertension is high blood pressure of the hepatic portal venous blood vessels. Blood vessels from the intestine, spleen, stomach and pancreas merge into the portal vein which then branches off into the liver. If the blood vessels in the liver become blocked due to disease or inflammation, blood cannot flow properly through the liver. The result is a build-up in pressure in the portal veins which become engorged with blood (varices). **Varices** can rupture and bleed profusely, resulting in a life-threatening medical emergency.

ACTIVITY 8.6: CASE STUDY

Rita is 64 and has a history of depression, excess alcohol intake and self-harm. Her liver function has deteriorated over the last week and she has now been moved to critical care for closer observation under your care.

Following your assessment, you note that Rita's skin appears yellow in colour and her abdomen is very swollen. You determine that Rita needs an urgent medical review and you take blood for urgent liver function tests (LFTs).

1. What is bilirubin?
2. What is the normal (reference) range for serum bilirubin?
3. What is ascites and how can it affect the person?

ACTIVITY 8.7: THEORY STOP POINT

Liver damage is the most common cause of ascites. The British Liver Trust has a case study for you consider with underpinning evidence resources. Please access the case study (Michael's story) on the following link: https://britishlivertrust.org.uk/what-is-ascites/ (accessed November 5, 2020)

CHAPTER SUMMARY

This chapter has supported your understanding of the following topics:

- The anatomy and physiology of the kidney and liver
- Some common renal and liver disorders that can occur in critical illness
- The application of this to commonly seen cases in critical care

---

GO FURTHER

Books

Tait, D. and Hanson, S. (2016) 'The patient with acute kidney injury', in D. Tait, J. James, C. Williams and D. Barton, *Acute and Critical Care in Adult Nursing* (2nd edition). London: Sage. pp. 191–218.

- This is helpful resource to develop your learning and understanding.

Porth, C.M. (2015) *Essentials of Pathophysiology* (4th Edition), Wolters Kluwer. Chapters 24–26 Kidney and Urinary Tract Function

- This book helps you understand pathophysiology and disease process (2015) `Interpreting Diagnostic tests', in L. Dougherty, S. Lister and A.West-Oram, (eds) *The Royal Marsden Manual of Clinical Nursing Procedures* (9th edition). London: Wiley Blackwell. pp. 435–494.
- This textbook chapter contains clinical procedures on how to take a urine samples and discusses normal renal/liver blood tests values.

Journal articles

Nhan, L.A. (2020) 'Acute kidney injury: Challenges and opportunities', *Nursing*, 50 (9): 44–50. doi. org/10.1097/01.NURSE.0000694776.10448.97

- This article explores the aetiology of acute kidney injury and management.

Li, G. and Grant, C., (2016) 'Hepatorenal syndrome: A nurse's guide to identification, management and advocacy', *Gastrointestinal Nursing*, 14 (5): s12–18. doi.org/10.12968/gasn.2016.14.Sup5.S12

- This article explores hepatorenal syndrome as a serious consequence of end stage liver disease (ESLD).

Taxbro, K., Kahlow, K., Wulcan, H. and Fornarve, A. (2020) 'Rhabdomyolysis and acute kidney injury in severe COVID-19 infection', *British Medical Journal*, 13 (9): 1–3. doi.org/10.1136/bcr-2020-237616

- This intriguing case report discusses a 38-year-old male with confirmed COVID-19 infection who was admitted to critical care and developed severe rhabdomyolysis and acute kidney injury 4 days later.

Useful websites

National Institute for Health and Care Excellence (NICE) (2018) 'Management of Cirrhosis', London: NICE. https://cks.nice.org.uk/cirrhosis (accessed November 5, 2020).

- This page covers assessing and managing suspected or confirmed cirrhosis in people who are 16 years or older.

National Kidney Federation: www.kidney.org.uk/ (accessed November 5, 2020)

- This website explores the experiences of people living with kidney disease.

British Liver Trust: https://britishlivertrust.org.uk/ (accessed November 5, 2020)

- This website contains supportive information to enhance your knowledge of liver conditions.

REFERENCES

Ahmad, J. (2020) 'Hepatitis B', *British Medical Journal Best Practice*. https://bestpractice.bmj.com/topics/en-gb/127 (accessed November 5, 2020).

Arici, M. (2014) *Management of Chronic Kidney Disease: A Clinician's Guide*. London: Springer.

Cohen, B.J., and Hull, K.L. (2015) *The Human Body in Health and Disease* (13th edition). London: Wolters Kluwer.

Cook, N., Shepherd, A. and Boore, J. (2021) *Essentials of Anatomy and Physiology for Nursing Practice* (2nd edition). London: Sage.

Cowley, B.D. and Bissler, J.J. (2018) *Polycystic Kidney Disease: Translating Mechanisms into Therapy*. London: Springer.

Dougherty, L., Lister, S. and West-Oram, A. (2015) *The Royal Marsden Manual of Clinical Nursing Procedures* (9th edition). London: Wiley Blackwell.

Ede, J., and Dale, A., (2016) 'A service evaluation comparing CVVH and CVVHDF in minimising circuit failure', *Nursing in Critical Care*, 22 (1): 52–7.

Kerr, M. (2012) *Chronic Kidney Disease in England: The Human and Financial Cost*. Redditch: National Health Service. www.england.nhs.uk/improvement-hub/wp-content/uploads/sites/44/2017/11/Chronic-Kidney-Disease-in-England-The-Human-and-Financial-Cost.pdf (accessed November 5, 2020).

National Health Service (NHS) (2018b) 'Hepatitis B vaccine overview', Redditch: National Health Service. www.nhs.uk/conditions/vaccinations/hepatitis-b-vaccine/ (accessed November 5, 2020).

National Institute for Health and Care Excellence (NICE) (2012) *Urinary Tract Infections in Adults*. London: NICE. Available from https://www.nice.org.uk/guidance/qs90/resources/urinary-tract-infections-in-adults-pdf-2098962322117 (accessed January, 10 2020).

National Institute for Health and Care Excellence (NICE) (2014) *Renal Replacement Therapy Services for Adults* (Quality Standard 72). London: NICE. Available from www.nice.org.uk/guidance/qs72 (accessed November 5, 2020).

National Institute for Health and Care excellence (NICE) (2018) *Pyelonephritis (Acute): Antimicrobial Prescribing*. (NICE Guideline 111). London: NICE. Available from https://www.nice.org.uk/guidance/ng111/ (accessed November 5, 2020).

National Institute for Health and Care Excellence (NICE) (2019) *Hepatitis A*. https://cks.nice.org.uk/hepatitis-a (accessed November 5, 2020).

O'Callaghan, C. (2009) *Renal System at a Glance*. London: Wiley-Blackwell.

Peate, I. and Wilde, K. (2018) *Nursing Practice: Knowledge and Care* (2nd edition). London: Wiley Blackwell.

Petejova, N. and Martinek, A. (2014) 'Acute kidney injury due to rhabdomyolysis and renal replacement therapy: A critical review', *Critical Care*, 18: Article #224.

Pollak, M.R., Quaggin, S.E., Hoeing, M.P. and Dworkin, L.D. (2014) 'The Glomerulus: The sphere of influence', *Clinical Journal of the American Society of Nephrology*, 9 (8): 1461–9.

Porth, C.M. (2015) *Essentials of Pathophysiology* (4th edition). Philadelphia, PA: Wolters Kluwer.

Sargent, S. (2009) *Liver Diseases: An Essential Guide for Nurses and Health Care Professionals*. London: Wiley-Blackwell.

Stewart, I.J., Faulk, T.I., Sosnov, J.A., Clemens, M.S., Elterman, J., Ross, J.D., [...] and Chung, K.K. (2016) 'Rhabdomyolysis among critically ill combat casualties: Associations with acute kidney injury and mortality', *Journal of Trauma and Acute Care Surgery*, 80 (3): 492–8. doi.org/10.1097/TA.0000000000000933

Tortora, G.J. and Derrickson, B. (2011) *Principles of Anatomy and Physiology*, Volume 2 (13th edition). Singapore: Wiley and Sons.

Waikar, S.S., Murray, P.T. and Singh, A.K. (2018) *Core Concepts in Acute Kidney Injury*. London: Springer.

World Health Organisation (WHO) (2019) 'What is hepatitis?', *World Health Organisation*. www.who.int/features/qa/76/en/ (accessed November 5, 2020).

THE COMPLEX PATIENT: SCENARIO 1

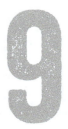

SAMANTHA FREEMAN, EMILY BRENNAN AND SALLY MOORE

> I really like working with an actual scenario, assessing and considering what I would do. It makes it more real and easier to apply what I have learned and I realise how much I have learned!
>
> **James, 2nd Year Student Nurse**

LEARNING OUTCOMES

When you have finished studying this chapter you will understand:

- How to link some of your previous learning to a complex scenario
- Some of the complex issues that can arise in critical care

INTRODUCTION

The aim of this chapter is to give you a complex case study for you to work through. The case will have an array of complex issues and you will need to navigate these to identify the evidence-based nursing assessment and care **intervention**s. You will need to ensure the values of person-centred care are maintained and consider the involvement of the wider multi-disciplinary team. You will also be asked to think about the impact of the admission on the person's family and visitors. Most of the information you need to guide your clinical decisions has been covered in the previous chapters. You may need some additional reading and the resources will be highlighted for you. The scenario has been written with the support of clinical experts from an Adult Critical Care Unit (ACCU). The reflective activities are designed in such a way that you can use them to support reflective discussions with colleagues or your practice supervisor or assessor. Once you have had the discussion, you can add these to your portfolio to support your development as a student or, if a newly registered nurse, they can support your revalidation evidence.

First, read the case study below and make some notes as you go.

THIS TOPIC IS ALSO COVERED IN CHAPTER 3

You have been on placement within a 14-bedded ACCU for two weeks and you are feeling a little more settled. You are allocated to work with Jane, a staff nurse with 5 years' experience. You walk over to the bed space you have been assigned to and receive handover of care from Danny who has just finished the night shift.

The handover of clinical information can be a stressful event for any member of the team. It is important all the key information is communicated. Danny used the SBAR and A-E format to help structure the handover.

SITUATION

Hi, this is Joyce; she is 72 years old and was admitted to us with **sepsis** following a chest infection. She has been ventilated and sedated for 5 days but despite changing her ventilation settings, her oxygenation was deteriorating and she was turned into the **prone** position 12 hours ago. Her ABGs have improved in this time but we have no plan at the moment to re-position her to a **supine** position.

Background

Joyce is a 72-year-old woman who was admitted to the hospital days ago with a community-acquired pneumonia. She was on Ward 10 for 4 days but despite non-invasive ventilation, she continued to deteriorate and was intubated and ventilated 5 days ago.

Assessment

Airway: Joyce has a size 7 **endotracheal tube** in, tied at 24cm at the teeth.

Breathing: She is being ventilated, her ventilator settings are charted below:

She was turned prone at the start of my night shift and like I say, she has improved but there is no plan as to when to turn her supine.

A sputum sample has been sent off and she has been prescribed Piperacillin.

Table 9.1 Joyce's ventilator settings

Time	05:00	06:00	07:00
MODE	Pressure Controlled Ventilation (PCV)	PCV	PCV
FiO$_2$	.75	.75	.75
Inspiratory pressure	28	28	28
PEEP	10	10	10
MV/TV	363mls	354	357
f set/meas	14		
I: E ratio	1:1		
Suction	Yes ++	No	Yes++
Sedation Score RASS	−4	−4	−4

Her last arterial blood gas taken at 06:20 is here.

pH	7.33
pCO$_2$	7.8 kPa
pO$_2$	9.8 kPa
Base Excess	+3.3 mmol/L
HCO$_3$	31 mmol/L
sO$_2$	95%

Her arterial blood gas before proning, taken at 18:00 yesterday, is here.

pH	7.32
pCO$_2$	7.9kPa
pO$_2$	8.9 kPa
Base Excess	+3
HCO$_3$	33 mmol/L
sO$_2$	90%

Circulation: She is in AF, but her heart rate is stable. Her BP is being maintained with Noradrenaline 8 mg/50mls infusion infusing at 5mls/hour which is ensuring her MAP stays above 65 and her CVP is 8.

Her urine output has been fine overnight averaging around 40mls per hour, however overall, in the past 24 hours she is a positive balance of 1000mls.

Disability: She is sedated with Propofol 2% with Alfentanil 0.5mg/ml or 1mg/ml concentration. and is scoring -4 according to RASS and this is what is prescribed. She was given cisatracurium when we turned her prone.

Exposure: She has had dressings applied to prominent points before she was turned prone to avoid skin damage, but her eyes are really swollen, her hands and feet are oedematous and damp to touch. We have repositioned her head and arms about an hour ago.

Recommendations

THIS TOPIC
IS ALSO
COVERED IN
CHAPTER 2

All her infusions are okay, you maybe have another hour before the first one runs out.

She needs to have a plan as to when she is going to be turned supine.

She has a daughter and I think two sons who visit, and they really need to be updated as to the deterioration by the doctors. Any questions?

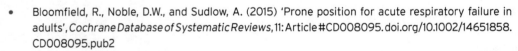

ACTIVITY 9.1: CRITICAL THINKING

1. What are your first thoughts?
2. Do you understand all that has been said to you in the handover?
3. What would your priorities of care be?
4. What other information would you need to know?
5. What questions would you want to ask the nurse handing over before they leave?
6. Do you understand all the above abbreviations?
7. Write these down and then check with our guide.
8. From what you have been told, what are the implications of her fluid balance?

WHAT'S THE EVIDENCE?

THIS TOPIC
IS ALSO
COVERED IN
CHAPTER 6

Read both the Cochrane review on prone positioning and the Intensive Care Societies 2019 updated proning guideline.

- Bloomfield, R., Noble, D.W., and Sudlow, A. (2015) 'Prone position for acute respiratory failure in adults', *Cochrane Database of Systematic Reviews*, 11: Article #CD008095. doi.org/10.1002/14651858. CD008095.pub2
- Faculty of Intensive Care Medicine and Intensive Care Society guidelines (2019) https://www. ficm.ac.uk/sites/default/files/prone_position_in_adult_critical_care_2019.pdf (accessed November 6, 2020)

It is now 40 minutes into your shift; you have made all the necessary checks and observations. Jane, the staff nurse you are working with, says Joyce's **sedation** and **inotropic** infusions will need replacing soon. She has asked you to chart Joyce's observations while she goes to the treatment room to draw up the medications. While Jane is away from the bedside, another nurse says two visitors have arrived asking to see Joyce and the nurse looking after her.

ACTIVITY 9.2: REFLECTIVE PRACTICE

Reflect on the situation above and consider your first concerns.

- The observations
- Talk with the family
- Leave the bedside and ask Jane to come back?

Discuss your thoughts with a colleague, as sometimes there is no right answer to these types of situations, but a discussion can help.

1. Do you feel you have enough knowledge to discuss Joyce with her visitors?
2. Reflect on how you would prepare them to see Joyce nursed in the prone position. If this was your relative what questions do you think would you ask?

It is helpful to consider this, and you can then maybe feel more prepared before speaking with distressed relatives.

3. Does the department you are in have open or restrictive visiting?
4. List the positives and negatives of both approaches from your perspective and then try to imagine this from the relatives' perspective and make a similar list.

Discuss these with a colleague.

Jane, the staff nurse, returns to the bed space and then speaks with the relatives. They are Joyce's son and daughter and are now sat beside their mum. Jane says the infusions she was preparing will run out very soon, so they need to be changed quickly. This is both Joyce's sedation and inotropic support.

ACTIVITY 9.3: CRITICAL THINKING

1. What potential medications risk can you think of in this situation?
2. What are the procedures applied to ensure we mitigate risk to avoid any errors?

I didn't want my patients' relatives to think I wasn't in control, but I've realised that being honest and saying I've got a couple of things to do and that I will speak to them as soon as I can is ok. They appreciate that I'm prioritising their loved one.

Claudette, Critical Care Staff Nurse

ACTIVITY 9.4: THEORY STOP POINT

Inotropic support, such as epinephrine infusions, cannot be stopped and swapped over. Look at your local policy on how these infusions are managed and then explore the current literature. Is the policy based on the most current evidence or are these infusions managed differently?

There is no template answer for this activity as the answer is based on your local policy.

You are now 2 hours into your shift and Joyce's condition is unchanged. She has yet to have a daily review by the medical team. Joyce's son seems to be becoming more anxious and asks why her hands and arms are wet and her eyes are so swollen. He also wants to know when she will be turned over.

ACTIVITY 9.5: REFLECTIVE PRACTICE

Consider the previous paragraph.

1. Do you feel you understand the physiology behind why Joyce's skin is damp and what the cause is? If not, take some time out to research this.
2. Consider how you would explain this to Joyce's son. What communication approaches could help you?

The multi-disciplinary team arrive and ask the relatives to wait in the visitors' room while they make an assessment and review Joyce's condition. The team asks for an update, which is provided by Jane.

Following an assessment and update the team decides that Joyce should be turned supine and they will return in an hour to do this. Jane says this will give you time to prepare.

ACTIVITY 9.6: REFLECTIVE PRACTICE

1. Who do you think would be part of the multi-disciplinary team and what input would they have on Joyce's care?

Write a list and compare this to our list. Discuss this with a colleague if you have any questions.

2. Before changing Joyce's position, what do you think you need to prepare and consider? Think of this in relation to the patient, the family, and the wider team.

Write down a list and then check this with our list and that of a colleague.

Joyce has been safely re-positioned on to her back. Before her family comes back to visit her hygiene needs must be met and a skin assessment needs to take place. Jane removes the hydrocolloid dressings that were applied to Joyce's pressure areas before her being turned prone to examine her skin underneath. All Joyce's bony prominences which were covered with protective dressings appear intact. Together you and Jane provide Joyce with a bed bath before changing her bed linen.

ACTIVITY 9.7: CRITICAL THINKING

1. What tools are used in your clinical area to help reduce the risk of pressure ulcers?
2. Based on your own experiences, think generally about the potential risk and benefits when repositioning critically ill patients.

List these and compare them to our ideas.

WHAT'S THE EVIDENCE?

It is common for patients who have been prone to develop pressure ulcers as a result.

Read Chapter 5 of the Faculty of Intensive Care Medicine and Intensive Care Society (2019) guideline on the nurse's role in reducing complications from prone positioning. Does the practice you have witnessed reflect these recommendations? If not, think about what potential barriers might exist to the implementation of these guidelines in practice.

Joyce's ET tube – which is currently secured with ties – now needs repositioning so that her mouth can be inspected and cleaned. Jane and another colleague work together to safely loosen and remove them whilst ensuring the ET tube does not move. The corners of Joyce's mouth appear damaged – Jane tells you she thinks the ties have caused pressure ulcers.

Jane now supervises you while you perform mouth care using Chlorhexidine toothpaste and apply lip balm to Joyce's lips.

ACTIVITY 9.8: CRITICAL THINKING

1. Write down what your initial action plan might be following the discovery of Joyce's pressure damage.
2. What MDT members would need to be involved?
3. What would you need to document?

Discuss your ideas with a colleague and take a look at our care plan.

THIS TOPIC IS ALSO COVERED IN CHAPTER 5

WHAT'S THE EVIDENCE?

Chlorhexidine toothpaste and mouthwashes are commonly used in critical care and are thought to play an essential role in the prevention of Ventilated Associated Pneumonia (VAP).

Read the systematic review by Hua et al. (2016) 'Oral hygiene care for critically ill patients to prevent ventilator-associated pneumonia'. doi.org/10.1002/14651858.CD008367.pub3

Think about how the author's recommendations relate to practice in your area.

The ward clerk informs you that Joyce's family is worried and has asked how much longer it will be until they can see her. Jane states that you both need ten more minutes to finish caring for Joyce as you have yet to perform eye care. Joyce's eyes are swollen and appear slightly red. Jane examines them with a pen torch before cleaning them with gauze and sterile water. She then applies ointment to each eye.

ACTIVITY 9.9: CRITICAL THINKING

1. Considering how unwell Joyce is, do you think providing eye care should be prioritised over her family returning to the bed space?

There is no right or wrong answer, but it might be useful to consider this from the point of view of both Jane and Joyce's family.

WHAT'S THE EVIDENCE?

Read the Royal College of Ophthalmologist's (2017) guideline on eyecare in the Intensive Care Unit, https://www.rcophth.ac.uk/wp-content/uploads/2017/11/Intensive-Care-Unit.pdf

1. Has reading the guideline changed your thoughts on the importance of eye care for Joyce?

There is no template answer to this activity as it is based on your own reflection.

You and Jane now tidy the bed area. Jane sits down to document the care you have given and asks you to collect Joyce's family from the relative's room.

ACTIVITY 9.10: CRITICAL THINKING AND REFLECTIVE PRACTICE

1. Would you feel apprehensive about doing this knowing that Joyce's family is likely to be anxious?
2. How would you provide reassurance?
3. Think about what questions they are likely to ask Jane when they return to the bedside. What might Jane need to explain?

Joyce's family are sat by the bedside and two hours have passed. Joyce suddenly experiences an episode of de-saturation. Jane carries out **suction** to remove secretions and this appears to resolve the situation, although Jane has also increased the amount of oxygen Joyce is receiving. After 30 minutes Jane obtains another ABG for analysis. This shows further deterioration. Jane speaks with the physiotherapist and they attend and carry out manual recruitment manoeuvres.

WHAT'S THE EVIDENCE?

Manual recruitment manoeuvres are carried out by an experienced member of the multidisciplinary team to improve gas exchange by 'opening' up areas of the lung field. There are a number of different methods used from supporting the person's breathing with a technique replicating sighing to providing a short interval of breathing using higher pressure.

It is not without risk and there is a disparity in the evidence base regarding its use.

Read the Systematic Review and Meta-Analysis by Cui et al. (2019) and discuss your thoughts with your practice supervisor or a colleague.

Over a couple of hours, Joyce's condition worsens, and the family asks if she can be turned back on to her front as this helped. The wider MDT agreed that in the end, this is not the most appropriate treatment and possibly, there needs to be a discussion about the limitation of the treatment Joyce is receiving. The family meeting has not yet taken place and you are coming to the end of your shift and need to prepare to hand over to the next shift. Jane asks you to provide the handover.

ACTIVITY 9.11: CRITICAL THINKING

1.   Who do you think should lead this discussion with the family and who should be there?
2.   What sort of questions do you think they will ask?
3.   How would you answer these if asked and what do you need to consider before this type of meeting?

Discuss your thoughts with a colleague.

ACTIVITY 9.12: CRITICAL THINKING

Using the SBAR and A-E structure write down your proposed handover.

1.   How confident would you feel to hand over this patient?
2.   If you don't feel confident, what could you do to improve this?

CHAPTER SUMMARY

In summary, you have worked through a complex case scenario and considered many elements of care. The activities aimed to prompt you to consider areas of your professional development. The activities may have highlighted gaps in some areas of your knowledge. Reflect on this and consider generating a personal development plan to support you to address these gaps. You can also add this to your professional profile or portfolio.

GO FURTHER

Books

Kraszewski, S. and McEwen, A. (eds) (2010) *Communication Skills for Adult Nurses*. Maidenhead: Open University Press.

* This book is a good general resource for you to read about how you can develop your communication and interpersonal skills.

Mallet, J., Albarran, J. and Richardson, A. (eds) (2013) *Critical Care Manual of Clinical Procedures and Competencies*. London: Wiley-Blackwell.

* This manual is an excellent resource on critical care clinical skills procedures.

Creed, F., Hargreaves, J. and Baid, H. (2016) *Oxford Handbook of Critical Care Nursing*. Oxford: Oxford University Press.

* This book focuses on the practical issues of nursing care and nursing procedures.

Journal articles

Small, J., Roberson, E., and Runcie, R. (2019) 'Care of the eye during anaesthesia and intensive care', *Anesthesia and Intensive Care Medicine*, 20 (12): 731–4. doi.org/10.1016/j.mpaic.2019.10.008

* This evidence explores the importance of eye care for the unconscious patient.

Pelosi, P., Gama de Abreu, M., and Rocco, P.R.M. (2010) 'New and conventional strategies for lung recruitment in acute respiratory distress syndrome', *Critical Care*, 14 (10): Article #210. www.researchgate.net/publication/42254516 (accessed November 6, 2020).

* This article discusses the definition, types and factors affecting recruitment manoeuvres.

Hudack, M.E. (2012) 'Prone positioning for patients with ARDS', *Nursing Critical Care*, 7 (2): 20–4. doi.org/10.1097/01.CCN.0000412309.28066.f0

* This informative article outlines the rationale and technique used to move critically ill adults into the prone position.

Bunker, D.L.J. and Thomson, M. (2015) 'Chin necrosis as a consequence of prone positioning in the intensive care unit', *Case Reports in Medicine*: Article #762956. doi.org/10.1155/2015/762956

- This paper looks a case study of a person who developed necrosis on their chin following prone positioning; such cases are rare but you may find the discussion interesting.

Useful websites

www.youtube.com/watch?v=FS4t5w1eCYw

- This YouTube clip gives a really good overview as to why we use the prone position.

www.ficm.ac.uk/sites/default/files/prone_position_in_adult_critical_care_2019.pdf (accessed November 6, 2020).

- This site offers a full set of guidance as to how to prone a person in critical care.

www.aci.health.nsw.gov.au/networks/icnsw/intensive-care-manual/statewide-guidelines/suctioning-an-adult-icu-patient (accessed November 6, 2020).

- This webpage has a lot of information about suctioning.

REFERENCES

Baile, W.F., Buckman R., Lenzi R. et al. (2000) 'SPIKES - A six-step protocol for delivering bad news: application to the patient with cancer'. *Oncologist*, 5 (4): 302–11.

Bamford, P., Denmade, C., Newmarch, C., Shirley, P., Singer, B., Webb, S. and Whitmore, D. (2019) *Guidance For: Prone Positioning in Adult Critical Care*. https://www.ficm.ac.uk/sites/default/files/prone_position_in_adult_critical_care_2019.pdf (accessed November 6, 2020).

Bloomfield, R., Noble, D.W. and Sudlow., A. (2015) 'Prone position for acute respiratory failure in adults'. *Cochrane Database of Systematic Reviews 2015*, Issue 11, Article CD008095. doi: 10.1002/14651858.CD008095.pub2 (accessed January 10, 2021).

Cui Y, Cao R, Wang Y, Li G. (2020) Lung Recruitment Maneuvers for ARDS Patients: A Systematic Review and Meta-Analysis. *Respiration*. 99(3):264 – 276. doi: 10.1159/000501045.

Hua, F., Xie, H., Worthington, H.V., Furness, S., Zhang, Q. and Li, C. (2016) 'Oral hygiene care for critically ill patients to prevent ventilator-associated pneumonia,' *Cochrane Database of Systematic Reviews*. doi.org/10.1002/14651858.CD008367.pub3

Royal College of Ophthalmologists (2017) Ophthalmic Services Guidance. Eye Care in the Intensive Care Unit (ICU). https://www.rcophth.ac.uk/wp-content/uploads/2017/11/Intensive-Care-Unit.pdf. Accessed April 2021.

CRITICAL CARE RELATED TO THE GASTROINTESTINAL SYSTEM

CLAIRE BURNS

10

> " I never realised patients on the ICU were allowed to eat. I remember caring for a patient on there who had been fed by a nasogastric tube for a few weeks. She was assessed by the speech and language therapist who said she could have something to eat. She was too weak to feed herself and I was able to give her the first food she had eaten in weeks. I gave her some yoghurt, she could only manage a few spoonfuls but the delight on her face of having that cold, sweet yoghurt in her mouth.
>
> **Shebah, 2nd Year Student Nurse** "

LEARNING OUTCOMES

When you have finished studying this chapter you will be able to understand:

- The overview of the anatomy and physiology of the gastrointestinal tract
- Assessment of nutritional requirement of the critically ill person and screening for malnutrition
- The routes of nutrition in the critical care area
- Any special considerations for the administration of nutrition
- The role of insulin in the glycaemic control of the critically ill person

INTRODUCTION

As you may have realised from reading other chapters in this book, adequate nutrition plays a vital role in the maintenance, functioning and healing of every system within the body. As can be identified from the opening quote of this chapter, eating is not only life-sustaining, it is an important part of daily life enjoyed, and taken for granted, by many people. Adequate nutrition is especially important in the person experiencing critical illness as the physiological stress experienced increases the calories required for their body to function at a time when the affected person may either be unable or unwilling to eat.

Poor nutrition has many negative effects on the person experiencing critical illness, these include: loss of body mass (this will include muscle, not just fat), increased infection risk, organ dysfunction, increased **mortality** and **morbidity** (Jordan and Moore, 2019), development of pressure ulcers and decreased healing (Coleman et al., 2014) all factors which can lead to increased morbidity, mortality and increased hospital length of stay. Some patients will already be malnourished on admission to the Adult Critical Care Unit (ACCU) whilst the condition of others will deteriorate during their stay. It is estimated that those experiencing critical illness will develop a 6000-kcal deficit within a week of admission to an Adult Critical Care Unit (ACCU) (Kuslapuu et al., 2015).

The aim of this chapter is to provide you with an overview of the relevant anatomy and physiology of the gastrointestinal system, signposting you where more detailed revision is required. The chapter will focus on the screening, assessment and nursing management linked to the nutritional care of the critically ill person.

OVERVIEW OF THE ANATOMY AND PHYSIOLOGY OF THE GASTROINTESTINAL TRACT

Structure and function

The gastrointestinal system has three main functions, these are digestion, absorption and elimination. It is composed of the alimentary canal and accessory organs.

Alimentary canal

The key anatomical structures of the **alimentary canal** include the mouth (oral cavity), the pharynx (throat), the oesophagus (gullet), stomach, small intestine (small bowel) which comprises of the duodenum, jejunum and ileum, large intestine (large bowel) and anus.

The first step in the process of digestion is the ingestion (eating) of food. As can be seen in Figure 10.1, when food enters the mouth, the processes of mechanical and chemical digestion begin. Mechanical digestion involves breaking down food into smaller pieces, this is normally done by the teeth when chewing. Enzymes are released by the salivary glands in the mouth and begin the process of chemical digestion. Once the food is sufficiently broken down, it is made into a ball known as a bolus and is moved by the tongue into the pharynx for swallowing.

The pharynx is the start of the continuous tube that is the alimentary canal. Upon swallowing the epiglottis closes the entrance to the larynx to prevent the bolus entering the airway. The bolus then travels to the oesophagus, which, by a coordinated process of contractions and relaxations called peristalsis, pushes the bolus to the stomach (Tortora and Derrickson, 2011) as seen in Figure 10.2.

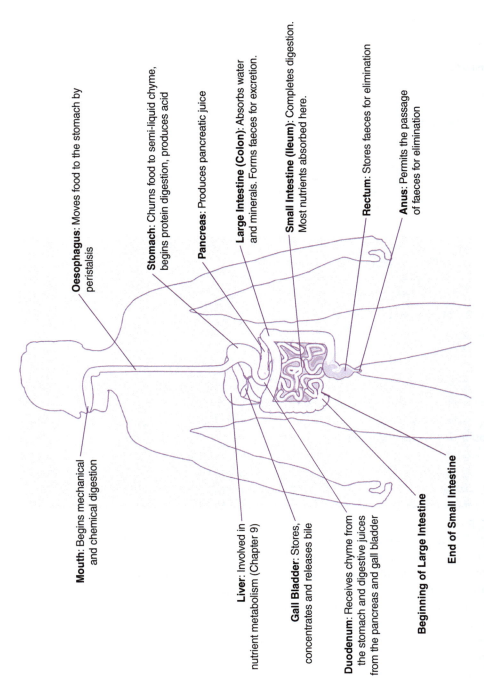

Oesophagus: Moves food to the stomach by peristalsis

Stomach: Churns food to semi-liquid chyme, begins protein digestion, produces acid

Pancreas: Produces pancreatic juice

Large Intestine (Colon): Absorbs water and minerals. Forms faeces for excretion.

Small Intestine (Ileum): Completes digestion. Most nutrients absorbed here.

Rectum: Stores faeces for elimination

Anus: Permits the passage of faeces for elimination

Mouth: Begins mechanical and chemical digestion

Liver: Involved in nutrient metabolism (Chapter 9)

Gall Bladder: Stores, concentrates and releases bile

Duodenum: Receives chyme from the stomach and digestive juices from the pancreas and gall bladder

Beginning of Large Intestine

End of Small Intestine

Figure 10.1 Components of the digestive system

Source: Cook et al. (2021).

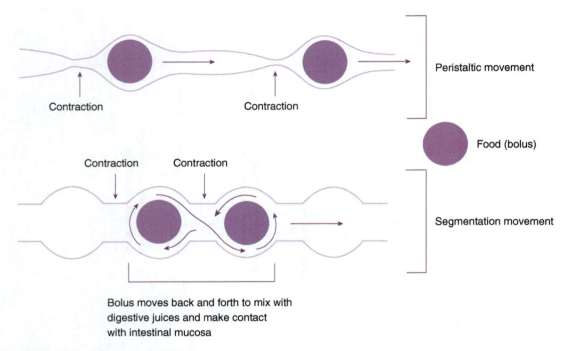

Figure 10.2 Movements of the gut

Source: Cook et al. (2021).

The stomach is a large muscular organ and it has several digestive functions. The stomach releases gastric juices which contain hydrochloric acid (HCl), pepsin and renin. These chemicals are essential in the chemical digestion of fats and proteins as well as facilitating the absorption of some vitamins; HCl is vitally important as it also kills bacteria (Tortora and Derrickson, 2011). Additionally, the stomach 'churns' the food using the process of peristalsis; this churning facilitates the mixing of food within the stomach with the digestive juices and breaks down (macerates) the food producing a liquid called chyme (Tortora and Derrickson, 2011). The chyme is then very gradually pushed into the duodenum.

Nearly all digestion and absorption of nutrients occurs in the small intestine (Tortora and Derrickson, 2011). Ducts that travel from the pancreas (minor duodenal papilla) and gallbladder (major duodenal papilla) empty bile and pancreatic juices into the duodenum. These juices, along with intestinal juices continue the chemical digestion of ingested food. After this process the chyme is pushed forwards into the large intestine where the last phase of digestion occurs. The large intestine is responsible for the breakdown of compounds with bacteria and the absorption of some vitamins and other useful nutrients and electrolytes as well as water (Tortora and Derrickson, 2011). Once the water has been absorbed and the chyme has become solid or semi-solid it is called faeces (Tortora and Derrickson, 2011). Peristalsis occurs in the large intestine at a much slower rate in comparison to the rest of the alimentary canal and the faeces is slowly moved into the rectum where, in the continent adult, it is released on voluntary relaxation of the external rectal sphincter (Waugh and Grant, 2009).

Accessory organs

The accessory organs of the gastrointestinal system include the liver, gall bladder and the pancreas. Below is a brief overview of these organs and their functions linked to the gastrointestinal system. You may find it useful to read about the liver, gall bladder and pancreas in an anatomy and physiology book to give you a more in-depth understanding of each of the organs.

Liver

The main functions of the liver within the digestive system are:

THIS TOPIC IS ALSO COVERED IN CHAPTER 8

1. Bile production
2. **Metabolism** of carbohydrate, fat and protein
3. Detoxification of harmful chemicals
4. Excretion of **bilirubin**, cholesterol, hormones and drugs

Gall bladder

The gallbladder is a small, green, muscular sac that lies behind the liver. Its main function is the storage and concentration of bile. Bile is important in the breakdown of fats to make them easier to digest.

Pancreas

The main functions of the pancreas include:

1. The secretion of insulin and glucagon to help regulate blood glucose levels
2. The secretion of pancreatic juices to help digest food

Screening and assessment of nutritional status

It is important to assess the nutritional status of the person experiencing critical illness and intervene appropriately as early as possible to prevent deterioration of their nutritional status (Lee and Heyland, 2019). A nutritional screen is a quick risk assessment used to identify those who are, or are at risk of becoming, malnourished and assist in the planning of **interventions** to improve nutrition. There are many ways in which nutritional status can be screened and assessed and the area in which you work is likely to have a preferred tool that is used. The European Society for Clinical Nutrition and Metabolism (ESPEN) recommend that general clinical assessment includes the patient's account of their medical history, whether the person has experienced any unintentional weight loss or a decrease in physical ability as well as a physical examination and general assessment of body composition, muscle mass and strength if possible (Singer et al., 2019). The National Institute for Health and Care Excellence (NICE, 2006) recommends that all inpatients receive nutritional screening on admission to hospital and weekly thereafter or when there is clinical concern.

The Malnutrition Universal Screening Tool (MUST) is commonly used to screen for malnutrition in practice. You can find the tool at the following link: www.bapen.org.uk/screening-and-must/must-calculator (accessed November 6, 2020). Activity 10.1 asks you to think about the advantages and disadvantages of using the MUST.

====== **ACTIVITY 10.1: CRITICAL THINKING** ======

a. What are the advantages of using MUST?
b. What are the disadvantages of using MUST?

Once a nutritional screen has been performed, a nutritional assessment must take place. The early input of specialists, such as a **dietician** or nutritional support nurse, is imperative in the assessment of nutritional status of those identified as being at risk of malnourishment. The British Association for Parenteral and Enteral Nutrition (BAPEN, 2016) suggest nutritional assessment improves clinical decision making, allows for a person-centred approach and revision of the plan as individual circumstances change. A nutritional assessment may include clinical examination as well as history taking and biochemical measurements and a review of the person's current medication (BAPEN, 2016). From this information, energy and fluid requirements will be calculated and a plan developed.

RE-FEEDING SYNDROME

During the assessment the person experiencing critical illness may also be assessed for their risk of developing re-feeding syndrome. Re-feeding syndrome occurs when a malnourished person begins feeding after a period of starvation or reduced food intake and potentially fatal shifts in fluids and electrolytes occur within the body (NICE, 2006). Re-feeding syndrome is most common in persons receiving enteral and parenteral nutrition but can also develop in those receiving oral diet (NICE, 2006). The risk factors for re-feeding syndrome include; low body weight, no or reduced food intake for more than 10 days, low levels of potassium, phosphate or magnesium before feeding and 'a history of alcohol misuse or drugs, including insulin, chemotherapy, antacids and **diuretics**' (BAPEN, 2016). If the person experiencing critical illness has any of these risk factors, it is important that they are assessed early by an appropriate healthcare professional so a tailored feeding regime can be developed. As with any intervention the effectiveness, indications, route, risks and benefits of nutritional support must be reviewed at regular intervals and a new plan developed as required (NICE, 2006). Activity 10.2 asks you to review the guidelines and consider how you would monitor someone receiving nutritional support in the ACCU.

====== **ACTIVITY 10.2: CRITICAL THINKING** ======

NICE (2006) developed Clinical Guidelines 32 *Nutrition Support for Adults: Oral Nutrition Support, Enteral Tube Feeding and Parenteral Nutrition*. These guidelines were reviewed in 2017 and no new evidence was found that affects the recommendations in this guideline: www.nice.org.uk/guidance/cg32 (accessed November 6, 2020).

1. After reading the guidance, how do you think a critically ill person receiving nutritional support should be monitored?

Oral diet and fluids

Oral food intake has many physiological and psychological benefits to the person experiencing critical illness. However, adequate oral intake can be prevented or inhibited by many factors including the person's consciousness level, swallowing disorders, psychological disorders, loss of appetite and alterations in taste (Massanet et al., 2015).

It is important to assess whether the person who is experiencing critical illness can be safely fed orally. This assessment will take into consideration many factors including the person's current medical condition and any pre-existing swallowing disorders (Massanet et al., 2015). Another factor than may impact on the person's ability to take oral diet is the presence of a tracheostomy tube. Not all patients with tracheostomy tubes will have swallowing problems (dysphagia) and research suggests that the underlying illness that led to tracheostomy is frequently the cause for dysphasia rather than the tracheostomy itself (Sharma et al., 2007). There is controversy surrounding the practice of giving oral diet to individuals with an inflated tracheostomy cuff. Some ACCUs will only give oral diet to individuals without a cuffed tracheostomy tube or when the tracheostomy cuff has been deflated. Research into this area is limited but the 'What's the evidence?' article below sheds some light onto the safety of this practice.

WHAT'S THE EVIDENCE?

Pryor, L., Ward, E., Cornwell, P., O'Connor, S. and Chapman, W. (2016) 'Patterns of return to oral intake and decannulation post-tracheostomy across clinical populations in an acute inpatient setting', *International Journal of Language and Communication Disorders*, 51 (5): 556–67. doi. org/10.1111/1460-6984.12231

A multi-disciplinary team (MDT) approach is necessary to assess the swallowing function of the person experiencing critical illness who is identified as being at risk of dysphasia. This will normally include referral to an appropriate professional such as a **speech and language therapist** (SLT) and a 'swallow test' being performed. Swallow tests can be performed at the bedside in several ways. Table 10.1 gives three examples.

Table 10.1 Examples of swallow tests

Test	Description
Swallow test using water and food	This test involves swallowing a range of substances starting with water and advancing to thickened liquids, pureed foods, soft foods and even regular foods if tolerated.
Evans Blue Dye Test (Cameron et al., 1973)	This test is performed by placing 4 drops of Evans blue dye on the tongue every 4 hours and then aspirating the tracheostomy regularly over 48 hours. If blue dye is seen, the test is positive for **aspiration.**
Fibreoptic Endoscopic Evaluation of Swallowing (FEES)	During a FEES, an endoscope is passed through the nose into the throat. Swallowing is then observed through the endoscope and an assessment of swallow function is made.

ACTIVITY 10.3: THEORY STOP POINT

What do you think are some of the potential advantages and disadvantages of each of the swallow tests detailed in Table 10.1?

Activity 10.4 asks you to put yourself in the position of a critically unwell person who is unable to eat.

ACTIVITY 10.4: REFLECTIVE PRACTICE

a. Consider how you would feel if you wanted to eat and drink but were told you could not. Imagine only being allowed teaspoons of fluids or if your favourite drink was thickened with a powder before you could drink it.
b. Do you think you would have much of an appetite if all your food was pureed?
c. Now consider if, as well as this, you can see the staff tea trolley where they are drinking cups of tea and sharing some biscuits. How would this leave you feeling?

Completing Activity 10.4 will have made you think about the psychological and sociological impacts of not eating. Oral diet is an important part of most people's lives and an important element of delivering person-centred care. Unfortunately, it is not always safe for those experiencing critical illness. Even when a person has been assessed as being able to swallow it is important that they are carefully monitored when consuming oral intake and reassessed if their condition changes. Simple steps you can take to assist safe oral intake are to ensure the patient is sat upright, preferably in a chair, though this can be done in a bed, with the chin flexed forward to the chest, and ensure the person is being the given the correct consistency of diet, e.g. pureed, if needed. During feeding, close monitoring of the person is essential. If any of the following occur stop feeding the person immediately and get help and specialist advice:

1. Signs of respiratory distress (e.g. decreased SpO_2, increased respiration rate)
2. The person becomes **fatigued**
3. The person coughs persistently
4. There is evidence of aspiration on tracheal **suction** (e.g. food, drink or stomach contents evident in tracheal suction)

Due to high caloric demands of being critically unwell it is difficult for the person experiencing critical illness to achieve their nutritional goals through the traditional 3 meals per day and it is recognised that those experiencing critical illness frequently do not meet their nutritional targets (Stewart et al., 2017). An MDT approach is necessary to assist in nutritional targets being achieved and the input of a dietician who can prescribe additional nutrition in the form of supplements or dual oral and enteral nutrition is often required.

ACTIVITY 10.5: CASE STUDY

Amara, a 68-year-old female, had been admitted to the ACCU for mechanical ventilation due to type II respiratory failure secondary to pneumonia. Amara received invasive mechanical ventilation for 3 weeks and had a tracheostomy tube inserted on day 8 of her stay to aid weaning from mechanical ventilation. Once Amara had been successfully weaned from ventilatory support her tracheostomy tube was removed and her swallow function was assessed by the speech and language therapist (SLT) the following morning. Amara's swallow was evaluated and the SLT prescribed a soft diet and thickened fluids for her.

That evening Amara started coughing and appeared to be choking at mealtime. The nurse stopped Amara from consuming any further oral intake and asked for a medical review.

1. What are the possible reasons for Amara displaying symptoms of aspiration when she was eating her evening meal?
2. What do you think should be the main considerations for Amara and her nutritional care?

ENTERAL NUTRITION (EN)

EN refers to any methods of feeding that use the gastrointestinal tract not including oral feeding. After oral diet EN is the preferred method of nutrition delivery in the ACCU as it supports the functional and structural integrity of the gut and can prevent changes in gut permeability which can increase the risk of **systemic** infection (Taylor et al., 2016) and subsequent organ failure (Jabbar et al., 2003). It is recommended that EN is considered for all persons staying in the ACCU for more than 48 hours (Singer et al., 2019).

EN feeding should be commenced within 48 hours of admission to the ACCU as this has been demonstrated to maintain gut integrity and reduce infectious complications (Singer et al., 2019; Taylor et al., 2016). If the critically ill person is unable to take oral diet, alternative forms of enteral feeding must be considered. This most often includes the passing of a tube into the stomach or small intestine. The three main types of enteral feeding tubes include:

1. Nasogastric tube (NGT) – a tube passed via the nose into the stomach
2. Orogastric tube (OGT) – a tube passed via the mouth into the stomach
3. Post-pyloric tube – a tube passed via the nose into either the jejunum or duodenum

Activity 10.6 looks at the importance of confirming NGT position.

ACTIVITY 10.6: CRITICAL THINKING

Take a moment to read the National Patient Safety Agency (NPSA, 2011) patient safety alert NPSA/2011/PSA002: 'Reducing the harm caused by misplaced nasogastric feeding tubes in adults, children and infants', which can be found using the following link: www.gbukenteral.com/pdf/NPSA-Alert-2011.pdf (accessed November 6, 2020)

(Continued)

1. Make a note of the clinical actions that should be taken to confirm the NGT is correctly positioned in the stomach on insertion
2. Make a note of the checks that should be made after initial correct placement of the NGT to ensure the tube has not been displaced
3. Familiarise yourself with your local policy; does it reflect the requirements set out in the NPSA (2011) document? How will this influence your practice?

There is no template answer to Question 3 as it is based on your local policy.

EN is most frequently administered via an NGT with post-pyloric feeding usually reserved for individuals who are at a high risk of aspiration or who cannot tolerate being fed into their stomachs. The feeding regimen is usually specified by a dietician who will calculate the nutritional requirements of the person experiencing critical illness and prescribe a prepared liquid feed along with the rate and/or volume to be administered. Although NG tubes are common within ACCU they are not without risk and a thorough risk assessment must be performed before the final decision to insert an NG tube is made.

Case Study 10.7 examines some potential risks of NG feeding.

ACTIVITY 10.7: CASE STUDY

It was midnight and Mark, a staff nurse who had been qualified and working on the ACCU for 6 months, admitted Ahmad, a 59-year-old male. Ahmad had experienced an in-hospital cardiac arrest with return of spontaneous circulation following 2 minutes of cardiopulmonary resuscitation (CPR) whilst in the emergency department (ED) after presenting with chest pain. He had a past medical history of asthma, **ischaemic stroke** and **hypercholesterolaemia**. Ahmad was sedated, intubated and placed on mechanical ventilation. He required minimal vasopressor therapy to maintain his blood pressure.

Once Ahmad was stabilised and a nutritional risk assessment had been completed, a nasogastric tube (NGT) was inserted by the **Specialist Trainee 6** (ST6). During the procedure the ST6 was called to assess an emergency in the ED. Mark was unable to aspirate gastric aspirates from the NGT so the Foundation Year 2 (FY2) doctor working on the ACCU requested an X-ray to confirm NGT position. The X-ray was performed and at 3.30am Mark contacted the FY2 to interpret the X-ray. The FY2 checked the X-ray and told Mark to commence feed. Mark commenced Ahmad's enteral feeding regime at the rate specified by local policy.

During handover to the day staff that morning Ahmad's oxygen saturations dropped from 95% to 88%. Upon **endotracheal tube** suctioning an aspirate resembling the nasogastric feed was observed. The feed was stopped immediately, and a chest X-ray was performed that showed the position of the NGT to be in the right lung and **pulmonary** aspiration. Ahmad went on to develop pneumonia secondary to pulmonary aspiration and died as a result 8 days later surrounded by his loving family.

Reflecting on the case study:

1. What events do you believe led to the death of Ahmad?
2. What interventions might have prevented the death of Ahmad?

Between 2005 and 2013 The National Patient Safety Agency (NPSA) published several safety alerts regarding NGT misplacement and risk of death and severe harm (NPSA, 2016). In the UK introducing fluids or medication into the lungs via a misplaced NGT or OGT is a never event, this means it is an entirely preventable event that should never happen (NPSA, 2016).

As you will have identified by completing your reflection on Activity 10.7, before commencing any feed via the nasogastric tube, it is vital that tube placement is checked by a competent person and that it is documented that it is safe to feed. This is to ensure that the tube has not been placed into the person's lungs on insertion or migrated out of the stomach after insertion (National Patient Safety Agency, 2011).

Guidance must be followed to ensure the safe administration of feed via any enteral feeding tubes. Placement confirmation is initially assessed by testing the pH of the contents aspirated from the NGT. If the pH of aspirates is less than 5.5 and there are no clinical concerns, feeding can commence. If the pH of aspirates is greater than 5.5 a chest X-ray may be indicated to confirm the position of the NGT. It is essential that this X-ray is interpreted by an appropriately competent person as misinterpretation and subsequent feeding into the lungs of the person can cause severe harm or be fatal. Wherever possible, patients receiving EN should be sat in an upright position, at a minimum of a 30-degree angle and monitored for signs of aspiration.

It is essential that once the enteral feeding tube has been inserted, it is secured at the nose with a fixation tape to reduce the risk of displacement and ensure comfort. When securing the tube, you must check it is not putting any pressure on the nose as this can cause nasal pressure injuries. It is good practice to observe for the potential of the tube to place pressure on the surrounding skin every time you use the enteral feeding tube. If this is the case, the fixation tapes will need to be replaced so the enteral feeding tube is in a position where it cannot cause a pressure injury.

A routine yet controversial practice in NG feeding is the monitoring of gastric residual volume (GRV). GRV refers to the amount of fluid aspirated via the NGT. This is typically done using a 50 ml syringe every 4-6 hours. It is thought that measurements of GRV can be used as a surrogate marker of gut function with high GRVs (usually exceeding 500ml) being associated with gut dysfunction. GRVs of 200–250ml are usually returned to the stomach via the NGT. Any volume exceeding this is often discarded and the infusion rate or volume of NG feed may be reviewed or a prokinetic medication added to the prescription of the person receiving the feed to improve gut motility.

Activity 10.8 asks you look at the some of the available evidence surrounding the monitoring of GRVs.

ACTIVITY 10.8: CRITICAL THINKING

Read Wang et al. (2019) 'Effects of not monitoring gastric residual volume in intensive care patients: A meta-analysis'. doi.org/10.1016/j.ijnurstu.2018.11.005

1. What are the possible implications of monitoring GRVs?
2. What are the possible implications of not monitoring GRVs?
3. Is the evidence presented in the meta-analysis robust enough to warrant a change in practice?

Enteral feeding tubes can also be used for the administration of medications. The route which the medication is to be administered must be documented on the prescription chart. It is important to understand that many medications are not licensed for administration via enteral feeding tubes and the professionals who prescribe, supply and administer them accept liability for their use (BAPEN, 2017). Consequently, input from the pharmacist is crucial to help ensure the safe administration of medications via an enteral feeding tube, particularly if this involves dissolving or crushing tablets or opening capsules.

Another important consideration when administering medication via an enteral feeding tube is the potential for some medications to interact with the enteral feed resulting in reduced drug or feed absorption (BAPEN, 2017), for example, some medications are required to be given on an empty stomach to ensure adequate absorption. It is essential that you understand how to correctly administer any medications via the enteral feeding tube and that the relevant members of the MDT are consulted before the administration of medications.

Enteral and parenteral feed and any medications administered via these routes are typically recorded on the fluid balance chart. Any discarded GRVs will need to be recorded as negative volume. Keeping an accurate record of nutritional support administered allows for the accurate calculation not only of fluid intake but also of calorie and nutrient intake, allowing any problems with the administration of nutrition to be detected and potentially resolved early.

All accessories associated with enteral feeding tubes have a specific design to prevent them from accidentally being connected to other systems, such as **intravenous** lines (which has resulted in several deaths in the UK). It is therefore imperative that you use the correct accessories when preparing or administering anything via an enteral device.

Additionally, enteral feeding tubes, particularly nasojejunal tubes, have the potential to become blocked. It is therefore essential that you follow your local protocol when administering medications via enteral tubes and ensure that you follow the instructions for flushing the enteral feeding tube in between giving individual medications (medications should never be mixed) as well as before and after administration of all medications is complete. This usually involves flushing the enteral feeding tube with 30mls of sterile water at the beginning and end of the administration of medicines and flushing with 10mls of sterile water between each medication (BAPEN, 2017).

Rate-based EN

In rate-based EN the critically ill person's nutritional requirements over a 24-hour period are calculated, usually by a dietician, and the feed is infused at a consistent hourly rate to achieve these requirements. Rate based infusions are typically commenced at a slow rate and increased gradually if there are no symptoms of intolerance such as abdominal distension or high gastric aspirates until the feed is at a rate where the critically ill person's nutritional needs are met.

One of the disadvantages of rate based EN is that there are often interruptions to enteral nutrition, for example, if the critically ill person needs to undergo a procedure. When the infusion is interrupted it is restarted at the original hourly rate, leading to inadequate nutrition and underfeeding resulting in poorer outcomes for those experiencing critical illness (McClave et al., 2015).

Volume-based EN

Volume-based EN involves the calculation of the total volume of feed to be infused over an entire period of time, allowing the healthcare worker to adjust the rate of feed as required to ensure the critically ill person receives the required volume of feed prescribed for them over a specific time period. For volume-based feeding to be effective it is important that you calculate the amount of feed infused hourly to ensure you can keep track of the volume of feed administered and the volume required by the individual. A study by McClave et al. (2015) demonstrated that administering volume based EN increased the number of calories administered when feeding was interrupted in comparison to rate-based EN.

EN intolerance

Some individuals experiencing critical illness may not be able to tolerate EN into their stomach. In individuals where intolerance is observed, or high gastric aspirates are present (i.e. >500ml/6h) prokinetic medications might be used or the feed rate might be reduced or stopped depending on the person's clinical condition. Post-pyloric feeding may also be considered.

Table 10.2 lists the European Society of Intensive Care Medicine (ESICM) (Blaser et al., 2017) recommendations for delaying early EN.

Table 10.2   ESICM recommendations for delaying early EN

1. Uncontrolled shock

2. Uncontrolled life-threatening hypoxaemia, hypercapnoea or acidosis

3. Overt bowel ischaemia

4. High output intestinal fistula if feeding distal to the fistula is not achievable

5. Abdominal compartment syndrome

6. Active upper gastrointestinal bleeding

7. Gastric aspirates greater that 500ml for 6 hours

PARENTERAL NUTRITION

Parenteral nutrition is nutritional support given via intravenous (IV) access, usually via a central line. Just like enteral nutrition, parenteral nutrition is started gradually so the possibility of adverse outcomes such as refeeding syndrome are reduced. As parenteral nutrition is administered intravenously, it increases the risk of infections such as **sepsis** and phlebitis and can also result in air **embolism**. Parenteral nutrition should only be used if EN is not appropriate or full dose EN is not tolerated during the first week of intensive care (Blaser et al., 2017). The risks and benefits of parenteral nutrition must be looked at on a case-by-case basis (Singer et al., 2019).

Parenteral nutrition contains lipids (fats) which can enable bacterial growth and lead to infection. Because of this it is essential that you comply with strict aseptic non-touch technique (ANTT) during the preparation and administration of parenteral nutrition. When caring for the person receiving parenteral nutrition, regular monitoring of blood chemistry is required to monitor for refeeding syndrome and to ensure the feed is made to the requirements of the person receiving parenteral nutrition. Additionally, it is important to continually assess the person receiving parenteral nutrition for any changes in their condition that will allow EN to commence. Parenteral nutrition will usually be stopped once the person is able to take in adequate EN.

GLYCAEMIC CONTROL

People experiencing critical illness may have deranged blood glucose levels (BGLs) for several reasons including diabetes and **stress-induced hyperglycaemia**. Studies have demonstrated that hyperglycaemia in the ACCU is associated with increased morbidity (Van den Berghe, 2006) and mortality (Godinjak et al., 2015). However, there is much debate around the optimal range for BGLs in the person experiencing critical illness.

It is important that you follow local guidelines regarding glycaemic control in the ACCU. These guidelines will typically advise on how regularly BGL monitoring should occur as well as when to initiate insulin and at what rate insulin should be administered to maintain BGLs within acceptable ranges. Along with monitoring for hyperglycaemia it is also vitally important that hypoglycaemia is avoided. Glycaemic control in the ACCU has been associated with moderate and severe hypoglycaemia, both of which are linked to increased morbidity and mortality of those experiencing critical illness (Finfer et al., 2012).

WHAT'S THE EVIDENCE?

The following is a meta-analysis looking at the evidence around glycaemic control in people experiencing critical illness:

Casilla, S. Jauregui, E. Surani, S. and Varon, J. (2019) 'Blood Glucose Control in the Intensive Care Unit: Where is the data?', *World Journal of Meta-Analysis*, 7 (8): 399–405. www.wjgnet.com/2308-3840/full/v7/i8/399.htm (accessed November 8, 2020).

> I remember when I first started eating in the ACCU. I did not have any appetite and all the food tasted like metal. I was given supplement drinks, but these were warm and tasted sickly sweet. The nurse brought me a menu, I didn't have much of an appetite and I am a vegetarian so that meant there wasn't much choice for me. My family had to bring me in food all the time because I didn't like what was on the menu. Then the dietician suggested I look at the Halal menu; the food was much better on there and there were more vegetarian options. This made me feel better as it meant I could stop asking my visitors to bring me food.
>
> **Mel, 46, under the care of ACCU for 35 days**

SPECIAL DIETS

In order to provide **holistic** care, it is important to understand and accommodate the dietary requirements of persons experiencing critical illness. Some people may have special requirements due to allergies, intolerance or medical needs whilst others may have dietary preferences due to religious, cultural or ethical beliefs. To ensure person-centred care it is important for you to find out the person's beliefs and preferences. Your clinical area may have a policy that can advise you on how to achieve the person's nutritional goals whilst respecting their choices. It is also useful to involve a specialist such as the dietician or nutritional nurse who may be able to offer advice to you and the person experiencing critical illness or their family.

CHAPTER SUMMARY

This chapter has supported your understanding of:

- The anatomy and physiology of the gastrointestinal system
- The nutritional screening and assessment of the person experiencing critical illness
- Oral, enteral and parenteral nutrition
- Glycaemic control in the ACCU
- Supporting special diets in persons experiencing critical illness

---

GO FURTHER

Books

Patton, K. and Thibodeau, G. (2018) 'Digestive System', in K. Patton and G. Thibodeau, *The Human Body in Health and Disease*. Toronto: Elsevier. pp. 492–520.

- This chapter explores the anatomy and common pathology of the gastrointestinal system.

Berger, M.M. (2018) *Critical Care Nutrition for Non-Nutritionists*. New York: Springer Science.

- This is a handbook on critical care nutrition.

Rajendram, R., Preedy, V. and Patel, V.B. (2015) *Diet and Nutrition in Critical Care*. New York: Springer Science.

- This book discusses the general aspects of nutrition in critical care.

Journal articles

Shankar, B., Daphnee, D.K., Ramakrishan, N. and Venkatataman, R. (2015) 'Feasibility, safety and outcome of very early enteral nutrition in critically ill patients: Results of an observational study', *Journal of Critical Care*, 30 (3): 473–5.

- This observational study explores the feasibility and safety of very early initiation of enteral feeding.

Fletcher, J. (2015) 'Giving nutrition support to critically Ill adults', *Nursing Times*, 111 (12): 12–16.

- This article discusses the nurse's responsibility when caring for individuals requiring nutritional support in the ACCU.

van Zanten, A.R.H., De Waele, E. and Wischmeyer, P.E. (2019) 'Nutrition therapy and critical illness: Practical guidance for the ICU, post-ICU, and long-term convalescence phases', *Critical Care*, 23: Article #368. https://ccforum.biomedcentral.com/articles/10.1186/s13054-019-2657-5 (accessed November 8, 2020).

- This journal article looks at the impact of adequate nutrition in the ACCU on the long-term outcomes of people experiencing critical illness.

Useful websites

www.bapen.org.uk/ (accessed November 8, 2020).

- The British Association for Parenteral and Enteral Nutrition is a charitable organisation that raises awareness of malnutrition and works to advance nutritional care.

www.esicm.org/ (accessed November 8, 2020).

- The European Society for Intensive Care Medicine website provides recommendations for nutrition in people experiencing critical illness as well as other useful resources.

www.espen.org/ (accessed November 8, 2020).

- The European Society for Clinical Nutrition and Metabolism disseminates good clinical practice in the field of clinical nutrition and metabolism.

REFERENCES

Blaser, A., Starkopf, J., Alhazzani, W., Berger, M.M., Casaer, M.P., Deane, A.M […] and Oudemans-van Straaten, H.M. (2017) 'Early enteral nutrition in critically ill patients: ESICM clinical practice guidelines', *Intensive Care Medicine*, 43 (3): 380–98. doi.org/10.1007/s00134-016-4665-0

British Association for Parenteral and Enteral Nutrition (BAPEN) (2016) 'Nutritional assessment', Redditch: British Association for Parenteral and Enteral Nutrition. www.bapen.org.uk/nutrition-support/assessment-and-planning/nutritional-assessment (accessed November 6, 2020).

British Association for Parenteral and Enteral Nutrition (BAPEN) (2017) 'Medications', Redditch: British Association for Parenteral and Enteral Nutrition. www.bapen.org.uk/nutrition-support/enteral-nutrition/medications (accessed November 6, 2020).

Cameron, J.L., Reynolds, J., and Zuidema, G.D. (1973) 'Aspiration in patients with tracheostomies', *Surgery Gynaecology Obstetrics*, 136: 68–70.

Coleman, S., Nelson, A., Kee, J., Wilson, L., McGinnin, E., Dealey, C. […] and Nixon, J. (2014) 'Developing a pressure ulcer risk factor minimum data set and risk assessment framework', *Journal of Advanced Nursing*, 70 (10): 2339–52.

Cook, N., Shepherd, A. and Boore, J. (2021) *Essentials of Anatomy and Physiology for Nursing Practice* (2nd edition). London: Sage.

Finfer, S., Blair, D., Bellomo, R., McArthur,D., Mitchell, I., Myburgh, J. […] and Wood, G. (2009) 'Intensive versus conventional glucose control in critically ill patients,' *New England Journal of Medicine*, 360 (13): 1283–97. https://www.nejm.org/doi/pdf/10.1056/NEJMoa0810625 (accessed November 8, 2020).

Godinjak, A., Iglica, A., Burekovic, A., Jusufovic, S., Ajanovic, A., Tancica, I. and Kukuljac, A. (2015) 'Hyperglycemia in critically ill patients: Management and prognosis', *Medical Archives*, 69: 157–60.

Heyland, D.K., Dhaliwal, R., Jiang, X. and Day, A.G. (2011) 'Identifying critically ill patients who benefit the most from nutrition therapy: The development and initial validation of a novel risk assessment tool', *Critical Care*, 15 (6): R268.

Jabbar, A., Chang, W.K., Dryden, G.W. and McClave, S.A. (2003) 'Gut immunology and the differential response to feeding and starvation', *Nutrition in Clinical Practice*, 18 (6): 461–82. doi. org/10.1177/0115426503018006461

Jarden, R.J and Sutton, L.J. (2014) 'A practice change initiative to improve the provision of enteral nutrition to intensive care patients', *Nursing in Critical Care*, 20 (5): 242–55. doi.org/10.1111/ nicc.12107

Jordan, E.A. and Moore, S.C. (2019) 'Enteral nutrition in critically ill adults: Literature review of protocols', *Nursing in Critical Care*, 25 (1): 24–30.

Kuslapuu, M., Jõgelaa, K., Starkopf, J., and Blaser, A.R. (2015) 'The reasons for insufficient enteral feeding in an intensive care unit: A prospective observational study', *Intensive and Critical Care Nursing*, 31 (5): 309–14. doi.org/10.1016/j.iccn.2015.03.001 (Accessed on April 6, 2020)

Lee, Z.Y. and Heyland, D.K. (2019) 'Determination of nutrition risk and status in critically ill patients: What are our considerations?', *Nutrition in Clinical Practice*, 34 (1): 96–111.

Massanet, P.L., Petit, L., Louart, B., Corne, P., Richard, C. and Preiser, J.C. (2015) 'Nutrition rehabilitation in the intensive care unit', *Journal of Parenteral and Enteral Nutrition*, 39 (4): 391–400.

McClave, S.A., Saad, M.A., Esterle, M., Anderson, M., Jotautas, A.E., Franklin, G.A., Heyland, D.K. and Hurt, R.T. (2015) 'Volume-based feeding in the critically ill person', *Journal of Parenteral and Enteral Nutrition*, 39 (6): 707–12.

National Health Service (NHS) (2016) *Nasogastric Tube Misplacement: Continuing Risk of Death and Severe Harm*. Redditch: NHS. Available from https://www.england.nhs.uk/2016/07/ nasogastric-tube-misplacement-continuing-risk-of-death-severe-harm (accessed November 6, 2020).

National Institute for Health and Care Excellence (NICE) (2006) *Nutrition Support for Adults: Oral Nutrition Support, Enteral Tube Feeding and Parenteral Nutrition*. (Clinical Guidelines 32). London: NICE. Available from www.nice.org.uk/guidance/cg32 (accessed November 6, 2020).

National Patient Safety Agency (NPSA) (2011) 'Patient safety alert NPSA/2011/PSA002: Reducing the harm caused by misplaced nasogastric feeding tubes in adults, children and infants', Redditch: National Patient Safety Agency. Available at www.gbukenteral.com/pdf/NPSA-Alert-2011.pdf (accessed November 6, 2020).

Sharma, O.P., Oswanski, M.F., Singer, D., Buckley, B., Courtright, B., Shekhar, S.R., Waite, P., Tatchell, T. and Gandaio, A. (2007) 'Swallowing disorders in trauma patients: Impact of tracheostomy', *The American Surgeon*, 73 (11): 1117–21.

Singer, P., Reintam-Blaser, A., Berger, M.M., Alhazzani, W., Calder, P.C., Casaer, M.P., [...] and Boschoff, S.C. (2019) 'ESPEN guideline on clinical nutrition in the intensive care unit', *Clinical Nutrition*, 38: 48–79. doi.org/10.1016/j.clnu.2016.09.004

Stewart, M.L., Biddle, M., Thomas, T. (2017) 'Evaluation of current feeding practices in the critically ill: A retrospective chart review', *Intensive and Critical Care Nursing*, 38: 24–30.

Taylor, B., McClave, S., Martindale, R., Warren, M., Johnson, D., Braunschweig, C. [...] and Compher, C. (2016) 'Guidelines for the provision and assessment of nutrition support therapy in the adult critically Ill patient: Society of Critical Care Medicine (SCCM) and American Society for Parenteral and Enteral Nutrition (A.S.P.E.N.)', *Journal of Parenteral and Enteral Nutrition*, 40, 2: 159–211. doi. org/10.1177/0148607115621863

Tortora, G. and Derrickson, B. (2011) *Principles of Anatomy and Physiology* (13th edition). Chichester: John Wiley and Sons.

Van den Berghe, G., Wilmer, A. M.D., Hermans, G., Meersseman, W., Wouters, P.J., Milants, I. [...] and Bouillon, R. (2006) 'Intensive insulin therapy in the medical ICU', *New England Journal of Medicine*, 354: 449–61.

Wang, Z., Ding, W., Fang, Q., Zhang, L., Liu, X. and Tang, Z. (2019) 'Effects of not monitoring gastric residual volume in intensive care patients: A meta-analysis', *International Journal of Nursing Studies*, 91. doi.org/10.1016/j.ijnurstu.2018.11.005

Waugh, A. and Grant, A. (2009) *Ross and Wilson Anatomy and Physiology in Health and Illness* (11th edition). Edinburgh: Churchill Livingston.

CRITICAL CARE RELATED TO NEUROLOGY, PHYSIOLOGY AND DISORDERS

GREGORY BLEAKLEY AND MARK COLE

> " It's a real challenge to nurse a patient with a head injury. There are various assessment tools that can be used to measure a patient's consciousness level. More specialist centres deal with complex neurological management such as ICP monitoring and neurosurgery. I know the goal is to prevent further neurological deterioration.
>
> **Aaliyah, Emergency Department Nurse** "

LEARNING OUTCOMES

When you have finished studying this chapter you will be able to understand:

- The basic structure and function of the brain and nervous system
- The key terms related to neurological assessment
- Some of the common types of head injury and neurological disorders seen in critical care
- The triggers for organ donation and role of the specialist nurse – organ donation

INTRODUCTION

This chapter will provide the reader with the evidence base surrounding the care of persons with neurological disorders. Topics to be covered include monitoring and observational assessment of neurological status, Cushing's signs and raised **intracranial** pressure, classification of head injury, and other complex neuromuscular disorders. It will discuss brain stem death testing and indications for organ donation.

The nervous system includes both the central nervous system and peripheral nervous system. The central nervous system is made up of the brain and spinal cord. The peripheral nervous system is made up of the somatic and the autonomic nervous systems. The brain and spinal cord are located within the dorsal body cavity and are encased in bone for protection. The brain can be divided into 3 main structures (Boore et al., 2016).

The *forebrain* is the largest section of the brain and consists of the cerebrum and the diencephalon. The *cerebrum* is the largest part of the brain and is responsible for higher functions like memory, speech, the senses and emotional response. The *diencephalon* is inside the cerebrum. This provides a structural connection between the midbrain and the cerebrum and includes the thalamus and hypothalamus. The diencephalon is associated with **homeostasis**, temperature, hormone production, thirst and water balance, appetite, sleep and regulation of the autonomic nervous system.

The *midbrain* forms the first part of the brain stem and in turn forms a structural connection between the diencephalon and the hindbrain.

The *hindbrain* is composed of the pons, the medulla oblongata and the cerebellum. Eye movement, auditory and visual stimuli, pain and regulating movement through the inhibition of the hormone dopamine are all functions of the hindbrain. The *pons* coordinates voluntary movements and regulates breathing. The *medulla oblongata* controls voluntary movement of the trunk, heart and breathing rate, reflexes for vomiting, swallowing, coughing, sneezing, hiccupping and yawning. The *cerebellum* regulates voluntary control of movement. It coordinates gait and maintains posture, controls muscle tone and voluntary muscle contraction.

The *spinal cord* is an extension of the brain and refers to the neural tissue encased within the spine. It is a long cylindrical structure that extends from the lower part of the brain stem and terminates, in adults, at the first lumbar vertebra. It contains important motor and secondary nerve pathways that exit and enter the cord through anterior and posterior nerve routes as well as spinal and peripheral nerves.

NEUROLOGICAL ASSESSMENT

Changes in a person's level of consciousness are the earliest and most sensitive indicator of a change in neurological status (Dougherty et al., 2015). While it may not be possible to directly assess someone's level of consciousness, it can be assessed by observing their behavioural response to different stimuli. There are multiple ways of assessing neurological status. Two will be considered here: ACVPU and the Glasgow Coma Scale (GCS). Neurological assessment consists of either a quick review of a patient's neurological state using the ACVPU scale, or the more comprehensive Glasgow Coma Scale.

ACVPU

ACVPU is quick and simple. It is particularly helpful when there is a need to make a rapid assessment of a person's gross level of consciousness, responsiveness, or mental status (Peate and Wilde, 2018).

Traditionally popular in the pre-hospital and emergency setting, ACVPU notes whether somebody is **A**lert, **C**onfused, responds to **V**oice, **P**ain or is **U**nresponsive (see Table 11.1). The assessment is completed in sequence and only one outcome is recorded. ACVPU can also have a vital role in Wards and critical care unit. It forms part of the National Early Warning Score (Royal College of Physician, 2017) and allows the nurse to detect changes in a person's physiologic status and recognise any potentially life-threatening issues that could have arisen during their hospital stay.

THIS TOPIC IS ALSO COVERED IN CHAPTER 3

Table 11.1   ACVPU

A	**A**lert	Are they alert?
C	**C**onfused	Are they confused?
V	Responds to **V**oice	Do they respond to verbal stimulation?
P	Responds to **P**ain	Do they respond to pain?
U	**U**nresponsive	Do they respond at all?

Glasgow Coma Scale

'The Glasgow Coma Score is a more comprehensive neurological scoring system. It has become the gold standard for the assessment, trend monitoring, classification and prognosis of, and clinical decision making about consciousness in patients with acute neurological conditions or brain injuries' (De Sousa and Woodward, 2016). It was devised by Teasdale and Jennet in 1974 and scores levels of neurological dysfunction in three components: motor, verbal and eye-opening responses. These are considered separately and combined into an overall score. A score of 15 is the highest score and this indicates a fully alert, responsive person, a score of 3 is the lowest possible score and represents a state of deep unconsciousness (see Table 11.2).

Table 11.2   Glasgow Coma Scale Assessment

Eye Opening		Verbal Response		Motor Response	
				6	obeys commands
		5	orientated	5	localising
4	spontaneous	4	confused	4	normal flexion
3	to sound	3	words/incoherent	3	abnormal flexion
2	to pressure	2	sounds/no words	2	extension
1	none	1	none	1	none
NT	not testable	NT	not testable	NT	not testable

Pupillary examination is a minimally invasive assessment that can detect subtle changes in the severity and progression of brain injury and **brainstem** function. Unlike other components of the neurologic examination that require consciousness, the pupillary examination is one of the few neurologic signs that can be assessed in an unconscious person, or in a person receiving neuromuscular blocking agents and **sedation** (Adoni and McNett, 2007). A normal pupil should be round and in adults, have a diameter of 2 to 4 mm in bright light and to 4 to 8mm when it is dark (Figure 11.1). When a light source is applied to the eye as part of a neurological assessment, the reaction of the pupils is recorded as brisk, sluggish, or nonreactive. A healthy response is a round pupil that has a brisk reaction that returns to its original size when the light source is removed. There should also be a consensual reaction, that is, the opposite pupil also constricts when the light source is applied to one eye. A sluggish or slow pupillary response may signal increased intracranial pressure, and nonreactive pupils is often associated with decreased blood flow to the brain stem and brainstem **ischaemia** (Majdan et al., 2015). A pupil that is not round but oval in shape may suggest early compression of the third cranial nerve and this is also indicative of increased intracranial pressure. If not treated, the oval-shaped pupil will become further dilated and eventually will become nonreactive to light.

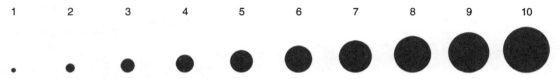

Figure 11.1 Pupil size assessment scale

Source: NHSBT, 2020b. Reproduced under the Open Government License. URL: www.nationalarchives.gov.uk/doc/open-government-licence/version/3/

Reflection

Before performing a GCS, you should understand your own local policies, guidelines and documentation. The NICE guidelines (2019) recommend that for patients with head injuries, GCS assessments should be undertaken every 30 minutes until a score of 15 is achieved. When this score is achieved, the minimum frequency for observations is 30 minutes for two hours, hourly for four hours and every two hours thereafter. Does this chime with your own unit's policy?

WHAT'S THE EVIDENCE?

In a critical review of the GCS Braine and Cook (2016) concluded that the GCS is the most universally used and validated consciousness scale worldwide. It has significant strengths, but it is not without its weaknesses and limitations. The majority of studies that have attempted to evaluate the GCS have been of poor quality. It has been argued that the components of the scale might hold greater reliability than the score itself; and that the inter-rater reliability (the degree of agreement between assessors) can be influenced by their education, training, experience and technique.

=== **ACTIVITY 11.1: CRITICAL THINKING** ===

Consider the following as best practice for recording a GCS:

Start at the top category of each component and work down

Documentation should reflect the clinical findings at the time of each assessment

Be consistent by asking the same questions in the same way

Improve inter-rater reliability by assessing GCS during handover

If unsure, ask for a second opinion

1.   How well does this describe the way that you undertake a GCS?

INTRACRANIAL HYPERTENSION

Intracranial **hypertension** occurs when high pressure builds up in the spaces that surround the brain and spinal cord. Normally, these spaces are filled with cerebrospinal fluid (CSF) which acts as a cushion against injury and removes waste products. Intracranial pressure can occur rapidly following a severe head injury, stroke (intracranial haemorrhage) or infection. Clinical signs of raised intracranial pressure include irritability, feeling drowsy, loss or partial loss of vision, continual throbbing headache or feeling nausea. A normal intracranial pressure (ICP) for an adult is 5–15 mmHg and this value can increase significantly following traumatic head injury (Ragland and Lee, 2016).

Intracranial hypertension is a common pathology in the critically ill and sustained ICP values greater than 40mmHg indicate profound, life-threatening intracranial hypertension. Typical critical care management for raised ICP include:

- Surgical evacuation and removal of new mass lesions where indicated
- Extra Ventricular Drainage (EVD) of CSF
- Sedation and/or paralysis
- Osmotherapy with either mannitol or hypertonic saline

MONRO-KELLIE HYPOTHESIS

Intracranial contents include the brain, spinal cord, blood and CSF. The skull encloses a total volume of 1700ml: 150 ml blood (10%), 150ml CSF (10%) and 1400ml brain tissue (80%). The Monro-Kellie hypothesis suggests that the sum of the intracranial content (blood, CSF and brain tissue) is constant, and that an increase in any one of these must be counterbalanced by an equal decrease in another. If these mechanisms fail, the Monro-Kellie hypothesis, or doctrine as sometimes called, proposes that intracranial pressure increases (Kim et al., 2012).

CEREBRAL DYNAMICS

Cerebral perfusion pressure (CPP) depends on **mean arterial** pressure (MAP) and ICP with the following calculation:

$$CPP = MAP - ICP$$

Essentially CPP is the net gradient pressure that drives oxygen delivery to cerebral tissue and is dependent on the ICP and MAP. The normal CPP range is 60 – 80 mmHg. The aim of critical care for a person with a severe head injury or other intracranial pathology is to maintain normal CPP values.

CUSHING REFLEX

Early signs of raised ICP include headache, nausea, amnesia or reduced conscious level/loss of judgement. Late signs and symptoms of raised ICP include dilated, non-reactive pupils, unresponsive, abnormal posturing and changes to respiratory pattern. A rise in ICP results in a rise in **systemic** blood pressure, fall in pulse rate and abnormal respiratory pattern. These collective signs and symptoms are known as Cushing's response triad. Abnormal posturing patterns are decorticate posturing (see Figure 11.2) where the limbs are drawn up towards the midline in response to deep pain stimuli and decerebrate posturing where the limbs are extended away from the midline in response to deep pain stimuli (see Figure 11.3).

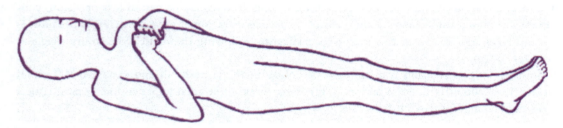

Figure 11.2   Decorticate posturing. Closed hands, arms are adducted and flexed against the chest, legs internally rotated, feet turned inwards

Source: Wikimedia Commons. https://commons.wikimedia.org/wiki/File:Decorticate.PNG Reproduced under the Creative Commons Attribution-ShareAlike 3.0 License.

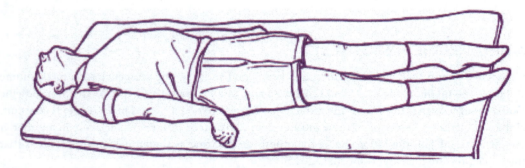

Figure 11.3   Decerebrate posturing . Head and neck arched, arms straight, extended and hands curled, legs straight and toes pointed downwards

Source: Wikimedia Commons. https://commons.wikimedia.org/wiki/File:Decerebrate.jpg Reproduced under the Creative Commons Attribution-ShareAlike 3.0 License.

INTRACRANIAL PRESSURE (ICP) MONITORING

In order to monitor CPP, both ICP and MAP require measuring. Typically, the MAP can be monitored through invasive cannulation of an artery such as the radial, brachial or femoral artery. Furthermore, MAP can be measured via non-invasive methods using a manual or automated sphygmomanometer. However, ICP is usually measured through insertion of an intracranial pressure transduction device. An intraventricular catheter is inserted into a sterile hole drilled into the cranium which advances directly into the underlying ventricle to measure intracranial pressure. The intracranial catheter can also be used to drain fluid and blood to help reduce ICP. An intraventricular catheter carries a risk of bleeding and infection and is often challenging to place if the ICP is very high. It is normal to have such a specialised catheter inserted within a neuro-critical care environment.

WHAT'S THE EVIDENCE?

The National Institute of Health and Care Excellence (NICE, CG 176; 2014 [updated 2019]) produced clinical guidelines to help practitioners in the assessment and early management of head injury. Explore this guidance and establish the criteria for transferring a patient with a head injury to a neuroscience unit.

www.nice.org.uk/guidance/cg176/chapter/1-recommendations#transfer-from-hospital-to-a-neuroscience-unit

---

CT HEAD SCAN

A computerised tomography (CT) scan of the head is an imaging scan that utilises X-rays to develop 3D images of the skull and intracranial contents. A CT scan of the head is routinely performed in patients with traumatic head injury, suspected intracranial haemorrhage or suspected brain tumour or other space occupying lesion (SOL). NICE (2014) guidance stipulates that a CT scan of the head should be performed within 1 hour of the following risk factors being identified:

- GCS less than 13 on initial assessment in the emergency department
- GCS less than 15 at 2 hours after the injury on assessment in the emergency department
- Suspected open or depressed skull fracture
- Any sign of basal skull fracture (haemotympanum, 'panda' eyes, cerebrospinal fluid leakage from the ear or nose, Battle's sign)
- Post-traumatic seizure
- Focal neurological deficit
- More than 1 episode of vomiting

(NICE, 2014; CG 176: 1.4.7)

MECHANISM OF INJURY (MOI) PREDICTIVE OF HEAD INJURY

Dewan et al. (2019: 1080) describe head injury as a 'silent epidemic' that contributes towards more death and disability worldwide than any other traumatic incident. The MOI following a road traffic collision, fall, assault, industrial accident, sporting accident or penetrating traumas are predictive of head injury. In addition, 30% of patients with a traumatic head injury will have at least one additional injury. The risk of cervical cord injury should always be considered with suspected head injury. Additional investigations may be required to exclude cervical cord damage including Magnetic Resonance (MR) imaging. MR imaging may add important information to that suggested by the X-ray, CT scan of the head or clinical findings (NICE, 2014).

Certain behaviours increase the risk of traumatic head injury including excess use of alcohol, illicit drug use, non or incorrect use of safety belts in motor vehicles, non-use of personal protective equipment (bicycle helmets) or participation in certain sports such as boxing/horse riding. Road traffic collision (RTC) is the most common cause of head injury and 60% of deaths from RTC are caused by head injury (Dewan et al., 2019). The major areas involved in head injury include:

- Scalp: outer covering of the skull (skin; **connective** tissue)
- Skull: cranial vault and base
- Meninges: three layers covering the brain (Dura mater [tough mother]; arachnoid mater; pia mater)
- Brain: cerebrum; cerebellum and brainstem
- Cerebrum: outer grey matter–cortex (neuron cell bodies); inner white matter–neuron axons
- Cerebrospinal fluid (CSF)
- Meningeal/cerebral blood vessels
- Tentorium: division between supra-tentorial compartment (anterior, middle, posterior fossa) and the midbrain that connects the cerebral hemispheres to the rest of the brainstem

Brain damage resulting from head injury is divided into two categories. Primary brain injury is the damage that occurs at the time of the impact and is unavoidable. There is often injury at the site of the impact (for example being hit by a baseball bat) or opposite side known as a 'contrecoup' injury. Secondary injury is brain damage resulting from the development of secondary complications including hypoxia, hypercapnia (high carbon dioxide), **hypotension**, hypoglycaemia, seizures, cerebral oedema, infection (brain abscess/meningitis) or intracranial haemorrhage. The goal of critical care in this context is to prevent secondary brain injury through evidence-based care strategies.

CEREBRAL BLOOD FLOW

A constant flow of blood is needed to provide the brain with oxygen and nutrients. Typically, the brain is 2% of body weight but consumes 20% of oxygen and nutrients from each cardiac output. Normal cerebral blood flow (CBF) is 50ml/100g/min of brain; or 750ml/min in a 1500g brain; 15% of cardiac output. A steady CBF is maintained by the brain's ability to autoregulate the flow by dilating or constricting cerebral blood vessels (altering cerebral vascular resistance) during normal activities of daily living (coughing/sneezing/straining).

Adequate CBF is dependent on adequate cerebral perfusion pressure (CPP). CPP is the difference between systemic MAP (MAP = Systolic BP + 2 (Diastolic BP)) and ICP (CPP = MAP minus ICP). These calculations appear complex but most critical care monitoring systems provide the numerical data needed to ascertain the CPP. A normal CPP is 80-100 mmHg and autoregulation maintains the steady CBF within the normal range of CPP. A minimum CPP of 60 mmHg is required for neuronal perfusion but a CPP below 70 mmHg may cause increased risk of ischaemia and is generally associated with a poor outcome in severe head injury.

Respiratory gases (oxygen and carbon dioxide) play an important role in regulation of cerebral blood flow. Increase in carbon dioxide (CO_2) causes cerebral smooth muscles relaxation, resulting in vasodilation. Conversely, decreased CO_2 levels cause **vasoconstriction**, thus lowering CBF. Changes in blood pH affects CBF in a similar manner to CO_2; a fall in pH (acidosis) results in cerebral **vasodilation**.

TYPES OF HEAD INJURY

Critical care settings observe many different types of head injury including patients with concussion, diffuse axonal injury, cerebral contusion/laceration, intracranial haemorrhage/haematoma and skull fracture.

Concussion is common in acceleration and deceleration force injury and divided into mild and classic categories. Mild concussion occurs following a diffuse brain injury but there is no identifiable lesion (on CT scan) and it is often experienced without loss of consciousness (LOC). The patient may experience some neurological dysfunction including headache, confusion, disorientation but without amnesia. Classical concussion is characterised by a diffuse brain injury and notable loss of consciousness. The LOC is often transient and reversible and occurs for no longer than 6 hours. Patients with classical concussion may experience post traumatic amnesia, confusion/disorientation, dizziness and memory loss.

Diffuse axonal injury is damage caused by mechanical shearing forces on the brain nerve fibres following deceleration. The shearing forces caused by movement of the brain against the cranium disrupt the function of neuronal axons. Depending on the severity of the diffuse axonal injury, immediate effects range from mild confusion to death. Clinical features include immediate unconsciousness (possible prolonged coma if brain stem and reticular activating systems involved), autonomic dysfunction hypertension (systolic BP 140–160 mmHg), hyperpyrexia (temp 40–40.5 C), excessive sweating and abnormal motor posturing: decorticate or decerebrate.

A contusion is a common focal brain injury in which tissue is bruised and damaged in a local area (usually associated with overlying subdural bleed: burst lobe). The vast majority occur in the Frontal and Temporal lobes. An intracerebral haematoma is caused by delayed haemorrhage or evolution of an intracerebral haematoma following rupture of a cerebral blood vessel or traumatic head injury. Early signs and symptoms of intracranial haematoma / haemorrhage include altered level of consciousness, unusual behaviour and abnormal motor posturing.

Extradural haematomas are collections of blood outside the dura but within the skull. Most often they are located in the temporal or parietal region and often result from tearing of the middle meningeal artery following a fracture. Signs and symptoms are decreased level of consciousness; they may follow a pattern of a patient presenting with the classic concussion. Extradural haematomas are characterised by a 'lucid interval' following the injury whereby a patient can 'talk and die' suddenly. Essentially there is an initial decrease in conscious level followed by return of consciousness followed by rapid LOC or a persistent decreased level of consciousness.

Subdural haematoma is more common, occurring in approximately 30% of head injury patients. It is a focal brain injury beneath the dura, resulting from acceleration, deceleration, or combination forces: tearing of bridging veins between the cerebral cortex and a venous sinus. The injury is more severe, and prognosis is worse than extradural haematoma. The high **mortality**

rate can be lowered by rapid neuro-surgical **intervention** and aggressive medical management. Onset of a subdural haematoma may be acute (within 48 hours) or chronic (up to 2 weeks after event). At risk groups include older people, those on anticoagulant therapy and chronic alcohol users. Signs and symptoms are variable but usually consist of a decline in LOC, hemiparesis or hemiplegia on opposite side of haematoma and/or unilaterally fixed and dilated pupil on same side as haematoma.

Fractures may be seen in the cranial vault or skull base. The significance of a skull fracture should not be underestimated as it takes a significant MOI to fracture the skull. Types of fracture:

Linear: Nondisplaced fracture of the cranium but underlying vessels may be lacerated. A linear vault fracture increases the risk of intracranial haematoma by x400 times in a conscious patient and x20 in a comatose patient.

Depressed: Extends below the surface of the skull and can cause compression and dural laceration, usually requires early surgical repair. Often depressed skull fractures are open with a palpable depression over the fracture site.

Basilar: Fractures of bones of the base of the skull. The presence of clinical signs should increase the index of suspicion and aid diagnosis. These clinical signs include headache, altered level of consciousness, raccoon's eyes: periorbital bruising (anterior fracture), battle's sign: mastoid bruising (posterior fracture), blood behind tympanic membrane (haemotympanum), facial nerve palsy (cranial nerve VII) and cerebrospinal fluid leakage from the nose and ear (rhinorrhoea or otorrhoea).

Importantly, displaced or nondisplaced fractures of the base of skull or craniofacial area may lacerate the dura mater, creating a passage for cerebrospinal fluid to exit from the nose or ear. An ancillary nursing test is to check the CSF with a glucose stick for positive (+ve) Halo Sign. The Halo Sign is a crude test to determine if leaking fluid from the ears/nose/mouth contains CSF. However, further confirmatory testing for CSF is needed as blood also contains glucose. Leakage of CSF is a potential entrance for infective pathogens, therefore places the patient at risk of meningitis, encephalitis and/or brain abscess.

General nursing observations for patients with head injury:

THIS TOPIC
IS ALSO
COVERED IN
CHAPTER 3

Adopt the structured A to E assessment (mentioned earlier in Chapter 3)

- **A**irway
- **B**reathing
- **C**irculation
- **D**isability
- **E**xposure

Check scalp for haematoma/laceration; craniofacial area bruising

Look in patient's ears, mouth and nose for signs of bleeding or CSF leakage

Peri-orbital bruising (racoon eyes, panda eyes)

Bruising around mastoid process (battle signs)

Assess extra-ocular movements; occlusion of mandible and maxilla

Palpable depressed skull fracture

Skin colour and sensation (clammy possible hypoglycaemia; hot, dry possible fever)

Odour: alcohol (never assume reduced LOC is due to alcohol; consider acetone (ketosis)

Urinary **incontinence** could follow seizure from head injury or other neurological problem

Check for needle marks which could suggest illicit drug use

ACTIVITY 11.2: CASE STUDY

You are on placement on the Emergency Admissions Unit (EAU) working closely with your practice supervisor, Nazir. You are admitting a patient from the Emergency Department who sustained a head injury following an assault. The patient is a 27-year-old female called Tina. Tina had a CT scan in the ED and has been admitted for regular neurological assessment and observation. On admission to EAU, Tina is drowsy but easily rousable. Nazir asks you to perform a set of neurological observations under his direct supervision.

Consider the following points:

1.   Which assessment tools can you consider using to support your neurological assessment?
2.   Why is Tina drowsy following her head injury?

BRAINSTEM DEATH AND BRAINSTEM TESTING

Brainstem death usually occurs following an unexpected, traumatic event including intracranial haemorrhage, traumatic head injury, meningitis or hypoxic brain injury (Bleakley, 2017). There are strict codes of practice that clinicians observe to arrive at a diagnosis of brain stem death (AOMRC, 2008). It is worth noting that different countries have independent guidelines to confirm brain stem death. UK practice focuses on the concept of brain stem death, but other countries concentrate on whole brain death. Essentially, UK legislation requires clinicians to confirm that brainstem function has ceased and is irreversible. The Academy of Medical Royal Colleges (2008) describe brainstem death as:

the irreversible loss of the capacity for consciousness combined with the irreversible loss of the capacity to breathe

(AOMRC, 2008: p 11)

Prior to brainstem death testing, potentially reversible causes of coma must be considered and excluded, including:

*   The action of sedatory and paralysing drugs have ceased and are not causing the unconscious state. Certain drugs like midazolam and thiopentone have a cumulative effect and persist in their action. Ancillary serum testing is often appropriate to ascertain levels of certain drugs prior to brainstem death testing

- The patient is not hypothermic
- There are no **metabolic** or endocrine disturbances causing the coma (hypernatraemia/hyper-glycaemia/hypokalaemia)
- Evidence of irreversible structural brain damage (usually detected by CT/**MRI** scan of the head)

Following the exploration of potential causes of the coma, brainstem reflexes are systematically tested to support the diagnosis and confirmation of brainstem death. In the UK, brainstem death tests are performed by two medical practitioners who must have been registered with the General Medical Council (GMC) for more than five years. One of the clinicians must be a consultant and both must be experienced in critical care and emergency medicine. The clinicians perform two sets of tests independently; doctor A completes the first set of tests closely observed by doctor B, then roles are reversed for the second set of brainstem death tests. Death cannot be confirmed until completion of the second set of tests, but the legal time of death is on completion of the first set of tests.

The clinical tests for brainstem death are as follows:

- **Corneal reflexes**: clinicians stimulate the corneas with a sterile gauze swap (mindful of the potential for tissue donation later). The normal response would be for the patient to blink but this reflex is absent in brainstem death.
- **Oculovestibular reflex**: 50mls of icy cold water is injected into clear ear canals and the eyes are observed closely for movement as the test begins. The normal response would be for the eye to move away from this stimulus (nystagmus) but there is no eye movement in brainstem death
- **Cough/gag reflex**: A suction catheter is placed down the endotracheal breathing tube. The normal response is coughing but this does not happen if the patient is brainstem dead.
- **Supraorbital motor response**: supraorbital pressure is applied to test cranio-facial nerve distribution. Grimacing is a normal response but is absent following brainstem death
- **Pupils**: If brainstem dead, the pupils do not respond to a bright light stimulus, they remain fixed and dilated
- **Confirmation of persistent apnoea**: the patient is disconnected from mechanical ventilation and passively oxygenated for a period of 5 minutes. Clinicians closely observe for chest wall movement (breathing) and arterial blood gas analysis is performed to ensure that $PaCO_2$ has increased above 6.5kPa, which would normally encourage respiratory drive. If, after 5 minutes, no respiratory effort is observed, mechanical ventilation is reconnected.

(Bleakley, 2017: 175)

Following completion of the brainstem death tests, clinicians are in a position to confirm the complete absence of brainstem reflexes and progress to reporting the legal death of the patient. Generally, clinicians record the outcome of the brainstem death tests in the medical notes and make plans to inform the family/significant others of the death.

WHAT'S THE EVIDENCE?

The Academy of Medical Royal Colleges (2008) produced *A Code of Practice for the Diagnosis and Confirmation of Death*. It is important that critical care nurses have knowledge and understanding of this guidance. Please access and inspect this document from: www.aomrc.org.uk/reports-guidance/ukdec-reports-and-guidance/code-practice-diagnosis-confirmation-death/ (accessed November 9, 2020).

ORGAN DONATION

The donation of an organ for use in transplant operations arrives from three types of patients. Deceased organ donation is subdivided into two distinct categories: Donation after Brainstem Death (DBD) and Donation after Circulatory Death (DCD). DBD is made possible from critically unwell patients whose death has been confirmed using neurological criteria. DCD (sometimes referred to as non-heart beating donation) refers to the donation of organs from patients whose death has been confirmed using cardio-respiratory criteria (AOMRC, 2008; Bleakley, 2019; NHSBT 2020a). Interestingly, there are 2 types of DCD, controlled and uncontrolled. The leading type is controlled DCD which occurs from a patient who dies following a planned withdrawal of life-sustaining treatment (WLST). Table 11.3 displays the types of DCD.

Table 11.3 The Maastricht classification of Donation after Circulatory Death

Category	Type	Circumstances	Typical location
1	Uncontrolled	Dead on arrival	Emergency Department
2	Uncontrolled	Unsuccessful resuscitation	Emergency Department
3	Controlled	Cardiac arrest follows planned withdrawal of life sustaining treatments	Intensive Care Unit
4	Either	Cardiac arrest in a patient who is brain dead	Intensive Care Unit

Source: NHSBT, 2020a. Reproduced under the Open Government License. URL: www.nationalarchives.gov.uk/doc/open-government-licence/version/3/

In addition, organs can be donated for use in transplant operations from patients who are alive. Live Donation (LD) kidney transplantation accounts for 98% of living donation activity in the United Kingdom. There are a few different types of living organ donation including directed donation, directed altruistic donation (DAD) and non-directed altruistic donation. Interestingly, a partial lobe of the liver can be donated from a live patient to help others, but this is much rarer than live kidney donation.

WHAT'S THE EVIDENCE?

There is strict legislative framework surrounding the donation of organs. Access the following Human Tissue Authority website and explore the different types of living organ donation:

www.hta.gov.uk/guidance-public/living-organ-donation (accessed November 9, 2020).

Every acute NHS hospital in the UK has an embedded Specialist Nurse – Organ Donation (SNOD) who is normally based within the critical care area. The SNOD supports potential donor families and critical care staff with the operational process of organ donation. They are specially trained in end of life care discussions and provide information for relatives/carers to make informed decisions about organ donation (Tocher et al., 2019).

NICE (2011) guidance stipulates that the on-call SNOD should be contacted at the earliest opportunity if there is a clinical plan to perform brainstem death tests or a planned WLST on a patient. Input from the SNOD is crucial to successful donation outcomes. Organ donation consent rates are significantly higher when the SNOD is involved in the donation request from distressed relatives (Tocher, 2019). See Figure 11.4 for the organ donation best practice flow chart.

The timing and language used during any donation conversation is an important consideration to secure successful donation outcomes. Early referral of the potential organ donor allows the SNOD to assess when the possibility of organ donation is best raised with the family. The breaking of bad news conversation should be carefully planned and include the lead clinician, bedside critical care nurse and SNOD working collaboratively. Some hospitals may have supportive bereavement services, and this should be explored to ensure optimal end of life care.

THIS TOPIC
IS ALSO
COVERED IN
CHAPTER 16

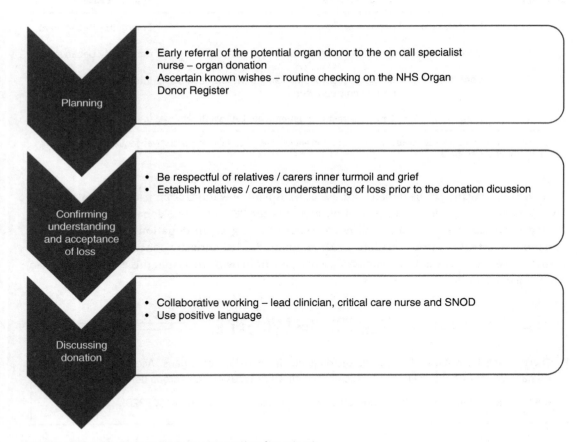

Figure 11.4   Organ donation best practice flowchart

Source: Adapted from NHSBT Best Practice Guidance. 'Consent and authorisation: The family approach'. http://odt.nhs.uk/pdf/family_approach_best_practice_guide.pdf

Reproduced under the Open Government License. URL: www.nationalarchives.gov.uk/doc/open-government-licence/version/3/

ACTIVITY 11.3: CRITICAL THINKING

Tissue Donation

Apart from the donation of organs for use in transplant operations, it is possible to donate tissue following death. Almost anyone can be considered for tissue donation, and donation needs to take place within 24–48 hours of death.

Consider the following:

1. Can you think of any tissues which can be donated following death to help other people with life enhancing and/or lifesaving transplants?
2. The following website link will support your critical thinking: www.organdonation.nhs.uk/helping-you-to-decide/about-organ-donation/what-can-you-donate/about-tissue-donation/ (accessed November 9, 2020).

ACTIVITY 11.4: CASE STUDY

You are a student nurse working with your practice supervisor on the critical care department. You have been caring for a 24-year-old gentleman called Ethan. This is his third day following admission with a traumatic head injury following a fall from a ladder. His sedation was stopped at midnight and there is no spontaneous respiratory effort on the ventilator. His pupils have been fixed and dilated since admission. A recent CT scan of the head confirms a Grade V subarachnoid bleed, subdural haematoma, and midline shift with tonsillar herniation of the brainstem through the foramen magnum. Neurosurgery was not indicated.

Following clinical assessment, clinicians decide to perform brainstem death tests and request the on-call specialist nurse – organ donation be informed and attend. His parents and partner are present in the relative's rest room waiting for an update.

Consider the following points:

1. How do you refer a potential organ donor to the on-call SNOD? What is the regional pager number and who is the embedded SNOD for your hospital? What information is needed to support the referral?
2. What are the pathophysiological changes in the brain injury that have contributed to an irreversible coma?
3. How can you establish known wishes regarding organ donation for the patient in your care? How can you access and check the NHS Organ Donor Register?
4. How will you prepare for a breaking bad news conversation with Ethan's family? Where will the discussion take place and which words will you use? Which members of the clinical team should be included in this conversation?

LONG TERM CONDITIONS IN CRITICAL CARE: GUILLAIN–BARRÉ SYNDROME AND MYASTHENIA GRAVIS

Guillain–Barré syndrome (GBS) and Myasthenia gravis (MG) are **autoimmune disorders** of the peripheral nervous system. They are probably the most common neuromuscular emergencies that require mechanical ventilation and critical care (Vellipuram, 2019). Autoimmune disorders have a complex pathology, where, in essence, the body's own immune system cannot distinguish between healthy tissue and potentially harmful antigens. As a result, the body sets off a reaction that destroys normal tissues. There are more than 80 types of autoimmune disorders.

ACTIVITY 11.5: THEORY STOP POINT

1. How many autoimmune disorders can you name that are a feature of people admitted to critical care?

GBS is usually preceded by infection or another kind of immune stimulation. This induces an aberrant autoimmune response that targets peripheral nerves and their spinal roots (Vellipuram et al., 2019). Symptoms often peak within 4 weeks, followed by a recovery period that can last months or years, as the immune response decays and the peripheral nerve undergoes an endogenous repair process. Patients with GBS need excellent multidisciplinary care to prevent and manage potential complications. 60% of them develop major complications like **sepsis**, pneumonia, and gastrointestinal bleeding. At any point they may require timely transfer to CCU. In the department the patient will require careful cardiac and **haemodynamic** monitoring, maintenance of respiratory function and the prevention of healthcare associated infections. According to Leonhard et al. (2019) routine measurement of respiratory function is advised, as not all patients with respiratory insufficiency will have clinical signs of dyspnoea. These respiratory measurements can include usage of accessory respiratory muscles, counting during expiration of one full-capacity inspiratory breath, vital capacity, and maximum inspiratory and expiratory pressure.

In MG the immune system antibodies block, alter, or destroy the receptors for acetylcholine at the neuromuscular junction. This leads to localized or generalised painless muscle **fatigue** and weakness that worsens after periods of activity and improves with rest. Approximately 20% of patients with MG will experience a myasthenic crisis, typically within 2 years (Vacca, 2017). Myasthenic crisis is a life-threatening complication that is characterised by severe weakness of the oropharyngeal and/or respiratory muscles. This can result in upper airway obstruction or severe dysphagia with **aspiration** which requires airway protection through intubation. Mechanical ventilation or non-invasive ventilation are often necessary (Bird and Levine, 2020). It is often unclear what the precipitating causes are for a myasthenia crisis, but factors seem to include respiratory infection, aspiration, immunosuppression, corticosteroids, pregnancy, stress and traumas. Appropriate **pulmonary** interventions are vital in these cases and you will need to apply or assist with aggressive physiotherapy, postural drainage and airway clearance through regular **suctioning**. Other complications that you should be mindful of are healthcare associated infections of the respiratory and urinary tract, bacteraemia and Clostridium difficile (Vacca, 2017).

CHAPTER SUMMARY

This chapter has supported your understanding of:

- Cranial anatomy and physiology
- Neurological assessment
- Mechanisms of injury that are predictive of head injury and types of head injury
- Brainstem death testing
- Types of organ donation and the significance of early integration of the Specialist Nurse – Organ Donation into care delivery

GO FURTHER

Books

Boore, J., Cook, N. and Shepherd A. (2016) *Essentials of Anatomy and Physiology for Nursing Practice*, London: Sage.

- This is an easily accessible and informative book that will help your understanding of neurological anatomy and physiology.

Powell, T. (2017) *Head Injury: A Practical Guide*. London: Routledge.

- This book contains contemporary information on how to care for someone with a head injury.

Silver, J.M., McAllister, T.W. and Arciniegas, D.B. (eds) (2019) *Textbook of Traumatic Brain Injury* (3rd edition). Washington, DC: American Psychiatric Association Publishing.

- This book will help you understand the **epidemiology** of traumatic brain injury and neurological assessment.

Journal articles

Bleakley, G. (2017) 'Understanding brainstem death testing', *British Journal of Neuroscience Nursing*, 13 (4): 172–7.

- This article will help you understand the concept of brainstem death and brainstem death testing.

Bleakley, G. and Cole, M. (2019) 'Organ donation: Reducing the risk of healthcare associated infection', *Nursing in Critical Care*, 24 (3): 149–52.

- This article discusses infections that may be present in the potential donor at the time of organ donation.

Waterhouse, C. (2020) 'The Glasgow Coma Scale Pupils score: A nurse's perspective', *British Journal of Neuroscience Nursing*, 16 (2): 86–9.

- This intriguing case report will help you understand the Glasgow Coma Scale assessment tool and associated prognostic dialogue with the relatives of patients who have sustained a severe brain injury.

Useful websites

www.odt.nhs.uk/

- The Organ Donation and Transplantation (ODT) clinical website provides a wealth of information about organ donation and best practice guidance.

www.organdonation.nhs.uk/

- The above weblink provides information on organ donation and the law in the UK.

www.nice.org.uk/guidance/cg176

- This website contains the NICE Clinical Guideline 176, Head injury: Assessment and early management.

REFERENCES

Academy of Medical Royal Colleges (AOMRC) (2008) *A Code of Practice for the Diagnosis and Confirmation of Death*. London: AOMRC. Available from www.aomrc.org.uk/reports-guidance/ukdec-reports-and-guidance/code-practice-diagnosis-confirmation-death/ (accessed November 9, 2020).

Adoni, A. and McNett, M. (2007) 'The pupillary response in traumatic brain injury: A guide for trauma nurses', *Clinical Care*, 14 (4): 191–6.

Bird, S. and Levine, J. (2020) 'Myasthenic crises', *UptoDate*. https://www.uptodate.com/contents/myasthenic-crisis (accessed November 9, 2020).

Bleakley, G. (2017) 'Understanding brainstem death testing', *British Journal of Neuroscience Nursing*, 3 (4): 172–7.

Bleakley, G. (2019) 'An overview of organ donation for support staff', *British Journal of Healthcare Assistants*, 13 (7): 350–3.

Braine, M. and Cook, F. (2016) 'The Glasgow coma scale and evidence-informed practice: A critical review of where we are and where we need to be', *Journal of Clinical Nursing*, 26 (1–2): 280–93. doi.org/10.1111/jocn.13390

Cook, N., Shepherd, A. and Boore, J. (2021) *Essentials of Anatomy and Physiology for Nursing Practice* (2nd edition). London: Sage.

De Sousa, I. and Woodward, S. (2016) 'The Glasgow Coma Scale in adults: Doing it right', *Emergency Nurse,* 24 (8): 33–9.

Dewan, M.C., Rattani, A., Gupta, S., Baticulon, R.E., Hung, Y., Punchak, M., Agrawal, A., Adeleye, A.O., Shrime, M.G., Rubiano, A.M., Rosenfeld, J.V., and Park, K.B. (2019) 'Estmating the global incidence of traumatic brain injury', *Journal of Neurosurgery*, 130 (4): 1039–408.

Dougherty, L., Lister, S. and West-Oram, A. (2015) *The Royal Marsden Manual of Clinical Nursing Procedures*. 9th edition. London: Wiley-Blackwell.

Kim, D.-J., Czosnyka, Z., Kasprowicz, M., et al. (2012) 'Continuous monitoring of the Monro-Kellie Doctrine: Is it possible?' *Journal of Neurotrauma*, 29 (7): 1354–63.

Leonhard, S., Mandarakas, F., Gondim, A., Bateman, K., Ferreira, M.L.B., Cornblath, D.R. [...] and Jacobs, B.C. (2019) 'Diagnosis and management of Guillain–Barré syndrome in ten steps,' *Nature Reviews Neurology*, 15: 671–83.

Majdan, M., Steyerberg, E., Nieboer, D., Mauritz, W., Rusnak, M. and Lingsma, H.F. (2015) 'Glasgow Coma Scale and pupillary reaction to predict six monthly mortality in patients with traumatic brain injury: Comparison of field and admission assessment', *Journal of Neurotrauma*, 32 (2): 101–8.

National Health Service Blood and Transplant (NHSBT) (2013) *Approaching the Families of Potential Organ Donors*. London: NHS Blood and Transplant. London. http://odt.nhs.uk/pdf/family_approach_best_practice_guide.pdf (accessed January 10, 2021).

National Health Service Blood and Transplant (NHSBT) (2020a) 'Deceased donation', www.odt.nhs.uk/deceased-donation/ (accessed November 9, 2020).

National Health Service Blood and Transplant (NHSBT) (2020b). *The Maastricht Classification of Donation after Circulatory Death*. Available from: https://www.odt.nhs.uk/deceased-donation/best-practice-guidance/donation-after-circulatory-death/ (accessed November 9, 2020).

National Institute for Health and Care Excellence (NICE) (2011) *Organ Donation for Transplantation: Improving Donor Identification and Consent Rates for Deceased Organ Donation* (Clinical Guideline 135). London: NICE. Available from www.nice.org.uk/guidance/cg135 (accessed November 9, 2020).

National Institute for Health and Care Excellence (NICE) (2014). *Head Injury: Assessment and Early Management* (Clinical Guideline 176). London: NICE. Available fromwww.nice.org.uk/guidance/cg176/ (accessed November 9, 2020).

Peate, I. and Wilde, K. (2018) *Nursing Practice: Knowledge and Care* (2nd edition). London: Wiley-Blackwell.

Ragland, J. and Lee, K., (2016) 'Critical care management and monitoring of intracranial pressure', *Journal of Neurocritical Care*, 9 (2): 105–12.

Royal College of Physicians (RCP) (2017) *National Early Warning Score (NEWS 2): Standardising the Assessment of Acute Illness Severity in the NHS*. London: RCP. Available from https://www.rcplondon.ac.uk/projects/outputs/national-early-warning-score-news-2 (accessed November 4, 2020).

Teasdale, G. and Jennet, B. (1974) 'Assessment of coma and impaired consciousness: A practical scale', *The Lancet*, 304 (7872): 81–4.

Tocher, J., Neades, B., Smith, G.D. and Kelly, D. (2019) The role of specialist nurses for organ donation: A solution for maximising organ donation rates? *Journal of Clinical Nursing*, 28 (9–10): 2020–7. doi: 10.1111/ jocn.14741.

Vacca, V. (2017) 'Myasthenia gravis and myasthenic crises', *Nursing Critical Care*, 12 (5): 38–46.

Vellipuram, A., Cruz-Flores, S., Chaudhry, M., Rawla, P., Maud, A., Rodriguez, G.J. [...] and Khatri, R. (2019) 'Comparative outcomes of respiratory failure associated with common neuromuscular emergencies: Myasthenia Gravis versus Guillain-Barré Syndrome', *Medicina*, 55 (7): 1–9.

CRITICAL CARE RELATED TO THE SKIN AND INTEGUMENTARY SYSTEM

CLAIRE BURNS

12

> " One of the most distressing things I've seen on my critical care placement was a man who had, like a burn but it was from his diarrhoea. He was in so much pain when we cleaned him but we had no choice, we had to keep him clean! "
>
> **Sam, 2nd Year Student Nurse**

LEARNING OUTCOMES

When you have finished studying this chapter you will be able to understand:

- The anatomy and physiology of the skin
- Nursing care of the person with Incontinence Associated Dermatitis
- Nursing care of the person who has, or is a at risk of, developing a pressure injury
- Nursing care of the burn-injured person

INTRODUCTION

In this chapter you are going to learn about the assessment and nursing **interventions** relating to some of the more commonly seen skin complications in the critical care environment. The chapter will provide you with an overview of the anatomy of the skin and discuss the nurse's role in the management of **incontinence**-associated dermatitis, pressure injuries and burn injuries.

The integumentary system comprises the skin, hair and nails. Just like every other organ in the body, the skin can suffer illness. Skin disorders are common within the Adult Critical Care Unit (ACCU) (Badia et al., 2013) and it is important to identify any existing and potential complications so you can develop an appropriate care plan. Skin disorders can increase **mortality**, affect the length of hospital stay, increase **morbidity** and cause pain and discomfort to the patient (Badia et al., 2013). Individuals experiencing critical illness may develop nail abnormalities and lose hair during critical illness. Although neither of these are life threatening, hair loss can result in an altered body image and lead to patients experiencing anxiety and **depression** (Aghaei et al., 2014).

ANATOMY AND PHYSIOLOGY OF THE SKIN

Structure

Examining the structure of the skin will help you to understand several of its homeostatic functions and the effects that damage to its structure can have on its ability to function effectively. The skin is the largest and heaviest organ of the body and provides a tough, waterproof layer that protects deeper, more fragile structures. The skin is composed of 2 distinct parts, the epidermis and dermis (Tortora and Derrickson, 2011). See Figure 12.1.

Epidermis

The epidermis is the layer of the skin that you can see. It does not contain any blood vessels or nerve endings, it is the thinnest part of the skin and is made up of stratified keratinised squamous epithelium. As the epidermis has no blood supply, it relies on the **interstitial** fluid in the dermis for a supply of nutrients and oxygen. The epidermis contains 4 main types of cell, these are keratinocytes, melanocytes, Langerhans cells and Merkel cells. Table 12.1 gives a brief overview of the main functions of each of these cells. The outermost layer of the epidermis is the stratum corneum; this is the main barrier between the body and the outside environment. A matrix layer of cornoecytes and lipids that lies below the stratum corneum helps to regulate the movement of water in and out of the stratum corneum ensuring the skin is correctly hydrated (Beeckman et al., 2015). Corneocytes contain natural moisturising factors that hydrate the skin and help to maintain the health of this flexible barrier (Voegeli, 2012). Additional to this barrier, the surface of the skin has an acid pH known as the acid mantle. The role of the acid mantle is to maintain the balance of bacteria on the skin and to maintain skin integrity. Damage or destruction of stratum corneum can lead to Moisture Associated Skin Damage (MASD) and other complications (Collier and Simon, 2016).

The deepest layer of the epidermis is the stratum basale. If this layer of the epidermis and its stem cells are destroyed, it cannot regenerate, and skin grafts are needed. This involves taking a healthy section of skin from a donor site, usually of the affected individual, and grafting it to the damaged area.

Table 12.1 Main function of the 4 types of cells in the epidermis

Name of cell	Function
Keratinocyte	These cells produce both keratin and lamellar granules. Keratin is a tough, fibrous protein, its main function is to protect the skin and its underlying structures from heat, chemicals and microbes. Lamellar granules give skin its waterproofing properties.
Melanocytes	These cells produce the brown/black pigment melanin. Melanin contributes to skin colour and protects the skin from harmful ultraviolet light.
Langerhans cells	These cells play a part in protecting the body from infection by mounting an immune response against microbes that attack the skin.
Merkel cells	Merkel cells function in the sense of touch.

Dermis

The dermis is the layer of skin situated directly below the epidermis. This layer is mainly comprised of **connective** tissue that contains **collagen** and elastic fibres; blood vessels, glands, nerves and hair follicles are also found here. The skin plays an important role in the regulation of body temperature (thermoregulation). The sweat glands in the dermis are activated by the sympathetic nerves when the body temperature rises or in response to fear. When sweat evaporates from the skin's surface it cools the body, helping with heat regulation. Another type of gland found within the dermis are sebaceous glands, these glands secrete an oily substance called sebum which has several functions including keeping the skin soft and hydrated and inhibiting bacterial growth. Sensory nerves within the dermis can sense pressure and changes in temperature, they also sense pain, an indicator of actual or potential tissue damage. In Activity 12.1 you will be asked to consider the key functions of the skin during critical illness.

ACTIVITY 12.1: CRITICAL THINKING

As can be identified from examining the structure of the skin it has several important homeostatic functions, these include:

- Regulation of body temperature
- Sense of touch
- Defence against microbes

1. Considering these key functions, how do you think critical illness might impact upon the health of skin?
2. What nursing interventions and precautions can be put in place to help maintain these functions in someone experiencing critical illness?
3. What might be the barriers to performing these interventions?

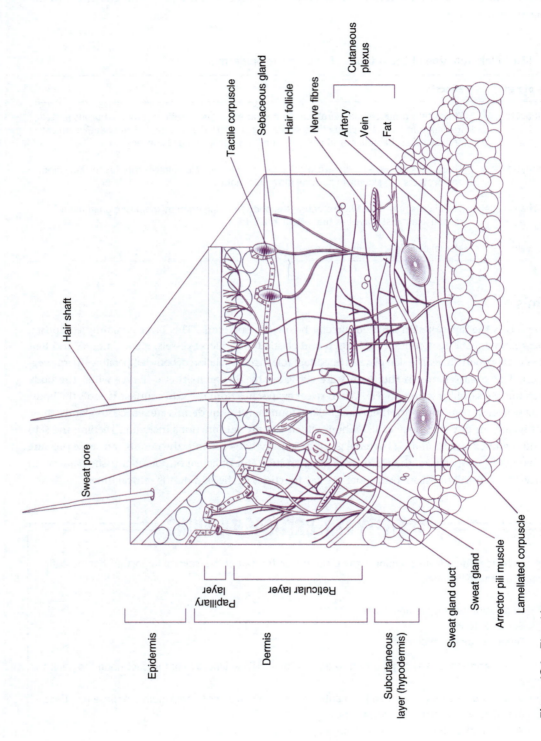

Figure 12.1 The skin

Source: Delves-Yates, C. (2018).

As you can see, critical illness increases the risk of developing complications relating to the integumentary system for many reasons. These include the severity of illness, multiple **invasive devices**, oedema and excessive sweating, lack of mobility, reduced sensation and the administration of medications such as **sedation** and **vasopressors** (Krupp and Monfre, 2015). It is important that you perform a thorough and structured skin assessment on admission to the critical care area (NPIAP, 2016) and regularly thereafter to identify the critically ill person at risk of developing skin complications. Activity 12.2 asks you to reflect on skin assessment in a healthcare environment.

ACTIVITY 12.2: CRITICAL REFLECTION

1. What risk assessments to assess skin integrity and to identify the critical ill person at risk of developing a pressure injury are available in the area where you work or are currently placed?
2. Are these assessments completed correctly?
3. What are the potential risks to the patient of not having an accurate risk assessment completed?
4. What are the risks to the nurse and the organisation in which they work?

There is no template answer to Question 1 as it is based on your own experience.

INCONTINENCE ASSOCIATED DERMATITIS (IAD)

From the activities you have just completed it is apparent that prolonged exposure of the skin to moisture, such as faeces, urine, wound exudate and even perspiration, can lead to skin damage. Overhydration of the epidermis can give rise to a group of conditions known collectively as MASD. IAD is a common form of MASD that you will encounter on the ACCU with prevalence being reported as between 32% and 95% (Coyer et al., 2017). As the name suggests, IAD is dermatitis caused by contact of the skin with urine and faeces (Beeckman et al., 2015). The predisposing factors of critical illness not only include lack of ability of the sedated person to maintain continence and personal hygiene but also the side effects of medications such as antibiotics and enteral nutrition which often include loose stools and **diarrhoea**.

You may notice the first signs of IAD as **erythema** (reddening) of the skin around the perineal area and the thighs and buttocks when you are assisting a person with their hygiene needs. Erythema can progress to swelling and blistering of the affected areas and cause severe discomfort as well as predisposing those affected to secondary skin infections and pressure injuries (Beeckman et al., 2015).

Care plan/prevention

The very nature of critical illness puts those persons admitted to critical care at risk of developing IAD and as an at-risk group they should have their skin assessed daily and at each episode of incontinence (Gates et al., 2019). Accurate assessment is necessary to ensure that correct prevention and treatment strategies are initiated. There are several risk assessment tools available for assessing IAD risk and the use of an IAD severity categorisation tool in conjunction with a care protocol is recommended to guide care (Beeckman et al., 2015).

The prevention and management of IAD consists of two key interventions (Beeckman et al., 2015). Firstly, continence needs to be managed. After careful assessment this may involve the insertion of an indwelling urinary catheter or the use of devices such as convenes to prevent skin contact with urine. Where faecal incontinence is an issue, attending promptly to hygiene needs and treating reversible causes of faecal incontinence is essential. A medication review that includes consideration of stopping or changing medications that cause diarrhoea or the excretion of metabolites that damage the skin is also beneficial. Other methods of managing faecal incontinence you might see include the use of faecal pouches. These are collection bags that adhere to the skin around the anus and collect the stool, thereby reducing the contact of faeces with skin. A faecal management system (FMS) can also be used; this is a soft, silicone catheter that is inserted into the rectum and retained by a low-pressure balloon. The faeces excreted is then collected into a drainage bag.

Secondary to the management of continence is the implementation of a structured skin care regime that preserves the skin's normal pH and maintains its integrity as an effective barrier (Beeckman et al., 2015; Collier and Simon, 2016). Both the prevention and treatment of IAD require a two-stage regime of cleanse and protect (Beeckman et al., 2015). A skin cleanser of similar pH to the skin is used to remove urine and faeces and other sources of soilage that could potentially lead to a MASD (Collier and Simon, 2016; Coyer et al., 2017). Once the skin has been cleansed and patted dry, an appropriate skin barrier is applied to any areas of skin that have the potential to be exposed to urine, faeces or other sources of moisture. Skin barriers come in several forms such as creams, pastes and films. Additionally, in some circumstances, you may find the use of moisturisers is required to maintain the integrity of the skin barrier (Beeckman et al., 2015). Activity 12.3 asks you to link your knowledge of the management of the integumentary system to the nursing process.

ACTIVITY 12.3: THEORY STOP POINT

Using the nursing process **Assess, Plan, Implement and Evaluate**, think about how you can support people experiencing critical illness to maintain healthy skin.

THIS TOPIC IS ALSO COVERED IN CHAPTER 15

It is important that you assess the effect of any interventions on a regular basis and document the results (Beeckman et al., 2015). If there is a deterioration of the skin, or no improvement in an identified IAD after 3–5 days of initiation of a structured skin care regimen, the care plan must be reassessed and referral to a specialist, such as a tissue viability nurse, considered (Beeckman et al., 2015). IAD can be very painful. It is thus important that you recognise when a person is in pain and ensure that adequate pain relief is administered. Chapter 15 explores pain and pain relief and can be used to help guide you in assessing and managing the pain experienced by people on the ACCU.

ACTIVITY 12.4: CASE STUDY

You have spent the last week caring for Joseph, a 67-year-old gentleman, who has been on the unit for almost 2 weeks. He was admitted to the critical care unit with **sepsis** secondary to community-acquired pneumonia and is currently being weaned from mechanical ventilatory support. Over the past 2 days, Joseph has experienced very loose and frequent stools. You have noticed that the area around his perineum is very red and it looks as though the top layer of skin is starting to peel off, he is also flinching in pain when you clean him after each episode of diarrhoea. When you look at his nursing notes you identify that Joseph has had diarrhoea 10 times in the last 24 hours.

1.   What steps should be taken to manage Joseph's skin integrity and prevent further deterioration?

PRESSURE INJURIES

The NHS (2018a: 7) define a pressure injury as

> localised damage to the skin and/or underlying tissue, usually over a bony prominence (or related to a medical or other device), resulting from sustained pressure (including pressure associated with shear). The damage can be present as intact skin or an open injury and may be painful.

Krupp and Monfre (2015) identified that individuals experiencing critical illness are more likely to develop pressure injuries due to the increased risks associated with critical illness. Treating pressure injuries costs the NHS more than £3.8 million every day (NHS, 2018a). Most pressure injuries, though not all, are preventable (NICE, 2014) and the occurrence of avoidable hospital acquired pressure injuries (HAPU) is seen as an indicator of care in the UK.

Pressure injury risk assessment

Your role in pressure care is prevention as well as cure. A pressure injury risk assessment tool should be used to predict individual risk factors for the development of pressure injuries and should consider issues such as skin integrity, nutritional deficiency, cognitive impairment and whether the individual currently has or has previously experienced a pressure injury (NICE, 2014).

Care planning

Once you have completed a comprehensive risk assessment, evidence-based interventions must be initiated to prevent the development of a HAPU or further pressure damage occurring, followed by regular evaluation of any actions implemented. Preventative measures will most often include repositioning of the person, offering nutritional support, good skin care and continence management and the use of pressure relieving devices such as pressure relieving mattresses. Continence management, as discussed earlier in this chapter, and the use of barrier creams should be considered to prevent skin damage in individuals who are at an increased risk of developing lesions due to MASD (NICE, 2014) as these are also a risk factor for developing pressure injuries (Beeckman et al., 2015).

Regular repositioning of individuals every 2 hours to relieve pressure on vulnerable tissue has been shown to be beneficial in reducing the number of early stage pressure injuries in surgical intensive care unit patients (Still et al., 2013). This must be done using correct moving and handling techniques to prevent skin damage caused by friction. You may find that there is a reluctance to turn individuals who are haemodynamically unstable due to concerns that this could cause their condition to deteriorate. The risks and benefits of not turning haemodynamically unstable individuals must be thoroughly considered before a decision not to turn is made. In cases of cardiovascular instability, Brindle et al. (2013) advocate slow, incremental turns to allow the patient time to adjust to the change in gravity on their body.

THIS TOPIC IS ALSO COVERED IN CHAPTER 10

Nutrition and hydration are essential to the maintenance of healthy skin and wound healing and individuals who have or are at risk of developing pressure injuries ought to receive a nutritional assessment by a **dietician** (NICE, 2014) and have a feeding regimen prescribed to support skin health. You can learn more about how to manage the nutritional needs of the critically ill person in Chapter 10.

Pressure injury wound assessment

Where a pressure injury is identified, an assessment of the wound must be performed to ensure appropriate treatment. Assessment involves the measurement of the pressure injury using a validated technique such as photography or **transparency tracing**, and categorisation of the injury. A common categorisation tool you might see being used is the National Pressure Ulcer Advisory Panel pressure injury staging tool (NPAUP, 2016). Assessment includes observation for clinical signs of infection. It is important to take a wound swab or pus sample for **microbial analysis** if evidence of infection is present, so appropriate treatment can be initiated if necessary.

Treatment of pressure injuries

Treatment of uncomplicated pressure injuries mainly involves implementation of the preventative measures as discussed above. Category 2, 3 and 4 pressure injuries may require the application of an appropriate dressing that encourages a warm and moist environment for healing (NICE, 2014). Many hospitals have specialist tissue viability teams who can offer advice on the treatment of pressure injuries and strategies to help prevent wounds from deteriorating. The team will be able to recommend the most appropriate treatment for the wound; they may also suggest other, more specialised therapies for more complex wounds that are difficult to heal.

ACTIVITY 12.5: CASE STUDY

Priscilla is a 76-year-old female who was admitted to the ACCU almost 4 weeks ago with an infective **exacerbation** of chronic obstructive pulmonary disease (COPD) and has been difficult to wean from mechanical ventilation. She has developed a category 2 pressure injury to her sacrum during her stay.

1. What factors should the initial assessment of Priscilla's wound include?
2. What factors should be considered when choosing an appropriate dressing for the wound?
3. What other factors would you consider important in the management of Priscilla's pressure injury?

BURNS AND SCALDS

Burns are caused by thermal, electrical, radioactive or chemical damage (Tortora and Derrickson, 2011); a scald is a burn caused by hot liquid or steam (NHS, 2018b). Both burns and scalds are treated in the same way (NHS, 2018b) and will be referred to collectively as burns throughout this chapter. The severity of a burn is dependent on the size and site of the injury, the depth of injury, the age of the person who has sustained the injury and any co-morbidities, as well as the presence of an **inhalation injury**. All these factors will predict the possibility for recovery. Severe burns can have negative effects on every organ system and expose the affected person to fluid loss and infection (Fagan et al., 2014). Although severe burns are cared for in specialist centres it is important that as a critical care nurse you have some knowledge of how to care for a burn-injured person.

Assessment

In order to care for a person with a burn effectively the severity of the injury must first be assessed. You may have heard burns being described in degrees or as full or partial thickness. Table 12.2 explains the different categories of burn injury.

Table 12.2 Different categories of burn injury

First-degree burn	This is a superficial burn that only affects the surface layers of the epidermis. This degree of burn causes discomfort. Peeling of the epidermis will usually occur 1–3 days after the initial injury. The skin will not blister, and tissue damage is minimal. An example of a first-degree burn is minor sunburn.
Second-degree burn	These burns involve both the epidermis and the dermis. Deep second-degree burns will damage sebaceous glands, sweat glands, and hair follicles. However, complete destruction of the dermis does not occur. These burns are more likely to blister and cause pain and swelling. If uncomplicated by infection, second degree burns usually heal within 2–4 weeks. First and second-degree burns are collectively referred to as partial thickness burns.
Third-degree burn	These burns involve complete destruction of both the epidermis and the dermis causing loss of skin function in the affected area. Tissue destruction includes the subcutaneous layer. These burns are usually less painful than first and second-degree burns due to the destruction of sensory nerve endings. Third degree burns can vary in appearance from white, to red, to charred. Skin grafting may be needed to promote healing.
Fourth-degree burn	This is the most serious category of burn. These burns extend below the subcutaneous layer and involve muscle and bone. Treatment may include skin grafting and some cases may require amputation. Third-and fourth-degree burns are collectively referred to as full thickness burns.

ACTIVITY 12.6: REFLECTIVE PRACTICE

Think of a time when either you or someone else experienced a burn or speak to someone who has experienced a burn injury.

1. What degree of burn was it?
2. Was the burn painful?
3. What treatments were administered?

There is no template answer to this activity as it is based on your own reflection.

As well as classifying the depth of the burn it is also important to assess the surface area of the body involved in the injury. A common method used for estimating the amount of skin surface affected is Wallace's 'rule of nines'.

The rule of nines method involves dividing the body into 11 areas, each of which represents 9% of the total body surface area (TBSA) and the genital area which represents 1% of TBSA. A burn is classed as major when more than 20% of TBSA has been affected.

When caring for the person experiencing burn-injury it is important that you are aware that they may have complex psychological and social needs. Burns can be one of the most severe forms of trauma, more severe burns and significant burns affecting areas such as hands, feet, face and genitalia require specialised treatment in a specialist burn centre. Being over the age of 60, having a TBSA >40% affected by burns and inhalation injury are all risk factors for death (Enoch et al., 2009). Initial assessment of burn categorisation and TBSA affected is frequently inaccurate and therefore regular reassessment is recommended.

ACTIVITY 12.7: CRITICAL THINKING

Familiarise yourself with the Thresholds for Referral to Burn Services found in the National Burn Care Referral Guidance (2012) www.britishburnassociation.org/wp-content/uploads/2018/02/National-Burn-Care-Referral-Guidance-2012.pdf (accessed November 10, 2020).
   After reading the National Burn Care Referral Guidance (2012) answer the following questions:

1. What is the minimum suggested threshold for referral to specialist burn care services?
2. Identify which specialist burn care unit your organisation refers individuals to and what the process is for the referral of individuals requiring specialist burn treatment.

There is no template answer to Question 2 of this activity as it is based on your own organisation's procedure.

Caring for someone who has suffered a significant burn-injury can be frightening. The person will need prompt intervention. As with all episodes of trauma an A-E assessment should be performed, and you should treat the patient according to your assessment findings. In Activity 12.8 you will be asked to consider areas of assessment using the A-E approach.

ACTIVITY 12.8: CRITICAL THINKING

Using the A-E assessment format as a guide jot down what you think will need assessing under each of the sections. Then read the next part of the chapter and compare your points.

Airway

The burn-injured person's airway may be compromised due to a reduced conscious level. Special consideration must be given to the possibility of the injured person having sustained an inhalation injury. Singed nasal hair, soot in the sputum or around the nose and mouth as well as burns to the face and neck and/or hoarseness of the voice present are all clues that a person may have an inhalation injury. In such cases, early referral to an anaesthetist and early tracheal intubation and mechanical ventilation must be considered (Henderson, 2015) as well as referral to adult burns services (NNBC, 2012).

THIS TOPIC IS ALSO COVERED IN CHAPTER 5

Breathing

Circumferential burns of the chest may lead to the formation of an eschar. An eschar is an area of tissue that has become scarred and inelastic. Eschars can arise in any areas of burned tissue. When they occur around the chest they can prevent adequate ventilation (Taveras, 2020) by inhibiting movement of the chest wall in addition to trapping extracellular and extravascular fluid within the chest. This may necessitate surgical removal of the eschar (escharectomy) to be performed to enable breathing and/or ventilation.

Inhalation of toxic gases can be fatal. Pulse oximetry cannot differentiate between oxygen and carbon monoxide (CO), this makes it unreliable in the case of CO poisoning. In cases of suspected CO poisoning an arterial blood gas analysis must be performed to determine CO levels. Carboxyhaemoglobin levels of 25–30 % indicate the requirement for mechanical ventilation with the administration of 100% oxygen to reduce the half-life of CO and increase the rate of dissociation of CO from haemoglobin (Trainor and McClure, 2014).

Circulation

Immediately post burn, circulatory changes occur resulting in what is termed 'burn shock'. Burn shock is caused by the release of inflammatory mediators that increase vascular permeability in both burn-injured and healthy tissues in the body (Guilabert et al., 2016) along with the loss of fluid through open body surfaces and blisters (Knighton, 2013) Clinical evidence of circulatory deficit or any burns covering more than 15% of TBSA in adults necessitates fluid resuscitation to prevent burns shock and ensure adequate oxygen delivery to the body's tissues (Guilabert et al., 2016).

If fluid resuscitation is required, 2 large bore cannulas should be inserted, preferably into areas of unburnt skin to facilitate fluid resuscitation (Trainor and McClure, 2014). There are several fluid resuscitation formulas and each specialist burns unit will have their own preference regarding which formula they use. There is no agreement regarding which fluid is best for circulatory resuscitation, but crystalloid solutions are preferred over colloids due to the potential risk of higher mortality and kidney injury posed by colloid use (Guilabert et al., 2016). Goal-directed fluid administration is recommended to avoid over resuscitation (sometimes termed 'fluid creep') as this can lead to raised compartment pressures and increased length of mechanical ventilation and hospital stay (Clarey and Trainor, 2017). Packed red cells and **coagulation** products may be required to replace blood lost from trauma or surgery (Clarey and Trainor, 2017). Consideration must also be given to obtaining blood samples to assess for electrolyte disorders, sepsis, hormonal changes and organ failure that can be caused by burn trauma (Jeschke, 2013).

Further considerations may include nursing the burn-injured person in a heated environment and measures to ensure **prophylaxis** of deep vein **thrombosis** must also be implemented.

Disability

THIS TOPIC
IS ALSO
COVERED IN
CHAPTER 3
AND 11

Assessment of the burn-injured person's consciousness level using either the Glasgow Coma Scale (GCS, 2014) or ACVPU scale (RCP, 2017) should be undertaken. A GCS of 8 or below, or an ACVPU assessment of voice, pain or unresponsive will require intubation.

Stress-induced hyperglycaemia is common due to the hypermetabolic state induced by burn injuries, and blood glucose levels must be monitored and controlled (Fagan et al., 2014). A nutritional assessment should be performed by a qualified health professional and, where appropriate, nutritional support commenced as soon as it is safe to do so (Lundy et al., 2016).

THIS TOPIC
IS ALSO
COVERED IN
CHAPTER 10

Pain increases the body's **inflammatory response** and increases the risk of **post-traumatic stress disorder** (Lundy et al., 2016). It is important that you assess pain levels and manage pain accordingly to prevent deterioration of the patient and patient discomfort.

Exposure

It is essential that you fully expose the body of the burn-injured person to appropriately assess the extent of injury including the TBSA affected and categorisation of burns. (Knighton, 2013; Trainor & McClure, 2014). You must observe carefully for circumferential wounds that can obstruct ventilation or impede limb perfusion and require escharectomy (Lundy et al., 2016). Contaminated burns should be irrigated and debrided early and any non-viable skin removed under anaesthetic by a surgeon to promote wound healing (Lundy et al., 2016; Trainor and McClure, 2014). Burn-injured individuals who cannot maintain their own body may need to be nursed in a thermally controlled cubicle (Trainor and McClure, 2014).

Wound care

Burns wound care aims to protect the surface of the wound, prevent infection and promote healing (Knighton, 2013). Burn wounds are initially sterile but are at risk of becoming infected and must be cleaned to remove debris (Trainor and McClure, 2014). Any adherent clothing should be gently soaked off the skin with normal saline (Knighton, 2013). There is no universal agreement on which dressings are most appropriate for each category or type of burn and the choice of dressing will vary between specialist units.

Initially, larger burns may be wrapped in cling film (Peate and Glencross, 2015) although circumferential dressings should be used with caution so as not to compress the affected tissues (Henderson, 2015). Dressings should be non-adherent and protect the wound from further damage whilst providing a moist environment for wound healing. Topical antiseptic treatments may be useful in the management of wounds and prevention of wound infection (Yoshino et al., 2016).

Due to the damage to the dermis caused by full thickness burns the skin is unable to heal satisfactorily on its own and will require surgical closure and/or skin grafting (Knighton, 2013). Before skin grafting and wound closure can take place, non-viable tissue must first be removed, which will involve surgical debridement and excision. Skin grafting often needs to be performed in stages, particularly in those with extensive burns where donor tissue is not abundant (Lundy et al., 2016; Knighton, 2013) or where there is excessive blood loss (Knighton, 2013). The burn-injured person requiring skin grafts will need several visits to theatre for the harvesting and grafting of donor skin. It is advisable that you leave skin grafts undisturbed for the first 5 to 7 days to promote optimal 'take' of the graft (Knighton, 2013). The term 'take' refers to the healing process where the graft connects with the local blood supply. Review of the skin graft should be undertaken sooner if there is reason to suspect a collection of blood or fluid under the graft as this will prevent the graft from taking. Again, there is no consensus regarding the most appropriate dressing to cover donor or graft sites. As with all wounds, when you are choosing a suitable dressing you must consider factors such as the stability of the wound, the amount of exudate and whether there are clinical signs of infection present. Nursing care includes adherence to strict infection control procedures, regular dressing changes and, if necessary, the administration of analgesia to reduce pain during dressing changes.

Infection control

THIS TOPIC IS ALSO COVERED IN CHAPTER 4

Infections are a leading cause of mortality and morbidity in individuals affected by burn-injuries (Lundy et al., 2016). This is due to loss of the protective skin barrier alongside immune dysfunction due to the body's inflammatory response and the insertion of invasive devices (Lundy et al., 2016). It is recommended that the burn-injured person is nursed in isolation to prevent infection with hospital-associated bacteria and that gloves and aprons are worn by all members of the healthcare team during all interactions (Clarey and Trainor, 2017). The administration of a **tetanus** vaccination is advisable if there is uncertainty around whether the affected individual has a full **vaccination** history.

Together with wound infection, burn-injured individuals are more likely to experience infections in central line catheters (Fagan et al., 2014; Lundy et al., 2016) and urinary catheters, as well as pneumonia and gastrointestinal infections (Lundy et al., 2016). As such, the health care team must always be alert to any changes in the burn-injured person's condition that may signify the presence of infection and the potential for the requirement of antibiotic therapy.

CHAPTER SUMMARY

This chapter has supported your understanding of:

- The anatomy and physiology of the integumentary system
- The management and prevention of pressure injuries
- The management and prevention of IAD
- The management of the burn-injured person

GO FURTHER

Books

Jeschke, M., Kamolz, L.P. and Sharokhi, S. (2013) *Burns Care and Treatment*. Vienna: Springer.

- This book offers a summary of the assessment and treatment of the burn-injured person.

Tortora, G. and Derrickson, B. (2011) 'The Integumentary System', in G. Tortora and B. Derrickson, *Principles of Anatomy and Physiology*, (13th edition). Chichester: Wiley. pp.153–181.

- Read this chapter of Principles of Anatomy and Physiology to improve your knowledge of the integumentary system.

Upton, D. and Upton, P. (2014) *Psychology of Wounds and Wound Care in Clinical Practice*. Berlin: Springer.

- This book uses research evidence to examine the psychological consequences of wounds and the psychological components of wound care.

Journal articles

Holden, J. (2015) 'Top tips for skin graft and donor site management', *Wound Essentials*, 10 (2): 7–13.

- Provides 10 tips for the care and management of donor and graft site wounds.

Yoshino, Y., Ohtsuka, M., Kawaguchi, M., Sakai, K., Hashimoto, A., Hayashi, M. [...] and Ihn, H. (2016) 'The wound/burn guidelines - 6: Guidelines for the management of burns', *The Journal of Dermatology*, 43: 989–1010.

- This article provides evidence-based guidance to support the appropriate diagnosis and initial treatment for patients with burns.

Beeckman, D., Campbell, J., Campbell, K., Chimentão, D., Coyer, F., Domanskky, R. [...] and Wang, F. (2015) 'Incontinence-associated dermatitis: Moving prevention forwards', *Wounds International*. Available from https://www.woundsinternational.com/resources/details/incontinence-associated-dermatitis-moving-prevention-forward (accessed November 9, 2020).

- This document offers useful practical guidance on the assessment, prevention and management of IAD.

Useful websites

National Institute for Health and Care Excellence (NICE) (2014) *Pressure Ulcers: Prevention and Management* (Clinical Guideline 179). Available from: www.nice.org.uk/guidance/cg179/evidence (accessed November 10, 2020).

- This NICE document offers guidance for the prevention and management of pressure ulcers

National Health Service (NHS) (2018) 'Pressure ulcers: Revised definition and measurement summary and recommendations'. https://improvement.nhs.uk/documents/2932/NSTPP_summary__recommendations_2.pdf (accessed November 10, 2020).

- This NHS document provides recommendations for the definition and measurement of pressure injuries along with a rationale for each recommendation.

https://npiap.com/page/PressureInjuryStages

- The NPIAP website has lots of useful information about the prevention and management of pressure injuries.

www.who.int/violence_injury_prevention/other_injury/burns/en/ (accessed November 10, 2020).

- The World Health Organisation website gives up-to-date information on the impact and incidence of burns globally.

http://nhs.stopthepressure.co.uk/How-To-Guides/howtogreatskinincontinencefinal.pdf (accessed November 10, 2020).

- This NHS guide looks at how to prevent pressure damage through the appropriate management of incontinence.

www.wounds-uk.com/ (accessed November 10, 2020).

- The Wounds UK website provides links to journals, continuing professional development activities, conferences and more.

REFERENCES

Aghaei, S., Saki, N., Daneshmand, E. and Kardeh, B. (2014) 'Prevalence of psychological disorders in patients with Alopecia Areata in comparison with normal subjects', *ISRN Dermatology*, 2014: Article# 304370. doi.org/10.1155/2014/304370 (accessed November 9, 2020).

Badia, M., Serviá, L., Casanova, J.M., Montserrat, N., Vilanova, J., Vicario, E., Rodriguez, A. and Trujillano, J. (2013) 'Classification of dermatological disorders in critical care patients: A prospective observational study', *Journal of Critical Care*, 28 (2): 220.e1–220.e8.

Beeckman, D., Campbell, J., Campbell, K., Chimentão, D., Coyer, F., Domanskky, R. […] and Wang, F. (2015) 'Incontinence-associated dermatitis: Moving prevention forwards' (Proceedings of the Global IAD Expert panel), *Wounds International*. Available from https://www.woundsinternational.com/resources/details/incontinence-associated-dermatitis-moving-prevention-forward (accessed November 9, 2020).

Clarey, A. and Trainor, D. (2017) 'Critical care management of severe burns and inhalalation injury', *Anaesthesia and Intensive Care Medicine*, 18 (8): 395–400.

Collier, M. and Simon, D. (2016) 'Protecting vulnerable skin from moisture-associated skin damage', *British Journal of Nursing*, 25 (20): S26–S32.

Coyer, F., Gardner, A. and Doubrovsky, A. (2017) 'An Interventional Skin Care Protocol (InSPiRE) to reduce incontinence associated dermatitis in critically ill patients in the intensive care unit: A before and after study', *Intensive and Critical Care Nursing*, 40: 1–10.

Delves-Yates, C. (2018) *Essentials of Nursing Practice* (2nd edition). London: Sage.

Enoch, S., Roshan, A. and Shah, M. (2009) 'Emergency and early management of burns and scalds', *British Medical Journal*, 338: B1307.

Fagan, S.P., Bilodeau, M.L. and Governan, J. (2014) 'Burn intensive care', *Surgical Clinics of North America*, 94: 765–79.

Gates, B.P., Vess, J., Long, M.A. and Johnson, E. (2019) 'Decreasing incontinence-associated dermatitis in the surgical intensive care unit', *Journal of Wound Ostomy Continence Nursing*, 46 (3S): S1–S70.

Glasgow Coma Scale (GCS), 2014. 'GSC Aid', *The Glasgow structured approach to assessment of the Glasgow Coma Scale*. Glasgow: Royal College of Physicians and Surgeons of Glasgow. www.glasgowcomascale.org/gcs-aid/ (accessed November 10, 2020).

Guilabert, P., Usua, G., Abarca, L. and Colomina, M.J. (2016) 'Fluid resusciation management in patients with burns: Update', *British Journal of Anaesthesia*, 117 (3): 284–96.

Henderson, R. (2015) Burns – Assessment and management', *Patient.info*. https://patient.info/doctor/burns-assessment-and-management (accessed November 10, 2020).

Jeschke, M.G. (2013) 'Critical Care of Burn Victims Including Inhalation Injury', in: M. Jeschke, L.P. Kamolz and S. Shahrokhi (eds.) *Burn Care and Treatment*. Vienna: Springer. pp. 67–89.

Knighton, K., (2013) 'Nursing management of the burn-injured person', in: M. Jeschke, L.P. Kamolz and S. Sharokhi, (eds.) *Burn Care and Treatment*. Vienna: Springer. pp. 111–48.

Krupp, A.E. and Monfre, J. (2015) 'Pressure ulcers in the ICU: An update on prevention and treatment', *Current Infection Disease Reports*, 17 (3): 1–6.

Lundy, J.B., Chung K.K., Pamplin J.C., Ainsworth, C.R. , Jeng, J.C., and Friedman, B.C. (2016) 'Update of severe burn management for the intensivist', *Journal of Intensive Care Medicine*, 31 (8): 499–510.

National Health Service (NHS) (2018a) 'Pressure ulcers: Revised definition and measurement summary and recommendations', Redditch: NHS. https://improvement.nhs.uk/documents/2932/NSTPP_summary__recommendations_2.pdf (accessed November 10, 2020).

National Health Service (NHS) (2018b) *Overview Burns and Scalds*. Redditch: NHS. www.nhs.uk/conditions/burns-and-scalds/ (accessed November 10, 2020).

National Institute for Health and Care Excellence (NICE) (2014) *Pressure Ulcers: Prevention and Management* (Clinical Guideline 179). London: NICE. Available from www.nice.org.uk/guidance/cg179 (accessed November 10, 2020).

National Network for Burn Case (NNBC) (2012) *National Burn Care Referral Guidance*. Redditch: NHS. www.britishburnassociation.org/wp-content/uploads/2018/02/National-Burn-Care-Referral-Guidance-2012.pdf (accessed November 10, 2020).

National Pressure Injury Advisory Panel (NPIAP) (2016) *NPAIP Pressure Injury Stages*. https://npiap.com/page/PressureInjuryStages (accessed November 9, 2020).

Peate, I. and Glencross, W. (2015) *Wound Care at a Glance*. Chichester: Wiley

Royal College of Physicians (RCP) (2017) *National Early Warning Score (NEWS2): Standardising the Assessment of Acute-Illness Severity in the NHS. Executive Summary*. London: Royal College of Physicians. Available from https://www.rcplondon.ac.uk/projects/outputs/national-early-warning-score-news-2 (accessed November 4, 2020).

Still, M., Cross, L.C., Dunlap, M., Rencher, R., Larkins, E.R., Carpenter, D.L. Buchman, T.G. and Coopersmith, C.M. (2013) 'The turn team: A novel strategy for reducing pressure ulcers in the surgical intensive care unit', *Journal of the American College of Surgeons*, 216 (3): 373–9.

Taveras, L.R., Jeschke, M.G., Wolf, S.E. (2020) 'Critical Care in Burns', in Jeschke, M.G. et al. (2020). *Handbook of Burns. Volume 1, Acute Burn Care* (2nd edition). Cham: Springer.

Tortora, G.J. and Derrickson, B. (2011) *Principles of Anatomy and Physiology* (13th edition). Chichester: Wiley.

Trainor, D. and McClure, J. (2014) 'Critical care management of inhalation injury and severe burns', *Anaesthesia and Intensive Care Medicine*, 15 (9): 415–19.

Voegeli, D., (2012) 'Moisture-associated skin damage: Aeteology, prevention and treatment', *British Journal of Nursing*, 21 (9): 517–21.

Yoshino, Y., Ohtsuka, M., Kawaguchi, M., Sakai, K., Hashimoto, A., Hayashi, M. […] and Ihn, H. (2016) 'The wound/burn guidelines – 6: Guidelines for the managment of burns', *The Journal of Dermatology*, 43 (9): 989–1010.

THE COMPLEX PATIENT: SCENARIO 2

13

GREGORY BLEAKLEY

I care for a patient with a high cervical cord injury at his home. He is quadriplegic and sustained a neck injury from sport. It is really difficult as he cannot care for himself but is fully aware of his surroundings.

Megan, 1st Year Nursing Student

LEARNING OUTCOMES

When you have finished studying this chapter you will understand:

- The initial management of a head and neck injury
- The significance of multi-disciplinary team (MDT) working
- Some of the complex issues that arise in critical care if a patient is unable to verbalise wishes

INTRODUCTION

This is the second complex case scenario and like the first the aim is to work through a complex case and activities. This complex case will contain a variety of key learning points for you to consider and align your thinking to evidence-based resources and policy documents. Every person that is admitted to critical care is 'complex', but a person who has sustained a neck injury and trauma is particularly challenging. These types of patients require robust team working and the ability to reflect, critically, on your nursing practice. Accessing resources to help plan your care delivery is important. The reflective activities within this chapter are constructed to support dialogue with your colleagues who work in critical care. Take time to discuss these reflections with other members of the MDT and retain copies for your professional portfolio. In doing so, a supportive culture develops and will strengthen your nursing knowledge.

Here is the scenario for you to work through:

THIS TOPIC
IS ALSO
COVERED IN
CHAPTER 6
AND 11

> You are a 2nd-year student nurse on placement with the adult critical care unit (ACCU). This was an elective placement and you wanted to gain knowledge and experience of critical care nursing. Your practice supervisor is called Mariam, and this is your third week of the placement. You are allocated to work with Mariam at bed 5. Declan is an 18-year-old who was admitted the previous evening with high cervical cord injury following jumping into shallow water from a 10-metre wall. He sustained multiple traumas to his right femur, pelvis, neck, and suffered a short cardiac arrest following a 5-minute submersion in the water. You had a brief handover of all patients in the ward seminar room and walk towards the bed space for a more detailed handover from the night shift bedside nurse. As discussed previously in Chapter 9, the bedside handover follows the SBAR and A-E assessment structure.

Situation

Good morning, this is Declan. He was admitted to us yesterday evening at 18:35 from the Emergency Department (ED). He was intubated and ventilated in the resuscitation room yesterday. We have struggled with his oxygenation and blood pressure overnight. We have increased his oxygen levels and added a noradrenaline infusion to support his blood pressure. His blood gases have deteriorated, and his pH is currently 7.21. Following orthopaedic review, there is a fractured pubic ramus which is stable and there is a closed fracture to the right femur which is currently stable. There is an abduction weight and splint attached to the right lower limb. There is apparent swelling and bruising to the right upper leg. A CT scan of the head and neck reveals a fracture to C3 spinal vertebrae. There is a supportive **C-spine** collar in-situ and he is fully immobilised.

Background

Declan has been previously fit and well. We do not have any further medical records at this stage and his family report he has no known allergies. Declan had been out at a reservoir with friends and wanted to cool off in the water from the heat. He jumped from a 10-metre wall into the water but did not realise the water was shallow. His friends had to wade in to recover his body from the water and they summoned help from the ambulance service. His friends state he was making a few occasional breaths, but the paramedic crew instigated full advanced life support measures upon arrival.

Assessment

A (Airway): Declan has a size 8 Endo-Tracheal Tube (ETT) inserted which is tied at 23cm at the lips. The ETT cuff pressure has been checked and is within acceptable parameters. There are no further secretions in the oral cavity upon examination.

B (Breathing): The ETT is attached to a ventilator and Declan is making no spontaneous respiratory effort. The ventilation settings are charted here:

Table 13.1 Declan's ventilator settings

Time	05:00	06:00	07:00
MODE	Pressure Controlled Ventilation (PCV)	PCV	PCV
FiO$_2$	.60	.65	.75
Inspiratory pressure	24	24	24
PEEP	7.5	7.5	7.5
MV/TV	640mls	632mls	633mls
f set/meas	20	20	20
I: E ratio	1:2	1:2	1:2
Suction	NO	No	Yes clear
Sedation Score RASS	−4	−4	−4

His last arterial blood gas is here.

pH	7.21
pCO$_2$	6.8 kPa
pO$_2$	9.4 kPa
Base Excess	−2.7 mmol/L
HCO$_3$	23 mmol/L
SaO$_2$	91%

His arterial blood gas the previous evening in Resus.

pH	7.29
pCO$_2$	7.5kPa
pO$_2$	12.6 kPa
Base Excess	+0.2 mmol/L
HCO$_3$	28 mmol/L
SaO$_2$	97%

There are no secretions from ETT **suctioning**, air entry appears equal and auscultation reveals no added sounds.

THIS TOPIC IS ALSO COVERED IN CHAPTER 5

C (Circulation): Declan is tachycardic and his heart rate is 118 beats per minute and regular. His blood pressure is 101/72 mmHg and is being supported by single strength noradrenaline (4mg/50 ml) at 15 mls/hr. This is achieving a **mean arterial** pressure (MAP) of 59 mmHg. His urine output is 35 mls for the previous hour and a total 840 mls for last 15 hours since admission to critical care.

D (Disability): Declan is sedated on 1% propofol which is infusing at 10 mls/hr. Additionally, Alfentanil (0.5mg/ml) is infusing at 4 mls/hr. Both pupils are equal in size and respond briskly to a bright light stimulus, GCS is 3/15. His Richmond Agitation-Sedation Scale (RASS) Score is –5.

E (Exposure): There is no evidence of head injury. There is a supportive C-spine collar in-situ. There is no obvious chest or abdominal injury. The right upper leg is swollen and bruised and there is an abduction weight attached to this limb. Orthopaedics do not advise any surgical repair at this stage due to **haemodynamic** instability and critical illness but wish to review. His recent temperature was 36.2°C and blood glucose was 5.1 mmol/L. Declan is being nursed in a **supine** position without head elevation due to his C3 vertebral fracture.

Recommendations

Declan is going for an urgent **MRI** scan of this neck this morning and the neurosurgical team are going to urgently review the case and scans. I think the orthopaedic surgeons also want to review his pelvic and right femur fractures.

All infusions are up to date and back up syringes have been prepared.

Declan's family consist of his girlfriend who states she is the next of kin and, with his mother and father, are waiting for an update in the relative's room. They are extremely anxious and tearful and asked the night shift nurse whether the fracture in Declan's neck will result in permanent disability. Any questions before I go?

ACTIVITY 13.1: CRITICAL THINKING

Jot down your immediate thoughts and consider what your nursing priorities may be.

1. Are there any aspects of the handover that you did not understand or anything that was not clear? Check all terms and abbreviations that are not clear with the guide in this book.
2. Is there anything else you need to ask the night shift nurse before they leave?
3. From what has been handed over so far, do you have concerns about Declan's ventilation and blood pressure?
4. What is the significance and implication of a cervical vertebral fracture and high cervical cord injury for the patient?

ACTIVITY 13.2: CRITICAL THINKING

Read the following NICE (2016b) NG 41 guidance on *Spinal Injury: Assessment and Initial Management*: www.nice.org.uk/guidance/ng41/resources/spinal-injury-assessment-and-initial-management-pdf-1837447790533 (accessed November 10, 2020).

How does this guidance help inform your nursing practice for patients with cervical/spinal injury?

You are now halfway through your shift and have an opportunity to talk with Mariam about your initial experiences. Mariam asks whether you would record the next set of physical observations on the chart under her direct supervision. The family had a brief spell at the bedside a few hours ago but are still waiting for an update. Diagnostic imaging has revealed a lesion to the spinal cord at C3< (see Figure 13.1 as an illustration of what this would look like) and the neurosurgeons/neurologist are involved in the care. Declan remains fully immobilised. The ward has taken a phone call from the local press who want an update on Declan's condition.

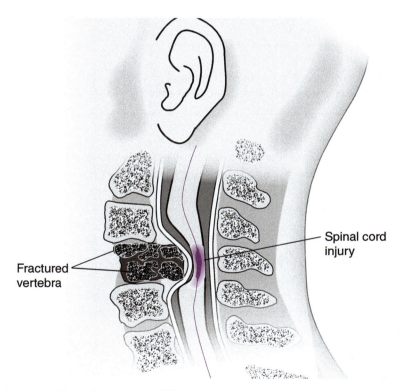

Figure 13.1 Lesion to the spinal cord at C3

Source: www.spire.org.au/spinal-cord-injury/what-is-spinal-injury/

ACTIVITY 13.3: REFLECTIVE PRACTICE

Reflect on the situation above and consider your first concerns.

1. How will you record the physiological observation and what do each of the values mean?
2. How are you going to plan to update the family and which words are you going to use to describe his high cervical cord injury?
3. Can you list all members of the MDT who would be involved in Declan's care at this point?
4. Although Declan's partner states she is the next of kin, you establish they are not married and do not have a civil partnership, so who is his next of kin?
5. Can information be released to the press about Declan's condition and how would you manage such a phone call?

ACTIVITY 13.4: CRITICAL THINKING

Read the following article by Ervin et al. (2018) about the importance of teamwork in the critical care unit: www.ncbi.nlm.nih.gov/pmc/articles/PMC6662208/pdf/nihms-1038414.pdf (accessed November 10, 2020)

After reading this article, consider the following points:

- Why is teamwork important in the critical care team?
- How can effective teamwork contribute to better patient outcomes and clinical decision making?

Following morning ward round, the duty consultant **intensivist** has asked that the sedation is stopped so the clinical team can assess neurological function. Mariam stopped the propofol and alfentanil 2 hours previously but there appears to be no spontaneous respiratory effort. All mandatory breaths are being delivered by the ventilator.

WHAT'S THE EVIDENCE?

High cervical cord injury/lesions can affect the nerves that control normal respiration. Injury of C1 to C4 cervical nerves can result in permanent paralysis of the arms, hands, trunk and legs. When all four limbs are affected, this is called tetraplegia or quadriplegia.

Read the following article by Waxenbaum et al. (2020) to fully understand cervical cord nerve distribution and function: www.ncbi.nlm.nih.gov/books/NBK538136/

You are nearing the end of the shift and Declan's blood pressure is starting to fall. His current arterial blood pressure is 85/64 mmHg. His noradrenaline infusion has been increased to 20 mls/hr.

Mariam alerts the duty Consultant Intensivist about her concerns regarding Declan's blood pressure. His MAP has deteriorated over the past few hours and is currently 51 mmHg.

ACTIVITY 13.5: CRITICAL THINKING

1. What could be causing Declan's blood pressure to fall?
2. Which inotropic therapies could be considered to improve his blood pressure?
3. Why is achieving a MAP of 60 – 70 mmHg significant?

WHAT'S THE EVIDENCE?

Fractures to the femur and pelvis can cause significant blood loss in critically ill patients. The estimated blood loss for a closed fracture of the femur is 1000-1500 mls. Active bleeding from the femur and pelvis is a clinical emergency and a blood transfusion could be necessary. Furthermore, inotropes need to be titrated to achieve an acceptable MAP.

Explore the following evidence sources to help inform your knowledge and practice:

- Bangash et al. (2011) about use of inotropes and vasopressor agents in critically ill patients: www.ncbi.nlm.nih.gov/pmc/articles/PMC3413841/pdf/bph0165-2015.pdf (accessed November 10, 2020)
- Wertheimer et al. (2018) which explores fractures of the femur and blood transfusions: https://doi.org/10.1016/j.injury.2018.03.007
- Read Section 10 (starting on p. 115) of the NICE (2016a) Guidelines 39 on *Major Trauma: Assessment and Initial Management*. Available from https://www.nice.org.uk/guidance/ng39 (accessed November 10, 2020)

The following day, you attend placement and are allocated to work with Mariam at Bed 5 again. Declan's blood pressure has improved and is currently 123/65 mmHg with a MAP of 68 mmHg. The family have difficulty coming to terms with his potential life changing injuries. They appear bewildered, tired, and confused. Declan has a morphine infusion in progress to manage pain. He is starting to open his eyes but is very groggy. There has been no spontaneous respiratory effort on the ventilator and no movement of upper/lower limbs.

13.6 ACTIVITY: CRITICAL REFLECTION

1. What strategy are you going to develop to explain Declan's injury to him once he is fully conscious?
2. What other services offer long term care and support for patients with high cervical cord injuries?

CHAPTER SUMMARY

This complex case scenario offered an opportunity consider and critically reflect on many important aspects of nursing a patient with a high cervical cord injury. The 'what's the evidence?' sections have directed you towards evidence sources and key policy documents to enhance your knowledge and practice. Take time to reflect on your own learning and consider the underpinning evidence to your clinical decisions. Importantly, this complex case chapter has focused on the importance of collaborative working within the MDT.

GO FURTHER

Books

Taylor, J. (2017) *The Cervical Spine: An Atlas of Normal Anatomy and the Morbid Anatomy of Ageing and Injuries*. Chatswood, NSW: Elsevier.

- This book explores the pathophysiology of cervical cord injury through in-depth discussion and use of illustrations and photographs.

Rodríguez-Merchán, E.C. and Rubio-Suárez, J.C. (2014) *Complex Fractures of the Limbs: Diagnosis and Management*. New York, NY: Springer.

- Chapters 5, 7 and 15 in this book will help your understanding of the limb and pelvic fractures associated with the complex case scenario.

Jevon, P. and Ewens, B. (2012) *Monitoring the Critically Ill Patient* (3rd edition). London: Wiley-Blackwell.

- Prior to you recording observations on the critical care chart, Chapter 3 (p. 39) will help you gain underpinning knowledge of the monitoring priorities of the ventilated patient.

Journal articles

Rozeboom, N., Parenteau, K. and Carratturo, D. (2012) 'Rehabilitation starts in the intensive care unit', *Critical Care Nursing*, 35 (3): 234–40. doi.org/10.1097/cnq.0b013e3182542d8c

- This article reveals that a delay in the transfer of patients with spinal injuries in critical care to specialist centres is significant. Furthermore, the article encourages early multidisciplinary team engagement to achieve optimal outcomes.

Bracht, H., Calzia, E., Georgieff, M., Singer, J., Radermacher, P. and Russell, J.A. (2012) 'Inotropes and vasopressors: More than haemodynamics!', *British Journal of Pharmacology*, 165 (7): 2009–11. doi.org/10.1111/j.1476-5381.2011.01776.x

- The article explores the use and efficacy of inotropic and vasopressor use in people experiencing circulatory shock.

Radomski, M., Zettervall, S., Schroeder, M.E., Messing, J., Dunnem, J. and Sarani, B. (2016) 'Critical care for the patient with multiple trauma', *Journal of Intensive Care Medicine*, 31 (5): 307–18. doi. org/10.1177/0885066615571895

- The article suggests that critical care practitioners should be familiar with various types of injury/trauma and their associated treatment strategies. The article adopts a logical A – E assessment of a person with polytrauma (multiple injuries).

Useful websites

British Association of Spinal Cord Injury Specialists: www.bascis.org.uk/ (accessed November 10, 2020).

- BASCIS is an association mainly of clinicians who are dedicated to the holistic management of patients with a spinal cord injury.

National Major Trauma Nursing Group: www.c4ts.qmul.ac.uk/nursing-and-ahp/national-major-trauma-nursing-group (accessed November 10, 2020)

- This group of trauma nurses aims to represent and develop national standards for trauma nursing from the point of injury through to rehabilitation.

NIH National Institute of Neurological Disorders and Stroke: 'Spinal cord injury – hope through research'. www.ninds.nih.gov/Disorders/Patient-Caregiver-Education/Hope-Through-Research/Spinal-Cord-Injury-Hope-Through-Research (accessed November 10, 2020).

- This website will provide an overview of the spinal cord structure and function, treatment, and diagnosis through to classification of spinal cord injury.

REFERENCES

Bangash, M.N., Kongm M., and Pearsem R.M. (2011) 'Use of inotropes and vasopressor agents in critically ill patients', *British Journal of Pharmacology*, 165: 2015–33.

Ervin, J.N., Kahn, J.M., Cohen, T.R. and Weingart, L.R. (2018) 'Teamwork in the Intensive Care Unit', *American Psychologist*, 73 (4): 468–77. doi.org/10.1037/amp0000247

National Institute for Health and Care Excellence (NICE) (2016a). *Major Trauma: Assessment and Initial Management*. (National Guideline 39). London: NICE. Available from https://www.nice.org.uk/guidance/ng39 (accessed November 10, 2020).

National Institute for Health and Care Excellence (NICE) (2016b). *Spinal Injury: Assessment and Initial Management* (National Guideline 41). London: NICE. Available from www.nice.org.uk/guidance/ng41 (accessed November 10, 2020).

Waxenbaum, J.A., Reddy, V. and Bordoni, B. (2020) 'Anatomy, head and neck, cervical nerves', StatPearls. www.ncbi.nlm.nih.gov/books/NBK538136/ (accessed November 10, 2020).

Wertheimer, A., Olaussen, A., Perera, S., Liew, S. and Mitra, B. (2018) 'Fractures of the femur and blood transfusions', *International Journal of the Care of the Injured*, 49 (4): 846–51.

CRITICAL CARE RELATED TO WOMEN DURING PREGNANCY AND CHILDBIRTH

GILLIAN SINGLETON AND KIM WILCOCK

14

> " I was struck by the vulnerability of the woman who arrived unexpectedly on the critical care unit having just given birth. She and her family were really scared. She told me she hadn't realised that this could happen. It felt really good to be able to listen to her fears and support her at such a difficult time. It was really nice to watch her with her new baby when she started to feel better. I felt that I made a difference to her.
>
> **Lucy, 3rd Year Nursing Student** "

> " The birth of my first baby should have been a really wonderful time. Things escalated really quickly and it was very frightening. I woke up on a critical care unit. The lights were bright, it was very noisy and there were a lot of strange people that I didn't recognise. My partner and baby were nowhere to be seen. I didn't know what had happened.
>
> **Helen, first time mum to baby Mia** "

LEARNING OUTCOMES

When you have finished studying this chapter you will be able to understand:

- Why women in the child bearing continuum may require critical care
- The obstetric emergencies that may result in an admission to an Adult Critical Care Unit
- How to monitor critically ill women during pregnancy or following childbirth
- How to recognise the deterioration of the critically ill obstetric woman
- The responsibilities of the health care professional when providing care for these women

INTRODUCTION

Pregnancy related complications including **sepsis**, venous **thromboembolism**, haemorrhage and **pre-eclampsia** can result in critical illness for childbearing women. Similarly, pre-existing medical conditions relating to increasing maternal age, obesity and comorbidities such as **hypertension**, cardiovascular disease and diabetes are all factors that can result in a woman becoming unwell during the childbearing continuum (**antenatal**, **intrapartum** or **postnatal** period).

Most women will remain healthy throughout pregnancy and childbirth and the United Kingdom has one of the lowest maternal **mortality** rates in the world (Knight et al., 2019). However, some women will become unwell and require transfer to an Adult Critical Care Unit (ACCU). It has been acknowledged that women who become unwell should have immediate access to critical care provided by multidisciplinary teams who are skilled in recognising and treating the acutely deteriorating obstetric patient (Royal College of Anaesthetists (RCOA), 2018).

Antenatal care is the care provided from the time of conception until the beginning of labour (Baston, 2014). 'Labour is the process where the foetus, placenta and membranes are expelled through the birth canal' (Jackson et al., 2014: 328). Most pregnancies last approximately 40 weeks, however labour can occur from 37 to 42 completed weeks of pregnancy (National Institute for Health and Care Excellence (NICE), 2017). The postnatal/postpartum period commences following birth of the placenta and membranes and continues for 42 days (Steen and Wray, 2014).

Few pregnancies are complicated by illness severe enough for the woman to warrant admission to critical care. In 2013 up to 83% of women requiring critical care were postnatal women with the main reason for admission being obstetric haemorrhage. Respiratory failure was the main reason for antenatal admissions in the remaining 17% of women (Intensive Care and National Audit Research Centre 2013). Maternity and critical care services should work in collaboration to ensure high quality evidence-based care is available to these women. The challenge of providing high quality critical care to women is ongoing due to the altered maternal physiology in pregnancy, consideration of the foetus and medical emergencies associated with pregnancy and childbirth (Guntupalli et al., 2015).

ACTIVITY 14.1: REFLECTIVE PRACTICE

Let's reflect on what a woman who has just given birth to a baby may need physically and psychologically and who might be involved in her care.

Now consider these factors should she be admitted to your critical care unit, she is ventilated and sedated.

1. What additional physical needs might she have?
2. What extra psychological support might she require?
3. Which specialities might need to be involved in her care?

Write these down and then repeat the exercise when you have worked through the chapter to compare your knowledge.

Management of the critically ill obstetric woman requires a multi-disciplinary team approach with active involvement from obstetricians, neonatologists, anaesthetists, physiotherapists, nurses and midwives. This list is not exhaustive. Stabilisation of the maternal condition is the priority when caring for a critically ill woman with foetal outcome being a further consideration. Priority should be given to keeping mother and baby together wherever possible. Below is an overview of conditions that may result in women being admitted to critical care units and the specialised care they may require.

COMMON CONDITIONS REQUIRING CRITICAL CARE

Haemorrhage

Antepartum Haemorrhage (APH) is defined as bleeding from the genital tract after 24 weeks of pregnancy but before the birth of the baby (Royal College of Obstetricians and Gynaecologists (RCOG), 2011). In Table 14.1 you can see different causes of APH.

Table 14.1 Different causes of antepartum haemorrhage

Type	Cause	Risk Factors
Placental abruption	Separation of a normally situated placenta	Hypertension, preeclampsia, multiparty, advanced maternal age, polyhydramnios, smoking, drug use, trauma, premature rupture of membranes, chorioamnionitis
Placenta praevia	Placenta is partially or fully covering the cervix which is in the lower uterine segment	Multiparty, advanced maternal age, previous caesarean section, uterine surgery.
Uterine rupture	Tearing of the uterine wall during pregnancy or delivery	Rupture of previous caesarean section scar, trauma, uterine anomalies, dystocia, use of uterotonic drugs
Other	Trauma, genital infections, vasa praevia, haematuria and cervicitis	

Primary Postpartum haemorrhage (PPH) is defined as bleeding from the genital tract in excess of 500 mls at any time following the baby's birth up to 24 hours postpartum (World Health Organisation (WHO), 2012). Secondary PPH can be defined as any abnormal bleeding from the genital tract occurring between 24 hours and 12 weeks postnatally, but is most likely to occur between 10 and 14 days after birth. Bleeding is usually due to a piece of retained placenta or membranes, or the presence of a large uterine clot (Begley, 2014).

A PPH can be minor (500–1000 ml) or major (more than 1000 ml). Major could be divided into moderate (1000–2000 ml) or severe (more than 2000 ml) (Mavrides et al., 2016).

There are many reasons why a PPH might occur. These relate to: Tone, Tissue, Thrombin or Trauma. The most common (69% of causes) being an atonic uterus (Tone), due to failure of the uterine muscles to contract following the birth, retained placenta or retained products (Tissue) which occurs in roughly 20% of cases (all or segments of the placenta or membranes are retained following the third stage of labour). Injury to the uterus, cervix or perineum (Trauma) accounts for 20% of cases and less than 1% of cases relate to blood **coagulation** disorders (Thrombin), preventing the arrest of bleeding following completion of the third stage of labour (Begley, 2014; Mavrides et al., 2016).

Figure 14.1 is a visual aid to help you understand the causes of PPH.

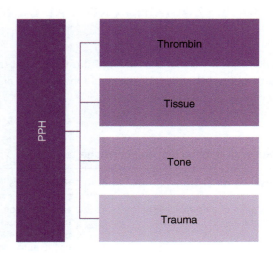

Thrombin	Preeclampsia (hypertension and organ damage)
	Placental abruption (Placenta separates from inner wall of uterus before birth)
	Protracted labour (labour that lasts longer than guidance recommends)
	Bleeding disorder
Tissue	Retained placenta (part of the placenta remains in the uterus)
	Placenta accreta (placenta deeply imbedded in uterine wall)
Tone	Placenta praevia (an abnormally situated placenta over the cervical opening)
	Over distended uterus (due to fibroids or the uterus inability to contract)
	Previous PPH
Trauma	Caesarean section (Surgical procedure to deliver a baby)
	Episiotomy (surgical incision between the vagina and the anus)
	Foetal macrosomia (large baby)
Other	Anaemia, obesity and induction of labour

Figure 14.1 The causes of PPH

A woman having a PPH will require urgent care and stabilisation. Table 14.2 indicates the care she will receive.

Table 14.2 Summarising the urgent care and stabilisation need during a PPH

Presenting Signs/ Symptoms of PPH	Immediate Care on Delivery Suite (undertaken by midwife)	Critical Care
• Blood loss • Visible pallor • Shock • Tachypnoea (>20 breaths/min) • Tachycardia (>90bpm) • Fall in BP (late sign of decline) • Rapid, thready pulse • Pale • Clammy • Maternal collapse • Some degree of compromise	• Communicate • Catheterise the bladder • Rub up a contraction to minimise bleeding • Resuscitate with IV fluids, maintain strict fluid balance • Administer oxytocic drugs according to protocol • Monitor, observations • Measure blood loss • **Possible sequela:** Balloon Tamponade, B-Lynch Suture, Uterine Artery ligation, hysterectomy • **Time** events and **document**	• May need to be transferred to ACCU • Consider CVP/Arterial Line • Observations • Urine (hourly) • Monitor lochia • Treat any infection Can lead to: • Acute Respiratory Distress Syndrome (ARDS) • Sheehan's (Necrosis Anterior Pituitary) • Common symptoms: no lactation, amenorrhea, hypothyroidism, hypoglycaemia • Daily obstetric/midwifery review • Psychological needs/counselling • Debrief • Accountability/record keeping

Source: Nursing and Midwifery Council, 2018.

WHAT'S THE EVIDENCE?

Read the evidence surrounding prevention and management of postpartum haemorrhage:

Mavrides, E., Allard, S., Chandraharan, E., Collins, P., Green, L., Hunt, B.J., Riris, S. and Thomson, A.J. (2016) 'Prevention and Management of Postpartum Haemorrhage (RCOG: Green-top Guideline 52)', *BJOG*, 124 (5): 106-49. Available from https://www.rcog.org.uk/en/guidelines-research-services/guidelines/gtg52/ (accessed November 11, 2020).

How does this compare to NICE (2017) guidelines recommendations for the management of postpartum haemorrhage?

www.nice.org.uk/guidance/CG190

You can also review any of the medications mentioned in the British National Formulary (BNF) available in paper copy or online via https://bnf.nice.org.uk/ (accessed November 11, 2020).

Hypertensive disorders

Hypertension can occur in a wide range of disorders. Complications can often result in admission to ACCU with women requiring critical care largely due to multi organ failure or seizures (Guntupalli et al., 2015). 8–10% of all pregnancies will be affected by hypertensive disorders (National Institute for Health and Care Excellence (NICE), 2019).

Hypertension in pregnancy can be divided into two groups: those that are unique to pregnancy and those that exist before pregnancy.

ACTIVITY 14.2: CRITICAL THINKING

Read the NICE guidance around hypertension in pregnancy. There is an interactive flow chart to help you. NICE (2019) *Hypertension in Pregnancy: Diagnosis and Management* (National Guideline 133). London: NICE. Available from www.nice.org.uk/guidance/ng133 (accessed November 11, 2020).

1. Write down the different types of hypertension
2. How might you diagnose them?

Whilst working on an ACCU you may be asked to care for women with preeclampsia or eclampsia. Preeclampsia is a condition that begins during pregnancy, usually after the 20th week, and is characterised by high blood pressure and protein in the urine. A severe complication of preeclampsia is eclampsia. This is the term used when seizures develop in a woman with severe preeclampsia. It is important to recognise the signs and symptoms of this potentially life-threatening condition which can escalate rapidly.

Signs and symptoms of preeclampsia include severe hypertension, proteinuria, epigastric pain, right upper quadrant discomfort and vomiting. Women will often complain of visual symptoms (floaters in front of the eyes), drowsiness, severe headaches and oedema. They will have impaired renal function, liver dysfunction and deep tendon reflex response. Women suffering from eclampsia will also have seizures (Stevenson and Billington, 2007). Care providers should be aware that preeclampsia increases the risk of placental abruption and stillbirth, so robust electronic foetal monitoring should be undertaken to monitor foetal wellbeing in the antenatal woman. (It is worth noting that preeclampsia and eclampsia can occur in the immediate postpartum period. In this case the baby will have already been born so welfare of the foetus is not a consideration.) In the case of placental abruption there is also the risk of maternal haemorrhagic shock and DIC (Disseminated Intravascular Coagulation), therefore delivery of the foetus should be considered (Dildy and Belfort, 2010).

THIS TOPIC
IS ALSO
COVERED IN
CHAPTER 6
AND 8

HELLP syndrome (Haemolysis, Elevated Liver enzymes and Low Platelets) is associated with pre-eclampsia or can occur on its own. Complications can include DIC, placental abruption, liver haematoma or bleeding, renal failure and **pulmonary** oedema (Boyce et al., 2014).

MATERNAL COLLAPSE

THIS TOPIC
IS ALSO
COVERED IN
CHAPTER 6

This is defined as an acute event involving the cardiorespiratory systems and/or brain resulting in a reduced or absent level of consciousness at any stage in pregnancy and up to 6 weeks postpartum (RCOG, 2014). This is rare and occurs in 0.14 – 6 per 1000 births (Long and Penna, 2018). Maternal collapse can be a direct result of a midwifery emergency, for example a massive obstetric postpartum haemorrhage. However, chronic causes may include cardiovascular disease (Knight et al., 2019). This is rising in the pregnant population due to increasing maternal age, rising levels of obesity and increasing fertility in women with pre-existing cardiac conditions. Acute coronary syndrome, peripartum cardiomyopathy and congenital heart disease need also to be considered during a maternal collapse. For these women, early **intervention**, early resuscitation and prompt transfer to the appropriate level of care such as the ACCU will improve outcomes.

Sepsis

Sepsis is a leading cause of maternal **morbidity** and mortality in the UK. During the childbearing continuum women may be more susceptible to a rapid deterioration of illness following an infection (Greer et al., 2020).

Factors that increase the risk of sepsis in pregnant women or those who have given birth in the past 6 weeks include women who have:

- Impaired immune systems because of illness or drugs
- Gestational diabetes or other comorbidities
- Undergone invasive procedures (e.g. caesarean section, **instrumental deliveries**, **manual removal of placenta**)
- Had prolonged rupture of membranes >24hrs
- Had exposure to group A streptococcal infection
- Had continued bleeding and offensive discharge

THIS TOPIC IS ALSO COVERED IN CHAPTER 7

Women who have undergone a traumatic delivery or experienced a midwifery emergency may also present with shock. It is important to have an understanding of the different types of shock that an obstetric patient may be susceptible to.

ACTIVITY 14.3: CASE STUDY

You are caring for Imogen who was admitted to your critical care department a few hours ago. She is a 29-year-old woman who had her third baby two days ago. She had a forceps delivery followed by a manual removal of placenta in the obstetric theatre. She lost 4 litres of blood during the procedure. They were unable to stabilise her blood pressure in theatre and she was admitted to the ACCU.

What is your immediate priority whilst caring for Imogen?

It is important that all health care professionals caring for women in the postnatal period are aware of the signs and symptoms of potentially life-threatening conditions that can occur up to 8 weeks after birth. In Table 14.3 the signs and symptoms of potentially life-threatening conditions of postnatal care are outlined which will help you recognise them.

Table 14.3 Signs and symptoms of potentially life-threatening conditions of postnatal care up to 8 weeks after birth

Signs and symptoms	Condition
Sudden and profuse blood loss or persistent increased blood loss Faintness, dizziness or palpitations/**tachycardia**	Postpartum Haemorrhage
Fever, shivering, abdominal pain and/or offensive vaginal discharge	Infection

(Continued)

Table 14.3   (Continued)

Signs and symptoms	Condition
Headaches accompanied by one or more of the following symptoms within the first 72 hours after birth: Proteinurea Visual disturbances Nausea, vomiting	Preeclampsia/Eclampsia
Unilateral calf pain, redness or swelling Shortness of breath or chest pain	Thromboembolism

Source: (NICE), 2015. Reproduced under the NICE UK Open Content License. URL: www.nice.org.uk/Media/Default/About/Reusing-our-content/Open-content-licence/NICE-UK-Open-Content-Licence-.pdf

ACTIVITY 14.4: CRITICAL THINKING

Explore NICE (2015) *Postnatal Care up to 8 Weeks after Birth.* (Clinical Guideline 37) Available from www.nice.org.uk/guidance/cg37 (accessed November 11, 2020).

Familiarise yourself with the normal pathway for postnatal women. This will help you to identify any deviations from the norm in women who present on an ACCU.

ACTIVITY 14.5: CASE STUDY

Doha's story: I went into labour with my first child and had long labour. My son was delivered by forceps. As soon as he was born I started to bleed and I began to feel really unwell. The next thing I remember was waking up in intensive care. I was scared and in pain and I didn't recognise anyone around me. I didn't know what had happened to my baby.

They told me I had suffered a massive obstetric haemorrhage and needed a lot of blood.

I felt so guilty that I had not been able to care for my son in those first few days. The staff were really good and encouraged my husband to bring the baby in to me for as long as I wanted although they weren't able to stay overnight. On day 3 my breasts became really engorged which I know now to be normal but it was so painful. My midwife brought a breast pump with her and taught me how to express milk. She helped me to fix the baby to the breast properly. Everyone was amazing and I felt so much better that I had started to develop a relationship with my son.

After a few days I was discharged back into the obstetric unit for the rest of my postnatal care. This made me feel more normal, just like any other Mum. I still have flashbacks to those first few days though. It was a really frightening and uncertain time for both me and my husband.

1.   What additional needs does Doha have specific to her just having had a baby?
2.   When performing a physical examination, what extra observations may you need to consider?
3.   Which members of the multidisciplinary team and different specialities could you liaise with to ensure Doha receives excellent evidence-based care?

THIS TOPIC
IS ALSO
COVERED IN
CHAPTER 15

MONITORING OF THE CRITICALLY ILL WOMAN DURING OR FOLLOWING PREGNANCY

As we have discussed in earlier chapters anyone deteriorating should be assessed using the structured ABCDE approach (RCUK, 2015). The assessment is no different from the assessment you would carry out when assessing a deteriorating person.

However, there are some key points that are specific to pregnancy. These are:

THIS TOPIC IS ALSO COVERED IN CHAPTER 3

C: Circulation

The uterus should be palpated to ensure it is contracted in order to minimise blood loss and the blood loss (lochia) assessed; a midwife will do this.

Blood pressure is an assessment of particular importance in pregnancy, and it has been identified that a raised blood pressure greater than 140/90mmHG could be associated with preeclampsia toxaemia (PET). As previously discussed, detailed assessment of PET, whereby blood pressure is assessed within the context of a urine test for protein, symptoms of epigastric pain, severe headache and visual disturbances is classed as a medical emergency and warrants immediate action.

During the antenatal stage of pregnancy, midwifery colleagues will be assessing for and considering uterine displacement by nursing the woman in a left lateral tilt to prevent compression of the inferior vena cava by the gravid uterus, thus preventing supine **hypotension** (Brewster, 2017). This could result in loss of consciousness for the woman and in extreme cases foetal death in utero.

Urine output should be closely monitored and catheterisation usually carried out to ensure accuracy. Catheterisation with measurement of hourly urine output is a useful gauge of perfusion, giving valuable information about wellbeing, fluid balance and response to treatment (Boyle and Bothamley, 2018). Urine output should be 0.5ml/kg/h–1 ml/kg/h. The urine should be tested for proteinuria, infection (leukocytes) and evidence of ketosis.

E: Exposure

Regular antenatal and postnatal checks should be performed by a midwife or obstetrician to identify improvement or deterioration of the woman. Growth and development of the foetus is dependent on the woman's health and monitoring of foetal wellbeing should also be undertaken after 24 weeks (Gaffney, 2014). Auscultation of the foetal heart or a **cardiotocography** (CTG) should be performed, the frequency of which should be determined on an individual basis and documented in the plan of care. Administration of corticosteroids for foetal lung maturation should be considered if a preterm birth is expected (Roberts et al., 2017).

Ongoing assessment is fundamental to the care of the critically ill woman during pregnancy or following childbirth. Failure to recognise the early deterioration of an obstetric patient has been a significant and recurring theme in cases of maternal mortality (RCOA, 2018). The clinical picture can change rapidly and observations are necessary to evaluate changes in status of the woman. Women who become unwell during pregnancy and birth often deteriorate quickly following a period of physiological compensation. A Maternity Early Obstetric Warning Score (MEOWS) should be used to record all observations performed on women who are pregnant or have given birth in the last 42 days (RCOA, 2018). Modifications have been made to support the physiological changes that occur in pregnancy. MEOWS charts have linked escalation protocols so abnormal physiological parameters follow a colour coded system that supports the need for more frequent observations or clinical review (Robbins et al., 2019). One or more abnormal observation in the red zone or two or more mildly abnormal parameters in the amber zone should be noted and trigger a prompt referral for appropriate management. All units will have a local policy, however there is currently no standardised MEOWS chart in maternity care (Boyle and Bothamley, 2018). There should be clear instructions in the plan of care for the required frequency of observations but in critical care they should be performed every four hours as a minimum.

ACTIVITY 14.6: REFLECTIVE PRACTICE

Take a look at the observations required in the MEOWS and compare them to the NEWS2.

1.   What are the differences?
2.   Which assessment tool do you think would support your practice?
3.   What do you think are the challenges of using different assessment tools in a clinical setting?
4.   How do you think a MEOWS chart would be useful during a PPH? What parameters of observations do you think would prompt clinical actions and why?

Discuss your thoughts with a peer, colleague or your practice supervisor.

Postnatal care

Lochia describes the vaginal loss after childbirth (Steen and Wray, 2014) and should be regularly assessed. The decidual lining of the uterus is shed in the lochia (Bick and Hunter, 2017). In the first few days following delivery it will be red and moderate. Any increase or blood clots should refer for senior review as they can be a sign of a secondary PPH which can occur from 24 hours post birth to 12 weeks. After birth the uterus gradually shrinks and descends into its prepregnancy position in the pelvis, known as involution.

Women with unilateral calf pain, redness or swelling should be evaluated for deep vein **thrombosis** (NICE, 2015). If the woman is unable to communicate with you it is important to assess her legs routinely for these signs and to escalate any concerns.

An additional consideration is required regarding the use of anti-D for rhesus negative mothers (Vincent and Frise, 2018).

Wound care

THIS TOPIC
IS ALSO
COVERED IN
CHAPTER 12

In the UK, 29% of births are performed by Caesarean section (National Health Service 2018). For women who have undergone a Caesarean section, wound care and observation should be performed regularly.

Breast care

It is important for all women to be offered advice and support on common breast and breastfeeding problems. Physical problems can include signs of engorgement when the breast feels hard and tight and cracked, or bleeding nipples. Breast engorgement on day 3 or 4 is a physiological condition as the body adapts to hormonal changes and milk is produced. It is common regardless of the feeding method. Support from midwives around the importance of feeding on demand where possible and hand expression should be sought. Regular analgesia should also be offered.

Mastitis (when the breast is painful, red and hot to touch) and thrush can also be common in the days after delivery. Please seek advice from your midwifery colleagues for support if you encounter problems with breast care.

Psychological support

Low mood postpartum is a normal reaction that occurs between 4 and 5 days after birth. This can affect up to 50% of women. This fluctuation of mood is transitory and should resolve within a short period of time (Royal College of Psychiatrists 2018). Women may be tearful and irritable with frequent mood changes, exacerbated by a traumatic experience such as admission to critical care. Health care professionals should reassure them that this will pass with further evaluation recommended if symptoms persist beyond 10–14 days (Bick and Hunter, 2017).

THIS TOPIC IS ALSO COVERED IN CHAPTER 15

Multi-disciplinary team approach to care

To reassure you, very few women have pregnancies complicated by severe illness. However, because of this, expertise in caring for these women and the ability to maintain and develop these skills can be limited. A multi-disciplinary team approach is essential to ensure women receive optimal care. Women should be reviewed by an obstetric team consisting of a consultant obstetrician, consultant anaesthetist and a midwife in conjunction with the critical care team at least once every 24 hours (RCOA, 2018). There should be a lead consultant obstetrician for all women who require critical care.

For women over 24 weeks gestation a plan for the regular assessment of foetal wellbeing should be in place. This can be performed by ultrasound imaging, foetal heart rate monitoring or cardiotochography (Vincent and Frise, 2018) and should be undertaken by trained professionals.

For antenatal women a plan should be in place for an emergency delivery, including peri mortem Caesarean section. Emergency drugs should be available, for example, **syntocinon** and **ergometrine**. Neonatal resuscitation equipment should also be easily accessible (Vincent and Frise, 2018).

Timing of delivery requires a multidisciplinary plan. Consideration should be given to whether delivery of the foetus will improve the maternal condition. The risks to the mother and the risks of a preterm birth for the foetus need to be carefully assessed (Roberts et al., 2017).

Infant feeding and care

Following birth admission to a critical care unit should not mean the automatic separation of woman and baby if the baby is well. Priority should be given where possible to keeping mother and baby together (RCOA, 2018). Contact between the woman and baby should be encouraged. Routine postnatal and neonatal care should be offered, for example breastfeeding support. Breastfeeding is often considered a return to normality for women who have undergone a traumatic birthing experience and should be encouraged as soon as the woman feels able to do so (Hinton et al., 2015). Establishing breastfeeding can be difficult for women who have been very unwell and milk production may be delayed. Infant bonding and attachment will also have been affected. You should encourage skin to skin contact. This has been proven to have many benefits for both the woman and the baby, least of all aiding the bonding and feeding processes which likely have been interrupted during the admission to ACCU. If the woman is too unwell to breastfeed, expression of breast milk should be facilitated to maintain lactation (Marino et al., 2019). Access to breast pumps and support staff to assist with this will be necessary. Women who have been acutely unwell perceive the ability to breastfeed their baby as a return to normality. Breastfeeding support therefore should be made available regardless of the location of care (NICE, 2015).

For women who have been unconscious it is important to document clearly the type and amount of feed that a baby has tolerated. Evidence of the care received by the baby will offer comfort and support to a woman who may be psychologically traumatised by the early separation (Spencer, 2007). For women whose babies are on the neonatal unit it is important to reunite them as soon as the physical condition of the woman allows. For those women who are unable to move from critical care it is important to have contact with their baby. Photographs or videos can be used to support this in the early days and regular verbal or written updates could be provided by neonatal staff or family (Knight et al., 2016).

Any medications given to a women who is breastfeeding or who intends to breastfeed should be checked to ensure they are safe to administer. Your midwifery colleagues will be able to support you with this. Clear records of any medications administered to the mother should be recorded for midwives to manage the suitability of any feed to be provided to the baby.

ACTIVITY 14.7: REFLECTIVE PRACTICE

You are looking after a woman who is sedated and ventilated.

1. Consider how you think this will impact on attachment and bonding
2. What steps could you take to support and improve this?
3. Who else could you ask to help you with this task?

Bereavement care

Sadly you may be asked to care for women who have suffered a neonatal loss. It is well documented that the care women receive at this time has long term implications for the parents' mental health and the support they receive is the single most crucial factor in their response to grief (Doherty et al., 2018). Women should be supported to spend time saying goodbye to their baby if facilities allow. Bereavement midwives are specially trained to provide ongoing support.

ACTIVITY 14.8: REFLECTIVE PRACTICE

THIS TOPIC IS ALSO COVERED IN CHAPTER 15

1. Consider how you would support a woman and her family who had experienced a stillbirth or neonatal loss
2. This can be a very emotional time. How can you manage your own feelings?
3. Think about what may worry you the most about this scenario.
4. Who could you ask to support you?

Ongoing support

All women should be offered a multidisciplinary postnatal review with clinicians with the necessary expertise, for example, midwives, clinical psychologists and other specialities as determined by the needs of the patient.

ACTIVITY 14.9: CRITICAL THINKING

Read Vincent, L.J. and Frise, C.J. (2018) 'Management of the critically-ill obstetric patient', *Obstetrics, Gynaecology & Reproductive Medicine*, 28 (8): 243–52.

www.sciencedirect.com/science/article/pii/S175172141830112X (accessed November 11, 2020).

1. What do you think women may experience during their critical care stay?
2. What strategies could you put in place to resolve some of the issues highlighted in the paper?

For many women finding themselves on a critical care unit comes as a complete shock. Some just wake up in a strange environment with no recollection of events that have led to the transfer. These women are more susceptible to **depression** and **post-traumatic stress disorder** (Desai et al., 2011). Opportunities should be given for women to debrief and ask questions (Hinton et al., 2015). Understanding the emergency and trail of events is important for women to come to terms with the events. Talking with clinicians involved and going through case notes will support this when the woman feels able (Knight et al., 2016). Ongoing counselling should also be considered once a woman has been discharged from critical care.

THIS TOPIC IS ALSO COVERED IN CHAPTER 15

Documentation provides a method of communication for both the woman and the professionals providing care. It should clearly demonstrate a sequence of events and should inform women of the care they have received, their needs and priorities. Healthcare professionals should use specific hand-held maternity records, the postnatal care plans and personal child health records, to promote this communication with women (NICE, 2015). For some women, particularly those who have been unconscious for a period of time, it might clarify their understanding of events of the care they received.

This is particularly important for women who find themselves in a multidisciplinary care environment where multiple disciplines may have input into her care (Kerkin et al., 2018). Women should be asked regularly about their emotional wellbeing, family and social support and whether they are feeling able to cope with daily routine, which may be very different in a critical care environment (NICE, 2015).

THIS TOPIC IS ALSO COVERED IN CHAPTER 17

CHAPTER SUMMARY

This chapter has supported your understanding of:

- Why women in pregnancy or following childbirth might require critical care
- Midwifery emergencies such as haemorrhage, hypertension, maternal collapse and sepsis which can result in the transfer of women to an ACCU
- A – E approach of assessment of the critically unwell obstetric patient
- Additional needs and support requirements of the antenatal or postnatal woman on an ACCU

GO FURTHER

Books

Marshall, J. and Raynor, M. (2014) *Myles Textbook for Midwives* (16th edition). Edinburgh: Churchill Livingstone.

- This basic midwifery textbook will provide you with an overall understanding of any aspect of midwifery care. A clear understanding of normal care and expectations will help you to support high risk women on the ACCU.

Baston, H. and Hall, J. (eds) (2018) *Midwifery Essentials: Emergency Maternity Care Volume 6.* Edinburgh: Elsevier.

- This basic text will give you further insight into the different midwifery emergencies that might result in a woman requiring critical care.

Boyle, M. and Bothamley, J. (2018) *Critical Care Assessment By Midwives.* Abingdon: Routledge.

- Following on from the previous text this will help you to recognise and understand deviations from the norm and help you to care for the acutely unwell woman.

Journal articles

Doherty, J., Cullen, S., Casey, B., Lloyd, B., Sheehy, L., Brosnan, M., Barry, T., McMahon, A. and Coughlan, B. (2018) 'Bereavement care education and training in clinical practice: Supporting the development of confidence in student midwives', *Midwifery, 66*: 1–9.

Gaffney, A. (2014) 'Critical care in pregnancy, is it different?' *Seminars Perinatology*, 38 (6): 329–40.

Hinton, L., Locock, L., and Knight, M. (2015) 'Maternal critical care: What can we learn from patient experience? A qualitative study', *BMJ Open*, 5 (4): e006676.

- The three articles listed above will provide you with an insight into critical care from different perspectives.

Useful websites

Royal College of Anaesthetists (RCOA) (2018) 'Care of the critically ill woman in childbirth: Enhanced maternal care'. London: RCOA. www.rcoa.ac.uk/sites/default/files/documents/2020-06/EMC-Guidelines2018.pdf (accessed November 11, 2020).

- This website will help you to understand why women in the childbirth continuum require critical care and how best this is facilitated.

National Institute for Health and Care Excellence (NICE) (2017) *Intrapartum Care for Healthy Women and Babies* (Clinical Guideline 190) London: NICE. Available from www.nice.org.uk/guidance/cg190 (accessed November 11, 2020).

National Institute for Health and Care Excellence (NICE) (2019a) *Caesarean Section* (Clinical Guideline 132). London: NICE. Available from www.nice.org.uk/guidance/cg132 (accessed November 11, 2020).

National Institute for Health and Care Excellence (NICE) (2019b) *Hypertension in Pregnancy: Diagnoses and Management* (NICE Guideline 133). London: NICE. Available from www.nice.org.uk/guidance/ng133 (accessed November 11, 2020).

• These three documents will give you an understanding of the pathways of care available to all pregnant women from the low risk pregnancy through to those with more complex needs.

REFERENCES

Baston, H. (2014) 'Antenatal Care', in J. Marshall and M. Rayno (eds), *Myles Textbook for Midwives*. Edinburgh: Churchill Livingstone Elsevier. pp. 179–202.

Begley, C. (2014) 'Physiology and care during the third stage of labour', in J. Marshall and M. Raynor (eds), *Myles Textbook for Midwives* (16th edition). Edinburgh: Churchill Livingstone. pp. 395–416.

Bick, D. and Hunter, C. (2017) 'Content and organisation of postnatal care,' in S. Macdonald and G. Johnson (eds), *Mayes Midwifery* (15th edition). Edinburgh: Elsevier. pp. 694–704.

Boyce, T., Dodd, C. and Waugh, J. (2008) 'Hypertensive Disorders', in S.E. Robson and J. Waugh. (eds) *Medical Disorders in Pregnancy: A Manual for Midwives*. Oxford: Blackwell Publishing.

Boyle, M. and Bothamley, J. (2018) *Critical Care Assessment by Midwives*. Abingdon: Routledge.

Brewster, J. (2017) 'Maternal and Newborn Resuscitation', in Boyle, M. (ed.) *Emergencies Around Childbirth: A Handbook for Midwives*. London: Routledge. pp. 19–36.

Desai, S.V., Law, T.J. and Needham, D.M. (2011) 'Long-term complications of critical care.' *Critical Care Medicine*, 39 (2): 371–9.

Dildy, G.A. and Belfort, M.A. (2010) 'Complications of preeclampsia', in M.A. Belfort, M.D. Saade, M.R. Foley, P. Phelan and D.A. Dildy (eds) *Critical Care Obstetrics* (5th edition). Oxford: Wiley-Blackwell. pp. 438–645.

Doherty, J., Cullen, S., Casey, B., Lloyd, B., Sheehy, L., Brosnan, M., Barry, T., McMahon, A. and Coughlan, B. (2018) 'Bereavement care education and training in clinical practice: Supporting the development of confidence in student midwives', *Midwifery*, 66: 1–9.

Gaffney, A. (2014) 'Critical care in pregnancy, is it different?' *Seminars in Perinatology*, 38 (6): 329–40.

Greer, O., Shah, N.M. and Johnson, M.R. (2020) 'Maternal sepsis update: Current management and controversies', *The Obstetrician & Gynaecologist*, 22 (1): 45–55.

Guntupalli, K.K., Hall, N., Karnad, D.R., Bandi, V. and Belfort, M. (2015) 'Critical illness in pregnancy, Part 1: An approach to the pregnant patient in the ICU and common obstetric disorders', *Contemporary Reviews in Critical Care Medicine*, 48 (4): 1093–104.

Hinton, L., Locock L., and Knight, M. (2015) 'Maternal critical care: What can we learn from patient experience? A qualitative study', *BMJ Open*, 5 (4): e006676.

Intensive Care and National Audit Research Centre (ICNARC) (2013) 'Female admissions (aged 16-50 years) to adult, critical care units in England, Wales and Northern Ireland, reported as "currently pregnant" or "recently pregnant"', London: ICNARC. https://www.oaa-anaes.ac.uk/assets/_managed/cms/files/Obstetric%20admissions%20to%20critical%20care%202009-2012%20-%20FINAL.pdf (accessed November 11, 2020).

Jackson, K., Marshall, J. and Brydon, S. (2014) 'Physiology and care during the first stage of labour,' in J. Marshall and M. Raynor (eds) *Myles Textbook for Midwives* (16th edition). Edinburgh: Churchill Livingstone. pp. 327–66.

Johnson, R. and Taylor, W. (2016) *Skills for Midwifery Practice* (4th edition). Edinburgh: Churchill Livingstone.

Kerkin, B., Lennox, S. and Patterson, J. (2018) 'Making midwifery work visible: The multiple purposes of documentation', *Women and Birth*, 31 (3): 232–9.

Knight, M., Acosta, C., Brocklehurst, P. et al (2016) *'Beyond Maternal Death: Improving the Quality of Maternal Care Through National Studies of 'Near-Miss' Maternal Morbidity*. Chapter 2. Unheard Voices: Women's and their partners' experiences of severe pregnancy complications. Programme Grants for Applied Research, 4 (9). pp. 5–18. Available from doi.org/10.3310/pgfar04090

Knight, M., Bunch, K., Tuffnell, D, Shakespeare, J., Kotnis, R., Kenyon, S. and Kurinczuk, J. (2019) *MBRRACE UK: Saving Lives, Improving Mothers Care – Lessons Learnt to Inform Future Maternity Care from the UK and Ireland Confidential Enquiries into Maternal Deaths and Morbidity 2015–2017.'* Oxford: NPEU.

Long, L. and Penna, L. (2018) 'Maternal Collapse', *Obstetrics, Gynaecology and Reproductive Medicine*, 28 (2): 46–52.

Marino, L.V., Kidd, C.S., Davies, N.J., Thomas, P.C., Williams, S.W. and Beattie, R.M. (2019) 'Survey of healthcare professional and parental experience in accessing support for breastfeeding during an acute hospital admission', *Acta Paediatrica*, 108 (1): 175–7.

Mavrides, E., Allard, S., Chandraharan, E., Collins, P., Green, L., Hunt, B.J., Riris, S. and Thomson, A.J. (2016) 'Prevention and management of postpartum haemorrhage (RCOG: Green-top Guideline 52)', *BJOG*, 124 (5): 106–49. Available from https://www.rcog.org.uk/en/guidelines-research-services/guidelines/gtg52/ (accessed November 11, 2020).

National Health Service Digital (NHS Digital) (2020) 'Maternity Services Monthly Statistics, Dec 2020, experimental statistics'. Leeds: NHS. Available from https://digital.nhs.uk/data-and-information/publications/statistical/maternity-services-monthly-statistics/september-2020 (accessed January 12, 2021).

National Institute for Health and Care Excellence (NICE) (2015) *Postnatal Care up to 8 Weeks after Birth* (Clinical Guideline 37), London: NICE. Available from https://www.nice.org.uk/guidance/cg37 (accessed November 11, 2020).

National Institute for Health and Care Excellence (NICE) (2017) *Intrapartum Care for Healthy Women and Babies* (Clinical Guideline 190). London: NICE. Available from https://www.nice.org.uk/guidance/cg190 (accessed November 11, 2020).

National Institute for Health and Care Excellence NICE (2019a) *Caesarean Section* (Clinical Guideline 132). London: NICE. Available from https://www.nice.org.uk/Guidance/cg132 (accessed November 11, 2020).

National Institute for Health and Care Excellence (NICE) (2019b) *Hypertension in Pregnancy: Diagnoses and Management* (NICE Guideline 132). London: NICE. Available from www.nice.org.uk/guidance/ng133 (accessed November 11, 2020).

Nursing and Midwifery Council (NMC) (2018) *The Code: Professional Standards of Practice and Behaviour for Nurses, Midwives and Aursing Associates.* London, NMC. https://www.nmc.org.uk/globalassets/sitedocuments/nmc-publications/nmc-code.pdf (accessed November 11, 2020).

Resuscitation Council UK (RCUK) (2015) *The ABCDE approach.* London: RCUK. Available from www.resus.org.uk/resuscitation-guidelines/abcde-approach/ (accessed November 11, 2020).

Robbins, T., Shennan, A. and Sandall, J. (2019) 'Modified early obstetric warning scores: A promising tool but more evidence and standardization is required,' *Acta Obstetricia et Gynecologica Scandinavica*, 98 (1): 7–10.

Roberts, D., Brown, J., Medley, N. and Dalziel, S.R. (2017) 'Antenatal corticosteroids for accelerating fetal lung maturation for women at risk of preterm birth', *The Cochrane Database of Systematic Reviews*, 3 (3): CD004454. doi.org/10.1002/14651858.CD004454.pub3

Robson, S.E., Marshall, J.E., Doughty, R. and McLean, M. (2014) 'Medical conditions of significance to midwifery practice', in J.E. Marshall and M. Raynor (eds) *Myles Textbook for Midwives* (16th edition). Edinburgh: Churchill Livingstone. pp. 243–86.

Royal College of Anaesthetists (RCOA) (2018) 'Care of the critically ill woman in childbirth: Enhanced maternal care', London: RCOA. https://www.rcoa.ac.uk/sites/default/files/documents/2020-06/EMC-Guidelines2018.pdf (accessed November 11, 2020).

Royal College of Obstetricians and Gynaecologists (RCOG) (2011) 'Antepartum haemorrhage (Green-top Guideline 63)', London: RCOG. https://www.rcog.org.uk/en/guidelines-research-services/guidelines/gtg63/ (accessed November 11, 2020).

Royal College of Obstetricians and Gynaecologists (RCOG) (2014) 'Maternal collapse in pregnancy and the puerperum (Green-top Guideline 56)', London: RCOG. https://www.rcog.org.uk/globalassets/documents/guidelines/gtg_56.pdf (accessed November 11, 2020).

Royal College of Physicians (RCP) (2017) *National Early Warning Score 2 (NEWS 2): Standardising the Assessment of Acute Illness Severity in the NHS*. London: RCP. Available from https://www.rcplondon.ac.uk/projects/outputs/national-early-warning-score-news-2 (accessed November 11, 2020).

Royal College of Psychiatrists (RCPSYCH) (2018) 'Postnatal Depression', London: Royal College of Psychiatrists. https://www.rcpsych.ac.uk/mental-health/problems-disorders/post-natal-depression (accessed November 11, 2020).

Spencer, L. (2007) 'Psychological Needs and Care of the Critically Ill Woman', in M. Billington and M. Stevenson (eds) *Critical Care in Childbearing for Midwives*. Oxford: Blackwell. pp. 257–70.

Steen, M. and Wray, J. (2014) 'Physiology and care during the puerperum', in J. Marshall and M. Raynor (eds) *Myles Textbook for Midwives* (16th edition). Edinburgh: Churchill Livingstone. pp. 499–514.

Stevenson, M. and Billington, M. (2007) 'Hypertensive Disorders and the Critically Ill Woman', in M. Billington and M. Stevenson (eds) *Critical Care in Childbearing for Midwives*. Oxford: Blackwell. pp. 91–117.

Vincent, L.J. and Frise, C.J. (2018) 'Management of the critically-ill obstetric patient.' *Obstetrics, Gynaecology & Reproductive Medicine*, 28 (8): 243–52.

World Health Organisation (WHO) (2012) *WHO Recommendations for the Prevention and Treatment of Postpartum Haemorrhage*. Geneva: WHO.

THE PSYCHOLOGICAL CARE OF THE CRITICALLY ILL

SAMANTHA FREEMAN

> " I was so frightened; at times I didn't know if I was dead or alive. I kept asking the nurses if I was in heaven.
>
> **Philip, 58-year-old, extended critical care stay following complications post-cardiac surgery** "

> " I couldn't understand why the staff didn't do anything about all the spiders over my bed and on the ceiling. I kept shouting but they couldn't hear me. After I realised it was a hallucination but at the time it's so real.
>
> **Aroush, 35-year-old, critical care stay following a car accident** "

LEARNING OUTCOMES

When you have finished studying this chapter you will be able to understand:

- The significant psychological effect a critical care stay can have on someone
- How to identify delirium, its assessment, and some management strategies
- The effects of sensory deprivation, sensory overload, and sleep disorder
- The potential longer-term impact of critical illness and some strategies for support
- How we can best support visitors to critical care

INTRODUCTION

In this chapter, will provide you with the evidence base surrounding the increased risk of psychological disorders following a critical care admission. Topics covered may have been mentioned earlier in the book but now we will be looking in more detail about the effect of sensory deprivation, sensory overload, and sleep disorder. We will explore the assessment and management of **delirium** using current guidelines, assessment tools, and **interventions**. We will also explore the possible longer-term effects of a period of critical illness on people's mental health. We will look at some potential strategies which may help support both those with a critical illness and their relatives/significant other during and following this period in their lives. In this chapter, we have also included the support required by visitors to the critical care unit.

THE PHYCOLOGICAL IMPACT OF CRITICAL ILLNESS

Critical care environments are stressful places and it's not surprising that a number of those who experience a critical illness experience fear, panic, depressed mood, and anger (Wade et al., 2018). Following a period of critical illness, some people may have positive emotions and feel grateful, however many experience negative feelings that can have a significant impact on their mental well-being. Symptoms that occur include intrusive memories, delusions, delirium, or panic nightmares. Conditions such as depression, anxiety, **post-traumatic stress disorder** (PTSD), and cognitive dysfunction are increasingly evident in people following a critical care admission and are described collectively as 'post-intensive care syndrome' (Clancy et al., 2015). Post intensive care syndrome and the subsequent symptoms experienced are major clinical concerns that can persist for several years after discharge from critical care and hospital (Vlake et al., 2020). There are several interventions to help prevent or reduce the psychological impact of critical illness, but the evidence is inconclusive regarding their effectiveness. This is possibly because there is such a diverse population requiring critical care each with individual needs, emphasising the need for person-centred care.

DELIRIUM

The presence of delirium during a period of critical illness is very common. It is important to remember that this is a reversible condition. It is an acute syndrome with disorders of attention and cognitive function and can have increased or decreased psychomotor activity with a disordered sleep-wake cycle (Borthwick et al., 2014). What you also need to be aware of is that there are three subtypes of delirium: hyperactive, hypoactive, and mixed delirium (Van Rompaey et al., 2008). The presence of delirium in any form has some serious short and possibly longer-term health consequences (van den Boogaard et al., 2011).

The National Institute for Health and Care Excellence (NICE, 2010) published guidelines covering the prevention, diagnosis and management of delirium. This document offers guidance around delirium management across healthcare settings, including Adult Critical Care Units (ACCU), helping to manage underlying causes and ensuring effective communication and re-orientation to time and place (NICE, 2010). The UK Intensive Care Society has also published guidance on the detection, prevention, and treatment of delirium (Borthwick et al., 2014). This provides guidance regarding the assessment of the critically ill, offering both non-pharmacological and pharmacological strategies for the prevention and management of delirium. Nurses in critical care have continuous contact with the critically ill person, and therefore are best placed to monitor fluctuations in delirium symptoms, ensure prompt recognition and instigate appropriate treatment (Zamoscik et al., 2017). However, there are still significant barriers to assessment and delirium remains underdiagnosed.

What are the risks of delirium?

Someone critically ill and experiencing delirium is at great risk of having a longer stay in critical care. In a meta-analysis looking at the presence of delirium in the ACCU population, Zhang et al. (2013) found the presence of delirium was associated with higher **mortality**, longer duration of mechanical ventilation, and longer hospital and ACCU stay. There are also longer-term implications with the presence of delirium linked to post-traumatic stress disorders and longer-term cognitive impairment (Hipp and Ely, 2012).

In the following activity, you will read a reflection about the experience of delirium from someone who has experienced this while in critical care.

ACTIVITY 15.1: REFLECTIVE PRACTICE

Read the reflections on delirium from the perspective of someone who has experienced this: https://journals.sagepub.com/doi/pdf/10.1177/1751143719851352 (accessed November 11, 2020).

1. Consider what you would find supportive if you were to experience a critical care stay. Discuss this with your peers, what are the differences and similarities in what you need?

Hyperactive delirium

The person experiencing hyperactive delirium, as you would expect, moves around a lot. They are hyperactively alert and agitated, experiencing delusions and hallucinations (van den Boogaard et al., 2011). They are generally easier to identify because of their actions, but clinical teams can find the behaviours more challenging to manage (Freeman et al., 2019). Self-extubation is related to the delirium subtype of 'hyperactive', when people demonstrate agitated behaviours (Zhang et al., 2013). The presence of agitation can mean that the person is inadvertently disconnecting their monitoring, infusion, and ventilation (Burk et al., 2014). It is very distressing for the person to experience this level of anxiety and it is also very distressing for the family to witness.

Hypoactive and mixed delirium

The person experiencing hypoactive delirium is lethargic and withdrawn but they may still be experiencing delusions and hallucinations. It is felt that this subtype is underdiagnosed. The mixed subtype is a fluctuation between both hyper and hypo delirious states (Borthwick et al., 2014). To distinguish between the subtypes of delirium the Richmond Agitation Sedation Scale (RASS) is commonly used (Ely et al., 2001).

Delirium assessment tools

Across the UK and globally there are several different tools to help support us to recognise delirium in the critically ill. The main two you will see and use are the Confusion Assessment Method for the Intensive Care Unit (CAM-ICU) and the Intensive Care Delirium Screening Checklist (ICDSC). The next activity asks you to consider the pros and cons of undertaking such an assessment.

ACTIVITY 15.2: CRITICAL THINKING

Assessing the presence of delirium using either of the tools mentioned above should take around 2-5 minutes and can be carried out by the nurse at the bedside.

1. What are the positives of such an assessment for both the person potentially experiencing delirium and the assessor?
2. What are the possible negative aspects of using such assessment tools?
3. What can the team put in place to support an effective assessment of delirium?

ACTIVITY 15.3: THEORY STOP POINT

Read the paper below that compares both assessment tools.

Nishimura, K. et al. (2016) 'Sensitivity and specificity of the Confusion Assessment Method for the Intensive Care Unit (CAM-ICU) and the Intensive Care Delirium Screening Checklist (ICDSC) for detecting post-cardiac surgery delirium: A single-center study in Japan', *Heart & Lung: The Journal of Cardiopulmonary and Acute Care*, 45 (1): 15-20. doi.org/10.1016/j.hrtlng.2015.11.001

1. What are the limitations of this paper's findings?
2. Discuss with your practice supervisor or peers about why the department you are in has selected a particular tool over the others available

There is no template answer to Question 2 as it is based on your own experience.

As explored in the previous activity, there are different tools to assess delirium. Once we have established that the person we are caring for is experiencing an episode of delirium, we need to reassure them and the family that this is a transient stage and outline the steps we will take to promote a quick recovery. The person's recovery from delirium can be supported via both pharmacological and non-pharmacological measures.

Agitation

Understandably, agitation is also common in those waking from a period of **sedation** during their critical illness. Agitation is not delirium but is often discussed together. The terms agitation, anxiety, and delirium are often used interchangeably, which sometimes is not helpful, particularly when trying to make sense of the evidence base. Agitation has been described as a psychomotor disturbance, characterised by an increase in motor and psychological activities (Chevrolet and Jolliet, 2007). This increase in activity can again result in accidental removal of vital equipment, causing harm or delay to recovery. Guidelines for the prevention and management of agitation are within the **P**ain, **A**gitation/sedation, **D**elirium, **I**mmobility, and **S**leep disruption international guidance, known as PADIS (Devlin et al., 2018). The working party that produced these guidelines consisted of 32 international experts, four methodologists, and four critical illness survivors. The guidelines are also endorsed by all key international critical care-related societies. The guidance offers 37 recommendations, two good practice statements, and 32 ungraded, nonactionable statements. Although agitation is in the title of the guideline, the recommendations related to agitation are found within other key areas such as sedation practice and the use of physical restraint. Summarised in Table 15.1 are the extracted recommendations related to agitation, alongside the type and quality of the evidence on which the recommendation is based.

Table 15.1   Summary of agitation related recommendations

Recommendation	Type	Quality of evidence
Light sedation (vs deep sedation) in critically ill, mechanically ventilated adults	Conditional recommendation	Low quality of evidence
Not using haloperidol or an atypical antipsychotic to treat subsyndromal delirium in critically ill adults	Conditional recommendation	Very low to low quality of evidence
Dexmedetomidine for delirium in mechanically ventilated adults where agitation is precluding weaning/extubation	Conditional recommendation	Low quality of evidence

Source: Adapted from Devlin et al. (2018). Reproduced by kind permission of Wolters Kluwer Health.

The limited number of recommendations directly addressing agitation could be due to the complexity of the reasons related to agitation and its development. The complex nature of agitation development can hamper recognition of the underlying causes; additionally, there are limited assessment tools to support this process (Kydonaki et al., 2019).

ACTIVITY 15.4: CRITICAL THINKING

1. Other than delirium, list the things that may make a person agitated during their critical illness
2. Now consider what strategies you and the clinical team could put in place to reduce the chances of agitation occurring

Discuss these with your practice supervisor or peers. What are their views and experiences?

MANAGEMENT OF DELIRIUM

Before we look at what medication may help, we need to consider that it is not just what is prescribed and what we administer that are important, but also whether there are any medications contributing to delirium. There are some drugs we use in critical care that can contribute to delirium development: ask a pharmacist to review the person's prescription, are there any medications that could contribute to delirium development, and can these be stopped?

Pharmacological management

Antipsychotics

Antipsychotics are frequently administered as a treatment of delirium, with haloperidol often being the drug of choice. However, there is limited data regarding the safety and efficacy of administering antipsychotics for the treatment of delirium in the critical care setting (Peitz et al., 2013). Benzodiazepines are also often used if the delirium is linked to alcohol or benzodiazepine withdrawal syndromes (Borthwick et al., 2014). As mentioned earlier, some of the medication we administer can contribute to delirium development and ironically the antipsychotics group of medications is one considered to contribute to delirium development.

Alpha-2 agonists

As a result of the increasing evidence linking the use of antipsychotics to delirium development in the critically unwell, there has been an increased interest in seeking different medications for sedation and analgesia. The group of medications known as alpha-2 agonists has shown some potential as a safe pharmacological therapeutic approach. Two common medications you will find within this group are clonidine and dexmedetomidine.

WHAT'S THE EVIDENCE?

Read the two papers below to support your understanding of the pharmacological agents mentioned. Borthwick et al. (2014) offer a summary of common medications we use in critical care that are actually linked to delirium development. Hipp and Ely (2012) provide a good comparison and overview of the pharmacology related to the medications mentioned. They also offer some suggestions for non-pharmacological approaches.

Borthwick, M., Bourne, R., Craig, M., Egan, A. and Oxley, J. (2014) 'Detection, prevention and treatment of delirium in critically ill patients (Version 1.2)'. London: The Intensive Care Society. https://www.wyccn.org/uploads/6/5/1/9/65199375/ukcpa_delirium_2006_1[1].pdf (accessed November 12, 2020).

Hipp, D.M. and Ely, E.W. (2012) 'Pharmacological and nonpharmacological management of delirium in critically ill patients', *Neurotherapeutics*, 9 (1): 158-75. doi.org/10.1007/s13311-011-0102-9

You can also review any of the medications mentioned in the British National Formulary (BNF) available in paper copy or online via https://bnf.nice.org.uk/ (accessed November 11, 2020).

Non-pharmacological approaches

There is evidence to suggest that in addition to considering the medications we are administering to the person there are non-pharmacological interventions that are effective in decreasing the incidence of delirium (Hshieh et al., 2015). Additionally, we currently do not have sufficient evidence to suggest that the medications previously mentioned are effective in hypodelirium. In the next activity, we consider what non-pharmacological interventions could be used.

We can all think about things that would aid our comfort and reassure us if we were unwell. The challenge we have when someone is critically unwell, we often cannot ask them what would help. Another challenge when trying to underpin our practice with the current evidence base concerning the use of non-pharmacological interventions, is the huge variability in the research as to what this entails. Often research studies have flaws, as we cannot account for a lot of the variables related to non-pharmacological interventions. Another factor to consider when you are reading the research is the lack of consent language when discussing non-pharmacological interventions. A lot of studies use phrases such as 'therapeutic measures' but may not offer a definition as to what these are. It seems logical that we would ensure the person is aware of where they are, what day it is and what time, as these factors can often be difficult for the person to remember or guess when in a brightly lit, highly technical department. The approaches to humanise critical care were covered in Chapter 2.

THIS TOPIC IS ALSO COVERED IN CHAPTER 2

The use of physical restraint

You may find the thought of using physical restraint upsetting or worrying and this is understandable, but to use, or not, is not a simple question to answer. We acknowledge that there is a huge ethical issue surrounding the restriction of someone's movement using physical restraint. Before reading this section, you may want to jot down your initial thoughts about it. You may or may not alter your view with further reading but you will need to understand that you will witness its use and you need to therefore consider how you will feel when this happens.

The use of physical restraint to prevent treatment interference remains prevalent in critical care departments worldwide (Perez et al., 2019), although the prevalence of use varies greatly between countries (Devlin et al., 2018). A clear, consistent, single definition of what constitutes physical restraint is lacking across the critical care community (Freeman et al., 2016). Definitions offered describe physical restraint as:

> all patient articles, straps, bed linen and vest, used as an intervention to restrict a person's freedom of movement or access to their own body

> (Martin and Mathisen, 2005: 134)

Additionally, restraint could be viewed as any device that was attached to the person to limit voluntary movement with the explicit inclusion of wrist and chest restraints, mittens and elbow splints, as well as bedsheets, whilst many studies exclude the use of bedside rails as a form of restraint (Mion et al., 2007). In the UK, physical restraints are manufactured products that are either padded gloves or 'mitts' (Treece and Baker, 2019). Internationally, four-point restraints are used (Luk et al., 2015). The focus of the above definitions fails to reflect the process of restraining people via chemical means; ensuring compliance with treatment by increasing sedation needs to be acknowledged as a form of restraint.

In addition to professional codes of conduct, clinical guidelines have been produced around physical restraint within critical care in the UK (Bray et al., 2004) and in America (Maccioli et al., 2003); both over a decade old. Across the guidance, the use of physical restraint when managing agitation in ACC is neither explicit nor supported by robust evidence. Recommendations from research have been that physical restraint should only be used once other therapeutic measures have proved ineffectual (Freeman et al., 2016; Jaber, 2005; Martin and Mathisen, 2005; Mion et al., 2007; Turgay et al., 2009). What is omitted across is the guidance is at what point therapeutic measures are deemed to be ineffectual, resulting in the use of either physical restraint or sedation. The use of physical restraint is a contentious issue that may generate disparate views both across and within professional groups. Additionally, the long-term psychological impact of the use of physical restraint during critical illness remains unknown.

ACTIVITY 15.5: REFLECTIVE PRACTICE AND CRITICAL THINKING

Consider the following statement as a definition of physical restraint:

> A way to use recognised and appropriate measures to control a person's movement, either with a device or holding, to purposefully stop them from causing harm to themselves or others even if this is against their will.

Reflect on this statement and discuss your thoughts with your peers.

1. When do you think 'holding' someone moves from comfort to restraint?

ACTIVITY 15.6: CASE STUDY

Rafaat is 67 years old and has been ventilated in the critical care department for four months following complications post cardiac surgery. During the day shift, he is withdrawn and sleepy and his family says he does not communicate with them. On the night shift, Rafaat becomes agitated and aggressive, trying to pull out his tracheostomy and succeeds in getting out of the bed. The nightshift staff administered haloperidol to re-sedate him and keep him safe. You are on the morning shift; the staff nurse you are shadowing say it's best to let Rafaat sleep.

1. What do you think is the risk in the day nurse's approach?
2. What assessment do you think is important to help support Rafaat's recovery?
3. How do you think you could support the family to help with Rafaat's recovery?

LONGER-TERM PSYCHOLOGICAL IMPACT OF CRITICAL ILLNESS

Depression

When reading the research around this topic of the longer-term psychological effect of a critical illness, what can be challenging is that anxiety, depression and PTSD are often studied together, and the terms used interchangeably across the literature. However, depression is a psychological illness characterised by continued feelings of sadness and disinterest as well as several physical symptoms such as problems with sleep. One study, exploring anxiety, found depressive symptoms occurred in around 29% of survivors at 3, 6 and 12 months following discharge from critical care (Nikayin et al., 2016). It has also been shown that when symptoms of one psychological condition are present, there is a 64% chance they will occur in parallel with other symptoms (Hatch et al., 2018). The psychological impact of critical illness is a major clinical concern that may persist for several years after discharge from critical care (Vlake et al., 2020). It has been suggested that depression could occur due to inflammation or neurotransmitter imbalances caused by sepsis (Battle et al., 2015). In addition to sepsis, several contributory factors can lead to the development of depression following critical care.

ACTIVITY 15.7: CRITICAL THINKING

1. List all the reasons you can think of as to why depression may develop post critical care.

Discuss these and any possible intervention or supportive measures you can think of with your practice supervisor or peers.

The UK National Institute for Health and Care Excellence guideline on rehabilitation from critical illness recommends that those experiencing high stress levels should be identified and offered psychological support as part of a recovery plan. In the next 'theory stop point' take a look at the NICE recommendations and consider how these can be embedded in our practice.

ACTIVITY 15.8: THEORY STOP POINT

Read the following guidance from NICE, noting the key elements of care and the focus on pre-care for critical care unit stay, and consider the limitations of these recommendations.

www.nice.org.uk/guidance/cg83 (accessed November 12, 2020).

1. Consider the current NHS system and how we discharge people from one department to another and then home. What challenges do you think there are to ensuring the person's rehabilitation needs 2–3 months after their discharge from critical care are met?
2. How could these challenges be overcome?

Post intensive care syndrome

THIS TOPIC IS ALSO COVERED IN CHAPTER 17

Any new or worsening physical, psychological, or mental health issue following critical care is referred to as post-intensive care syndrome (PICS). The physical elements of this syndrome are covered in Chapter 17.

Here we will discuss the psychological and mental health of patients post critical care. Depression, anxiety, and post-traumatic stress disorder (PTSD) are the group of mental illnesses that are encompassed within PICS.

As a consequence of critical illness, family members of the critical illness survivor can also be adversely affected. This is referred to as PICS-Family (Rawal et al., 2017). The psychological conditions experienced in families include anxiety, depression, acute stress disorder, PTSD, and complicated grief (Inoue et al., 2019).

THIS TOPIC IS ALSO COVERED IN CHAPTER 3

One of the most important roles for us as nurses is to ensure we provide support and effective communication at all times to both the unwell person and their family. We must ensure continuous implementation of measures to prevent the development of PICS via the use of the ABCDE care bundle covered in Chapter 3

Also, diaries may be a useful tool to support incomplete memories or help families discuss how they felt. The effectiveness of diaries as a psychological tool remains unproven. Another support strategy that can help is the establishment of follow up clinics and services to support ongoing rehabilitation, and discuss and support psychological or mental health symptoms.

THIS TOPIC IS ALSO COVERED IN CHAPTER 17

Supporting visitors and family

It is important that families are also a focus of our care in the critical care environment. The critical care environment can be incomprehensible to the individual waking from sedation (Meriläinen et al., 2013). Having family connection during critical illness has been linked in previous research to feelings of security and a way to alleviate stress (Al-Mutair et al., 2014; Cutler et al., 2013). The promotion of family visitation is also meaningful for the visitors who often express feelings of distress when excluded (Blom et al., 2013). Family members carry intimate knowledge of the person in your care that could support their re-orientation to reality, whilst providing reassurance from a familiar contact (Mitchell et al., 2017). Family-centred critical care should include nursing interventions that promote the health needs of family caregivers (Dale et al., 2020). Supporting families when visiting is essential and any involvement needs to be appropriate for both the family member and the critically unwell person (Mitchell et al., 2017). To facilitate and promote family involvement and person-centred visitation, families need to be prepared. Most critical care departments have family information resources and the charity ICUsteps provides a guide for families and those experiencing critical illness which you can look through in the next activity. After the activity there is a link to a short editorial on how we can best support children when they visit adult intensive care.

ACTIVITY 15.9: REFLECTIVE PRACTICE AND CRITICAL THINKING

ICUsteps is a charity organisation that supports people and their families following a critical illness. Take a look at their website: https://icusteps.org/home/patients (accessed November 12, 2020).
This is an excellent resource developed by people who have been in critical care.

1. Do you think we should depend on such a charity or should all of this information be provided by the National Health Service?
2. Do you think any sections of society may not be able to access such a resource? Who do you think this may be and how do you think we can overcome this?

WHAT'S THE EVIDENCE?

When families visit there is often a discussion about children visiting either due to the person in critical care being the parent or the visitor lacking childcare. In an attempt to protect children, some staff within critical care try to limit children visiting, but we need to remember that person-centred care extends to the family and to that child. What can be helpful and supportive for one child may have a negative effect on another child.

Read the short editorial by Hersov (2014) and then discuss with your peers what the local policy is on supporting children visiting in critical care.

Hersov, K. (2014) 'Supporting children with relatives in the intensive care unit', *Journal of the Intensive Care Society*, 15 (3): 188–9. https://journals.sagepub.com/doi/pdf/10.1177/175114371401500302 (accessed November 12, 2020).

ICUsteps have developed an activity booklet for children:

https://icusteps.org/information/visiting-the-icu (accessed November 12, 2020).

ACTIVITY 15.10: CASE STUDY

Dala is a 47-year-old man who has been discharged home. He spent four months in the critical care department and then three weeks on the ward after pituitary tumour complications following a stem cell transplant. He is back with you for his follow up visit eight weeks after he left the hospital. He becomes tearful saying has not slept and he keeps having dreams. He says, in the dream, 'It's dark and I'm strapped up to these wires and tubes and there was someone running around the room purposefully hitting my ventilator and then stopping it'. He also says he can't stop thinking of the noises of the sounds of the machines: 'it's as though they are talking to you all the time saying my name over and over'. His wife and son are also with him. His wife expresses concern that he is still not back to his normal self and needs to go back to work as his sick pay will run out.

1. What assessment could he have had before he was discharged home?
2. What other potential symptoms could you ask him about?
3. What support may the family need?
4. Who within the multidisciplinary team can you refer Dala and his family to?

THE POTENTIAL IMPACT OF COVID

Severe Acute Respiratory Syndrome Coronavirus 2 (SARS-CoV-2), the virus responsible for the Covid-19 (WHO, 2020) pandemic was declared by WHO in March 2020, and data regarding the increased occurrence of agitation is clearly limited. The virus destroys the respiratory tract but also has a significant impact on the person's neurobiology (Kotfis et al., 2020). In addition to the factors ever-present in critical care contributing to agitation development, some of the recommended treatments for Covid-19 require deeper levels of sedation. In China, 16 expert clinicians caring for those with Covid-19 generated 46 recommendations for management. The quality of the evidence underpinning each recommendation was assessed using the **G**rade of **R**ecommendation, **A**ssessment, **D**evelopment, and **E**valuation (GRADE). The early use of **prone** positioning and Extra Corporeal Membrane Oxygenation (ECMO) were both based on strong (Grade 1) evidence (Shang et al., 2020). Both interventions required deeper levels of sedation. It was also commented on that in Wuhan, 'deep sedation was extremely important for reducing oxygen consumption and developing tolerance to mechanical ventilation' (Shang et al., 2020: 15). Light sedation was recommended where possible due to the increased risk of agitation and delirium; this recommendation was based on expert opinion (Shang et al., 2020). In addition to these factors, the pandemic has created a circumstance of reduced human contact and distancing from family (Kotfis et al., 2020). The facilitation of the non-pharmacological interventions discussed above may be extremely limited. Ensuring families stay connected via novel technological options for communication needs to be considered (Kotfis et al., 2020).

The initial focus during the pandemic was the organisational issues such as creating critical care space and ensuring adequate personal protection equipment. We now need to consider how humanised, person-centred care can be safely supported. The longer-term effect of a critical care admission due to Covid-19 can only be speculated upon, but it appears that the risk of complications such as depression and PTSD or post-intensive care syndrome may be exacerbated (Kotfis et al., 2020). This risk could be particularly heightened if those with a critical illness experience agitation or delirium while separated from their families.

One thing you need to consider as we are coming to the end of this chapter is that a lot of research studies exploring the experiences of critical illness handle the phenomena of critical illness as a central point. However, the entire critical illness experience requires attention, encompassing the time spent in the critical care department, as well as the surrounding events (Cutler et al., 2013). Critical care research needs to span the entire critical illness trajectory to help understand the longer-term implications of the care delivered.

CHAPTER SUMMARY

This chapter has supported your understanding of:

- The significant impact critical illness has on the person's psychological wellbeing
- The incidence of delirium, its assessment, and some management strategies
- The potential longer-term impact of critical illness and some strategies for support

GO FURTHER

Books

Page, V.J. and Ely, E.W. (2015) *Delirium in Critical Care*. Cambridge: Cambridge University Press.

- This book is probably one of the best books to give you all the information about delirium prevention, diagnoses, and management.

Stevens, R.D., Hart, N. and Herridge, M.S. (eds) (2014) *Textbook of Post-ICU Medicine: The Legacy of Critical Care*. Oxford: Oxford University Press.

- Although quite medically focused, it is written by an interdisciplinary group. The book is an excellent reference point for nurses caring for long term ICU survivors as well as specialists in intensive care medicine, neurology, psychiatry, and rehabilitation medicine.

White, S.J. and Tait, D. (2019) *Critical Care Nursing: The Humanised Approach*. London: Sage.

- This book explores critical care cases with a holistic approach.

Journal articles

Freeman, S., Yorke, J., and Dark, P. (2019) 'The management of agitation in adult critical care: Views and opinions from the multi-disciplinary team using a survey approach', *Intensive and Critical Care Nursing*. https://doi.org/10.1016/j.iccn.2019.05.004

- This article explores the views of the multi-disciplinary team on how agitation is managed in critical care.

Inoue, S., Hatakeyama, J., Kondo, Y., Hifumi, T., Sakuramoto, H., Kawasaki, T. [...] and Nishida, O. (2019) 'Post-intensive care syndrome: Its pathophysiology, prevention, and future directions', *Acute Medicine & Surgery*, 6 (3): 233–46. https://www.ncbi.nlm.nih.gov/pmc/articles/PMC6603316/ (accessed November 12, 2020).

- This is a review article covering post-intensive care syndrome.

Rawal, G., Yadav, S., and Kumar, R. (2017) 'Post-intensive care syndrome: An overview', *Journal of Translational Internal Medicine*, 5 (2): 90–2.

- This article provides a good overview of post-intensive care syndrome.

Useful websites

www.nice.org.uk/sharedlearning/think-delirium-in-intensive-care (accessed November 12, 2020).

- This is a link to the NICE resources around delirium and its management.

https://www.bbc.co.uk/news/av/health-15881720 (accessed November 12, 2020).

- This is a link to a podcast by the Times journalist and commentator David Aaronovitch who has written vividly about a spell in an intensive care unit after complications set in for him after a routine operation.

www.youtube.com/watch?v=7yeDTmyMYIw (accessed November 12, 2020).

- This is a link to a brief video demonstrating how to perform the CAM-ICU test created by Manchester University NHS Foundation Trust Critical Care.

REFERENCES

Al-Mutair, A.S., Plummer, V., Clerehan, R. and O'Brien, A. (2014) 'Needs and experiences of intensive care patients' families: A Saudi qualitative study', *Nursing in Critical Care*, 19 (3): 135–44.

Battle, C., James, K. and Temblett, P. (2015) 'Depression following critical illness: Analysis of incidence and risk factors', *Journal of the Intensive Care Society*, 16 (2): 105–8.

Blom, H., Gustavsson, C. and Sundler, A.J. (2013) 'Participation and support in intensive care as experienced by close relatives of patients – A phenomenological study', *Intensive and Critical Care Nursing*, 29 (1): 1–8. doi.org/10.1016/j.iccn.2012.04.002

Borthwick, M., Bourne, R., Craig, M., Egan, A. and Oxley, J. (2014) *Detection, Prevention and Treatment of Delirium in Critically Ill Patients (Version 1.2)*. London: The Intensive Care Society. https://www.wyccn.org/uploads/6/5/1/9/65199375/ukcpa_delirium_2006_1[1].pdf (accessed November 12, 2020).

Bray, K., Hill, K., Robson, W., Leaver, G., Walker, N., O'Leary, M., Delaney, T., Walsh, D., Gager, M. and Waterhouse, C. (2004) 'British Association of Critical Care Nurses position statement on the use of restraint in adult critical care units', *Nursing in Critical Care*, 9: 199–212. www.ncbi.nlm.nih.gov/pubmed/15462118 (accessed November 11, 2020.

Burk, R.S., Grap, M.J., Munro, C.L., Schubert, C.M. and Sessler, C.N. (2014) 'Agitation onset, frequency, and associated temporal factors in critically ill adults', *American Journal of Critical Care*, 23 (4): 296–304. https://www.ncbi.nlm.nih.gov/pmc/articles/PMC4451814/ (accessed November 11, 2020).

Chevrolet, J.-C. and Jolliet, P. (2007) 'Clinical review: Agitation and delirium in the critically ill--significance and management', *Critical Care*, 11 (3): Article #214.

Clancy, O., Edginton, T., Casarin, A. and Vizcaychipi, M.P. (2015) 'The psychological and neurocognitive consequences of critical illness. A pragmatic review of current evidence', *Journal of the Intensive Care Society*, 16 (3): 226–33.

Cutler, L.R., Hayter, M. and Ryan, T. (2013) 'A critical review and synthesis of qualitative research on patient experiences of critical illness', *Intensive and Critical Care Nursing*, 29 (3): 147–57. doi.org/10.1016/j.iccn.2012.12.001

Dale, C.M., Carbone, S., Istanboulian, L., Fraser, I., Cameron, J.I., Herridge, M.S. and Rose, L. (2020) 'Support needs and health-related quality of life of family caregivers of patients requiring prolonged mechanical ventilation and admission to a specialised weaning centre: A qualitative longitudinal interview study', *Intensive and Critical Care Nursing*, 58: Article #102808. doi.org/10.1016/j.iccn.2020.102808

Devlin, J.W., Skrobik, Y., Gélinas, C., Needham, D.M., Slooter, A.J.C., Pandharipande, P.P., [...] and Alhazzani, W. (2018) 'Clinical practice guidelines for the prevention and management of pain, agitation/sedation , delirium, immobility, and sleep disruption in adult patients in the ICU', *Critical Care Medicine*, 46 (9): e825–e873. doi.org/10.1097/CCM.0000000000003299

Ely, E.W., Inouye, S.K., Bernard, G.R., Gordon, S., Francis, J., May, L., Truman, B., Margolin, R., Hart, R.P. and Dittus, R. (2001) 'Delirium in mechanically ventilated patients: Validity and reliability of the Confusion Assessment Method for the Intensive Care Unit (CAM-ICU)', *JAMA*, 286: 2703–10. http://jama.ama-assn.org/content/286/21/2703.short (accessed November 11, 2020).

Freeman, S., Yorke, J. and Dark, P. (2019) 'The management of agitation in adult critical care: Views and opinions from the multi-disciplinary team using a survey approach', *Intensive and Critical Care Nursing*, 54: 23–8. doi.org/10.1016/j.iccn.2019.05.004

Guyat, G.H., Oxman, A.D., Vist, G.E., Kunz, R., Falck-Ytter, Y., Alonso-Coello, P. and Schunemann, H.J. (2008) 'GRADE: An emerging consensus on rating quality of evidence and strength of recommendations', *BMJ*, 336: 924. doi: https://doi.org/10.1136/bmj.39489.470347.AD

Hersov, K. (2014) 'Supporting children with relatives in the intensive care unit', *Journal of the Intensive Care Society*, 15 (3): 188–9.

Hipp, D.M. and Ely, E.W. (2012) 'Pharmacological and nonpharmacological management of delirium in critically ill patients', *Neurotherapeutics*, 9 (1): 158–75. doi.org/10.1007/s13311-011-0102-9

Hshieh, T.T., Yue, J., Oh, E., Puelle, M., Dowal, S., Travison, T. and Inouye, S.K. (2015) 'Effectiveness of multicomponent nonpharmacological delirium interventions a meta-analysis', *JAMA Internal Medicine*, 175 (4): 512–20.

Inoue, S., Hatakeyama, J., Kondo, Y., Hifumi, T., Sakuramoto, H., Kawasaki, T., Taito, S., Nakamura, K., Unoki, T., Kawai, Y., Kenmotsu, Y., Saito, M., Yamakawa, K. and Nishida, O. (2019) 'Post-intensive care syndrome: Its pathophysiology, prevention, and future directions', *Acute Medicine & Surgery*, 6 (3): 233–46.

Kotfis, K., Williams Roberson, S., Wilson, J.E., Dabrowski, W., Pun, B.T. and Ely, E.W. (2020) 'COVID-19: ICU delirium management during SARS-CoV-2 pandemic', *Critical Care*, 24 (1): 1–9.

Kydonaki, K., Hanley, J., Huby, G., Antonelli, J. and Walsh, T.S. (2019) 'Challenges and barriers to optimising sedation in intensive care: A qualitative study in eight Scottish intensive care units', *BMJ Open*, 9 (5): 1–9.

Luk, E., Burry, L., Rezaie, S., Mehta, S. and Rose, L. (2015) 'Critical care nurses' decisions regarding physical restraints in two Canadian ICUs: A prospective observational study', *Canadian Journal of Critical Care Nursing*, 26 (4): 16–22.

Maccioli, G.A.G., Dorman, T., Brown, B.R., Mazuski, J.E., McLean, B.A., Kuszaj, J.M., Rosenbaum, S.H., Frankel, L.R., Devlin, J.W., Govert, J.A., Smith, B. and Peruzzi, W.T. (2003) 'Clinical practice guidelines for the maintenance of patient physical safety in the intensive care unit: Use of restraining therapies-American College of Critical Care Medicine Task Force 2001-2002', *Critical Care Medicine*, 31 (11): 2665–76.

Martin, B. and Mathisen, L. (2005) 'Use of physical restraints in adult critical care: A bicultural study', *American Journal of Critical Care*, 14: 133–42.

Meriläinen, M., Kyngäs, H. and Ala-Kokko, T. (2013) 'Patients' interactions in an intensive care unit and their memories of intensive care: A mixed method study', *Intensive and Critical Care Nursing*, 29 (2): 78–87. doi.org/10.1016/j.iccn.2012.05.003

Mion, L., Minnick, A., Leipzig, R.M., Catrambone, C.D. and Johnson, M.E. (2007) 'Patient-initiated device removal in intensive care units: A national prevalence study'. *Critical Care Medicine*, 35(12): 2714–20.

Mitchell, M.L., Kean, S., Rattray, J.E., Hull, A.M., Davis, C., Murfield, J.E. and Aitken, L.M. (2017) 'A family intervention to reduce delirium in hospitalised ICU patients: A feasibility randomised controlled trial', *Intensive and Critical Care Nursing*, 40: 77–84. doi.org/10.1016/j.iccn.2017.01.001

National Institute for Health and Care Excellence (NICE) (2010 [updated 2019]) 'Delirium: Prevention, diagnosis and management (Clinical Guideline 103)'. London: NICE. Available from https://www.nice.org.uk/guidance/cg103 (accessed November 11, 2020).

National Institute of Mental Health (2020) Post Traumatic Distress Disorder. U.S. Department of Health and Human Services, National Institutes of Health NIH Publication No. 20-MH-8124. https://www.nimh.nih.gov/health/publications/post-traumatic-stress-disorder-ptsd/20-mh-8124-ptsd_38054.pdf (accessed January, 14 2021).

Nikayin, S., Rabiee, A., Hashem, M.D., Huang, M., Bienvenu, O.J., Turnbull, A.E. and Needham, D.M. (2016) 'Anxiety symptoms in survivors of critical illness: A systematic review and meta-analysis', *General Hospital Psychiatry*, 43: 23–9. doi.org/10.1016/j.genhosppsych.2016.08.005

Nishimura, K., Yokoyama, K., Yamauchi, N., Koizumi, M., Harasawa, N., Yasuda, T. […] and Uchiide, Y. (2016) 'Sensitivity and specificity of the Confusion Assessment Method for the Intensive Care Unit (CAM-ICU) and the Intensive Care Delirium Screening Checklist (ICDSC) for detecting post-cardiac surgery delirium: A single-center study in Japan', *Heart & Lung: The Journal of Cardiopulmonary and Acute Care*, 45 (1): 15–20. doi.org/10.1016/j.hrtlng.2015.11.001

Peitz, G., Balas, M.C., Olsen, K.D., Pun, B.T. and Wesley Ely, E. (2013) 'Top 10 Myths Regarding Sedation and Delirium in the ICU', *Critical Care Medicine*, 41 (9): S46–S56. https://sites.duke.edu/micu/files/2015/11/Ten-Myths-Regarding-Sedation-in-the-ICU-Crit-Care-Med-2013.pdf (accessed November 11, 2020).

Perez, R.N. Peters, K. Wilkes, L. Murphy, G. (2019) 'Physical restraints in intensive care-An integrative review', *Australian Critical Care*, 32(2): 165–74. https://doi.org/10.1016/j.aucc.2017.12.089

Rawal, G., Yadav, S. and Kumar, R. (2017) 'Post-intensive care syndrome: An overview', *Journal of Translational Internal Medicine*, 5 (2): 90–2.

Shang, Y., Pan, C., Yang, X., Zhong, M., Shang, X., Wu, Z., Yu, Z., Zhang, W., Zhong, Q., Zheng, X., Sang, L., Jiang, L., Zhang, J., Xiong, W., Liu, J. and Chen, D. (2020) 'Management of critically ill patients with COVID-19 in ICU: Statement from front-line intensive care experts in Wuhan, China', *Annals of Intensive Care*, 10 (1): 1–24. doi.org/10.1186/s13613-020-00689-1

Treece, A. and Baker, J. (2019) 'Identifying determinants for the application of physical or chemical restraint in the managment of psychomotor agitation on the critcal care unit', *Journal of Clinical Nursing*, 29: 5–19.

Turgay, A., Sari, D. and Genc, R. (2009). 'Physical restraint use in Turkish Intensive Care Units'. *Clinical Nurse Specialist*, 23 (2): 68–72. 10.1097/NUR.0b013e318199125c.

van den Boogaard, M., Kox, M., Quinn, K.L. et al. (2011) 'Biomarkers associated with delirium in critically ill patients and their relation with long-term subjective cognitive dysfunction: Indications for different pathways governing delirium in inflamed and noninflamed patients', *Critical Care*, 15: R297. https://doi.org/10.1186/cc10598

Van Rompaey, B., Schuurmans, M.J., Shortridge-Baggett, L.M., Truijen, S. and Bossaert, L. (2008) 'Risk factors for intensive care delirium: A systematic review', *Intensive & Critical Care Nursing*, 24 (2): 98–107. doi.org/10.1016/j.iccn.2007.08.005

Vlake, J.H., van Genderen, M.E., Schut, A. et al. (2020) 'Patients suffering from psychological impairments following critical illness are in need of information', *Journal of Intensive Care* 8 (6). https://doi.org/10.1186/s40560-019-0422-0

Wade, D., Als, N., Bell, V., Brewin, C., D'Antoni, D., Harrison, D.A. [...] and Rowan, K.M. (2018) 'Providing psychological support to people in intensive care: Development and feasibility study of a nurse-led intervention to prevent acute stress and long-term morbidity', *BMJ Open*, 8 (7): 1–12.

Zamoscik, K., Godbold, R. and Freeman, P. (2017) 'Intensive care nurses' experiences and perceptions of delirium and delirium care', *Intensive and Critical Care Nursing*, 40: 94–100. doi.org/10.1016/j.iccn.2017.01.003

Zhang, Z., Pan, L. and Ni, H. (2013) 'Impact of delirium on clinical outcome in critically ill patients: A meta-analysis', *General Hospital Psychiatry*, 35 (2): 105–111. doi.org/10.1016/j.genhosppsych.2012.11.003

SUPPORTING THOSE AT THE END OF LIFE IN CRITICAL CARE

KAREN HEGGS

> " Cure sometimes, relieve often, comfort always.
>
> **Bion and Coombs (2015: 289)** "

LEARNING OUTCOMES

When you have finished studying this chapter you will understand:

- What end of life care means
- How care in the last days of life is managed in the critical care setting
- The role of the **multi-professional team** in end of life care
- The role of the nurse in supporting the patient and their family carers at end of life, in the last days of life and into bereavement
- The need to ensure your own emotional health and wellbeing

INTRODUCTION

Despite developments and advances in **interventions** and extensive support for the patient in the critical care environment, recovery is not always possible, and, in this situation, there is acknowledgement that the patient will die and that they are approaching the end of their life. It is important that we acknowledge death as part of life; but this can be challenging in a care environment where the focus is to provide 'life-sustaining therapies with the goal of restoring or maintaining organ function' (Mercadante et al., 2018: 1). In our society, we have an increasingly ageing population, who are living with multiple complex co-morbidities. The developments in advancing treatment options for many conditions and diseases leads to a greater risk of complexity and this also bring with it many challenges in the management of the patient in the critical care setting and with this, the possibility that the person may die in the critical care setting.

Between 2018 and 2019, over half of admissions to critical care settings in the UK were unexpected or transfers following a complex planned surgical procedure for those with additional health needs and co-morbidities (NHS Digital, 2019). It has been identified that over the last 2-year period in England, approximately 8% of patients admitted to the critical care setting died during their stay in critical care unit. Alongside this population, many younger people who have been involved in trauma such as road traffic accidents or assaults will be cared for and die in the critical care setting. This brings with it a range of complex issues including organ and tissue donation.

THIS TOPIC IS ALSO COVERED IN CHAPTER 3

This chapter will provide an outline of the provision of end of life care in the critical care setting, including an overview of how end of life care is managed. We will consider some of the nuances specific to critical care; the role of the multi-professional team and, importantly, the central role of the nurse in the delivery of end of life care for the critically ill person and their family. We will also consider the challenges of the delivery of **palliative care** in critical care and the importance of self-care for the nurse working in this area in order that end of life care provision is effective for the person as well as the nurse.

The following activity will help you to begin to consider your own perceptions of end of life care and what this means to you as an emerging practitioner.

ACTIVITY 16.1: REFLECTIVE PRACTICE

1. What does end of life care mean to you?
2. Have you cared for a person at the end of their life?
3. Was this in a critical care setting or in another care setting?
4. What differences do you think you may find in the delivery of end of life care in a critical care setting?

There is no template answer to this activity as it is based on your own reflection. However, do note down your thoughts to these questions - they will support you as you move through this chapter.

DEFINING END OF LIFE

There have been many developments over recent years with regards to defining 'end of life' with a drive to raise awareness of the need to identify those felt to be approaching the end of their life, in order that they and their family can be involved in decision-making and delivery of care. It has also been suggested that effective identification of those at the end of their life can lead to greater opportunity for open dialogue about death, clear communication with all involved and, subsequently, better care planning.

In recent years, there was a suggested change in nomenclature and how the term 'end of life care' was utilised, in order to facilitate more open communication between patients, their families and healthcare professionals and support with care planning. The North West end of life care model (North West Strategic Clinical Networks, 2015) present this in a linear framework. There is acknowledgement that end of life care is the last 12 months of life (or beyond), care in the **last days of life** and then into the bereavement, which can be extended.

For the purpose of this chapter, we will continue to use this language.

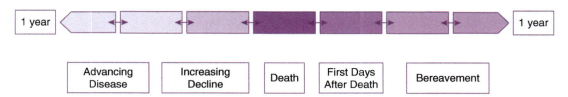

Figure 16.1   The North West End of Life Care Model

Source: North West Strategic Clinic Networks (2015). Contains public sector information licensed under the Open Government Licence v3.0. License.

DECISION-MAKING AT END OF LIFE

There are a number of factors that need to be considered in the identification of someone who is felt to be in the last year of their life. In 2000, Kerry Thomas strived to develop a tool that may support this process in order to initiate a systematic change to how people in the last year of their life are supported. The Gold Standards Framework (GSF) sought to break down barriers with the introduction of a simple process. The 'surprise question' (Thomas et al., 2011) is used as a trigger by clinicians to help them to identify those whose condition may be deteriorating following their assessment, by asking 'would you be surprised if this person died in the next 12 months?' If the answer to the question is 'no' this would then be a prompt for the practitioner to open dialogue with the person and their family and begin communication with others involved in the delivery of their care. The GSF has its roots firmly grounded in primary care; with community practitioners engaging in regular meetings to discuss those identified to be in the last year of life, and to ensure that appropriate services are in place for them. It is important that this information is communicated across care settings; and many areas of the UK now have electronic communication systems where this can be shared across primary and secondary care, including ambulance services. It is important that we have an awareness of this in the critical care setting, to help aid discussion and care planning for the people in our care.

It is acknowledged that diagnosing end of life is not an exact science and can be influenced by many factors, including disease and the typical trajectory that this may follow. The variations of this are demonstrated in Figure 16.2, where the sudden and rapid deterioration often seen in those with a cancer diagnosis contrasts significantly with the gradual and stepped deterioration of those living with organ failure such as heart failure or Chronic Obstructive Pulmonary Disease (COPD). This may be further complicated by the fact that many people now live with a number of co-morbidities, so there may be blurring of these identified disease trajectories and one may supersede the other. The use of clinical judgement alongside supporting prognostic indicator guidance can support healthcare professionals in the identification of deterioration and whether a person may be at the end of their life.

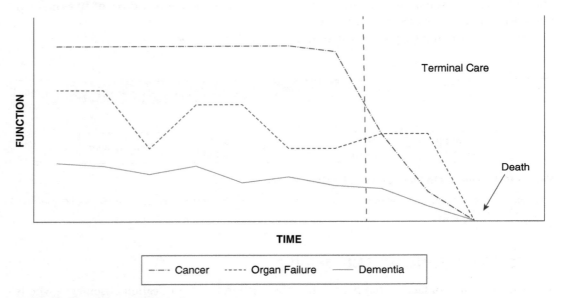

Figure 16.2 Disease trajectory

The opportunity to identify the stage of disease and end of life allows for the facilitation of discussion and the opportunity to consider advance care planning options with the person and their family. This may in turn reduce the need for critical care admission with planning in the event of deterioration and the need for critical care input. There is also the opportunity here for early engagement of palliative care services, which may lead to facilitated discussion about care needs and effective **holistic** care and support, which we will discuss in more detail later in this chapter (Ma et al., 2019). As complexity continues to be an issue and to facilitate decision-making, a possible solution to this could be the development and use of decision-making tools to support critical care clinicians in identifying when to consider palliative care and when to seek specialist input to care. Adler et al. (2019) suggest that there is limited evidence in the use of decision-making tools in critical care to support this important aspect of care; and that the development of such trigger tools must be developed at grass root level.

The need to address decision-making, uncertainty and end of life care in the critical care setting was acknowledged by The Faculty of Intensive Care Medicine by the publication of a key paper 'Care at the end of life: A guide to best practice, discussion and decision making in and around critical care' in

September 2019 (Cosgrove et al., 2019) with the proactive development of a number aide memoires in the form of decision-making. The key tools developed are designed to support critical care practitioners in their decision-making process, when it is identified that someone is at the end of their life. These tools have a specific focus for care in the last days of life, in addition to the need to consider a change of focus in treatment through an achieved consensus.

The following activity will allow you to begin to consider some of the challenges of end of life care and care in the last days of life in the critical care setting and how communication is central to this.

ACTIVITY 16.2: RESEARCH AND EVIDENCE-BASED PRACTICE

Review the tools developed in the publication by The Faculty of Intensive Care Medicine (Cosgrove et al., 2019) 'Care at the end of life: A guide to best practice, discussion and decision making in and around critical care'.

Look at the following tools:

- Dealing with dilemma on p. 9
- Aide memoire for end-of-life care on the critical care unit on p. 15
- Aide memoire for achieving consensus on p. 27

Consider how these tools could support decision-making for those at the end of their life and also those in the last days of life

1. Do you feel that they would facilitate communication?

CARE IN THE LAST DAYS OF LIFE IN THE CRITICAL CARE SETTING

The critical care setting allows for the opportunity for excellence in the delivery of care in the last days of life. Often people may have been in the setting for a long period; allowing for the development of an effective therapeutic relationship between the patient, family and the nurse and healthcare team (Stokes et al., 2019). In addition to this, the high ratio of staff to patients lends itself to the delivery of individualised and intensive care in the last days of life and for continuity of care from the team.

But the complexity of the cases that require critical care and the intensity of the care interventions, with ongoing developments of what can be achieved in the drive to save lives, can lead to often complex and challenging decision making for practitioners and the people that they care for and their families. One of the significant challenges is the shift of care from lifesaving care to care in the last days of life (Kisorio and Langley, 2016). This can involve the withdrawal and withholding of life sustaining treatments and situations where a person may lack capacity due to their condition and the use of medications to facilitate **sedation** (Mercadante et al., 2018). Critical care nurses are often at the forefront of these care decisions and are active in the changes in care delivery; they are the face that the family see and engage with at a time of great vulnerability and emotional distress.

Nurses in the critical care setting may also provide care in the last days of life for people who are organ donors following diagnosis of brain stem death. Interestingly, over the last 2 years less than 0.5% of those who have died in the critical care setting have been organ donors (both heartbeat and non-heartbeat or cadaveric donation) (NHS Digital, 2019). With this in mind and minimal occurrence the opportunity for nurses to experience caring for a person at the end of life in this situation is limited and requires the input of specialist support. The implementation of the role of the Specialist Nurse for Organ Donation (SNOD) has ensured that the critically ill person, their family, and critical care nurses are supported with this often complex and challenging area of end of life care, with the key role of the SNOD (Noyes et al., 2019) including:

- Education
- Support for family
- Support for staff
- Consent

THIS TOPIC
IS ALSO
COVERED IN
CHAPTER 11

The change to UK law in 2020 and the move to an opt-out system for organ donation may lead to an increase in the number of **organ donation** cases and increased opportunity for critical care nurses to engage in this end of life care delivery.

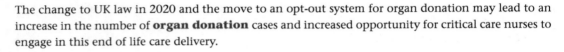

WHAT'S THE EVIDENCE?

There is a developing evidence base looking at the role of the nurse in both decision-making and delivery of care for people in the last days of life. It is suggested that although this is a significant part of their role, there is the need to develop knowledge and skills for critical nurses to support them in the delivery of care in the last days of life (Jang et al., 2019; Kisorio and Langley, 2016; Todaro-Franceschi, 2013). As interventions advance and develop and complexity of health increases, there will be a continued need and drive to ensure that critical care nurses continue their own professional development in the delivery of end of life care.

However, in 2013 the European Association for Palliative Care presented a white paper that identified a three-tier approach to support in the delivery of education (Gamondi et al., 2013). The three tiers are presented here in Table 16.1.

Table 16.1   Three tier approach to support the delivery of education

Palliative care approach	Integrating the ethos of palliative care into all settings
	Education provided to all staff across a range of care
	Staff access education in pre-registration programmes and also post-registration education
General palliative care	Education accessible to all healthcare professionals who regularly provide palliative care as part of their work
	Staff access education in pre-registration programmes and also post-registration education
Specialist palliative care	Palliative care for patients with complex and challenging needs
	Accessed when generalist input and treatment plans have not been effective
	Higher level of education required due to the complexity of the care requirements

Source: Based on the work of Gamondi et al. (2013).

It would be interesting for you to consider here where there may be a merge in the educational requirements of the nurse working in the critical care setting.

1. Do you feel that nurses in critical care would require education targeted at both general and specialist palliative care?
2. Do you feel that the level of complexity of cases that nurses working in critical care are managing would impact this?

There is no template answer to this activity as it is based on your own reflection.

Nurses working in critical care require advanced communication skills to ensure that they can communicate effectively in complex situations, transferring often complex information to the patient, their family and to members of the wider multi-professional team, in order that effective care can be delivered. There is also the challenge for the critical care nurse to ensure that communication to the patient and their family is clear, easy to understand and readily available at the time that this is needed. A study published by Nelson et al. (2010) sought to hear the voices of patients and their families in the critical care setting. The findings identified that communication was central to their entire experience, with a need for information that was consistent and delivered in a compassionate and considered way. Communication has also been identified as a key priority by Cosgrove et al. (2019) who have highlighted the need to ensure transparency in communication to reduce the potential for confusion and conflict between healthcare teams, the patient and family members.

ACTIVITY 16.3: CASE STUDY

Elizabeth is a 62-year-old woman who has a diagnosis of COPD and type 2 diabetes. She has a good quality of life and continues to work in her local library 3 days each week. She is active and enjoys attending the gym and walking with a local walking group – she does this following her recent diagnosis and after a recent admission to hospital with an **exacerbation** of her COPD and a programme of respiratory rehabilitation.

Elizabeth is the main carer for her husband Reginald, who has early stage Lewy Body dementia. He lives at home with her and is able to manage many activities of daily living with support. Elizabeth and Reginald have 2 adult children who live locally, and they have 3 young grandchildren. Elizabeth performs childcare for her grandchildren 2 days each week. They are a close family unit and are supportive of each other.

Elizabeth has been admitted to hospital via the acute medical admissions unit where she has presented with a severe exacerbation of her COPD. She was reviewed by the medical consultant on call and was then transferred to the critical care unit after her condition deteriorated further. She has been diagnosed with pneumonia and required intubation and ventilation. She also required **inotropic** support and haemofiltration. Elizabeth has been in the critical care unit for the last 6 weeks and was initially showing signs of improvement; however, she has developed a further infection, and this is not responding to treatment as her team would have hoped.

Despite these interventions Elizabeth's condition continues to deteriorate and following review by her medical teams, the decision has been made to withdraw supportive interventions.

(Continued)

Think about the shift in care focus here.

1. How would the nurse in the critical care environment manage the transition of care to care in the last days of life?
2. What do you feel would be the nurses' main priorities?
3. How would the nurse support Elizabeth's family?
4. What feelings do you feel the nurse may be experiencing in this situation? How would they manage their own emotions in this situation?

PALLIATIVE CARE IN THE CRITICAL CARE SETTING

The involvement of the palliative care team earlier in the trajectory of admission can have a positive impact, including initiation of discussions with family carers at an earlier point and facilitation of communication to support effective decision making for the critical care team (Mercadante et al., 2018). In addition to this the ethos of care delivery from a critical care and palliative care perspective are inextricably linked, with many similarities in their approach and principles such as multiprofessional working and a person-centred and holistic approach to care delivery (Bion and Coombs, 2015; Matthews and Nelson, 2019). There may not be the disparity that was suggested in the introduction at the opening of this chapter; but it is acknowledged that there is a need to identify a sense of balance between the drive to treat and the need to ensure that we consider the wishes of a person who is at the end of their life (Bloomer, 2019).

Only 0.6% of critical care patients are transferred to a palliative care provider (i.e. a hospice) over last 2 years (NHS Digital, 2019). There are a number of reasons that this may be the case, including the complexity of care and the issue of rapid deterioration once life-sustaining treatments such as inotropic and ventilator support are removed; often it is not safe, practical or in the best interests of the person to move them at this stage. A study by Ma et al. (2019), identified that early intervention of specialist palliative care services in the critical care environment led to increased access to hospice care provision and also advance care planning such as 'do not attempt CPR' and also decisions about future care plans. This also led to more effective utilisation of critical care provision and appropriate management of person-centred care. But this does not preclude the delivery of effective palliative care in the critical care setting (see Figure 16.3).

Palliative care is defined as the care of a person living with and dying from a life-limiting condition; the World Health Organisation (2013) provides a detailed insight into its view of palliative care with a clear vision on the importance of person-and family-centred holistic care that is both life and death affirming:

- Provides relief from pain and other distressing symptoms
- Affirms life and regards dying as a normal process
- Intends to neither hasten nor postpone death
- Integration of emotional and spiritual care
- Offers a support system to help families cope throughout disease and into bereavement
- For the affected person to live the best quality of life they can

- Using a team approach, care and interventions are utilised to enhance quality of life alongside life prolonging treatments
- Ensures that investigations are considered to support in the management of symptoms and to enhance quality of life

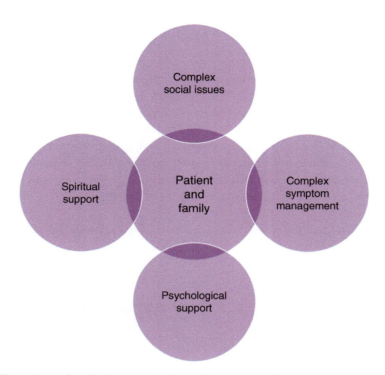

Figure 16.3   The ethos of palliative care in the critical care setting

The delivery of palliative care is the responsibility of every healthcare professional and in the UK, recent policy development is ensuring that the profile of palliative care is raised and that initiatives such as advance care planning are promoted. In 2015, the National Palliative and End of Life Care Partnership published a positive and ambitious national framework to raise the profile of palliative care across a range of care settings, ensuring that everyone has access to palliative and end of life care when they need this.

A National Framework for Palliative and End of Life Care – The six key aims

- Each person is seen as an individual
- Each person gets fair access to care
- Maximising comfort and wellbeing
- Care is coordinated

- All staff are prepared to care
- Each community is prepared to help

Source: adapted from National Palliative and End of Life Care Partnership, 2015: 11.

THE ROLE OF THE MDT IN THE PROVISION OF END OF LIFE CARE

As we have already identified, care delivery in the critical care setting can be complex due to a number of multifaceted issues. With a number of key teams engaged in decision-making and in the delivery of care, the nurse plays a significant role in ensuring communication across teams and the co-ordination of care delivery in response to this. It is essential that the patient and their family are central to this and that this is facilitated to ensure that the complexity is managed. It will also ensure that a team approach to delivery of palliative care, as indicated by the World Health Organisation, is facilitated. In addition to this, it has been advised that there is a significant need to work in a joint manner to ensure the co-ordination of care delivery for people at the end of their life (The Choice in End of Life Care Programme Board, 2015).

The following activity will encourage you to reflect on your appreciation of multi-professional working in the context of critical care.

ACTIVITY 16.4: REFLECTIVE PRACTICE

Consider your own experiences from practice.

1. How can multi-professional working be effectively facilitated?
2. What actions and interventions have you observed that could facilitate this in the critical care setting?

There is no template answer to question 2 as it is based on your own reflection.

In 2003 Skilbeck and Paye developed an understanding of the difference between generalist and specialist palliative care; their work allowed greater clarity in this field. However, since the publication of their work, there have been many advances in healthcare interventions, and we have many people now living with multiple complex needs requiring critical care input. Ryan and Johnston (2018) provide further and more current discussion about the differentiation between generalist and specialist palliative care. With the drive to ensure that palliative care is delivered alongside potentially curative or intensive treatments and management, there is a real need for team working, and the specialist teams contribute significantly to the delivery of this care by the main care team (see Figure 16.4). It is suggested that this may need to be reconsidered for the critical care setting as all patients who require critical care input will also have a higher level of complexity and thus need for specialist palliative

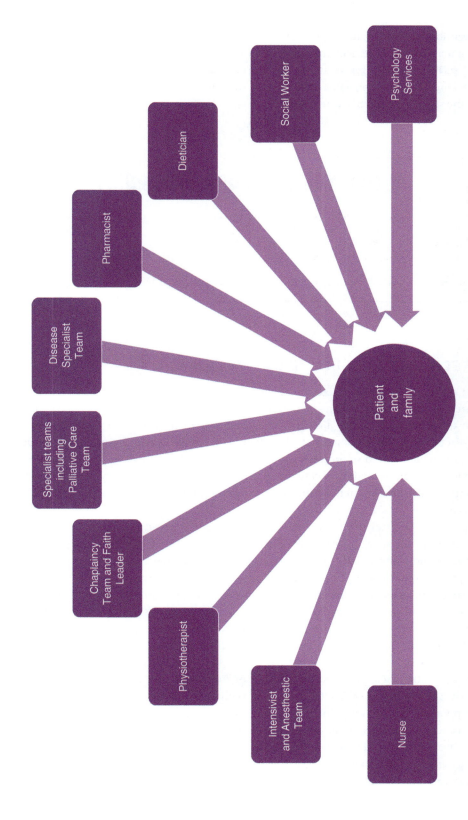

Figure 16.4 The wider multi-professional team engaged with a patient and their family in the delivery of end of life care

care intervention. In contrast to this, the level of intensity of nursing and medical care in the critical care setting may preclude the need for specialist palliative care input; we will consider the role of the **specialist palliative care team** later in this chapter. The next activity will encourage you to reflect on the differences between generalist and palliative care; understanding this can help in your decision to engage the specialist palliative care team.

ACTIVITY 16.5: THEORY STOP POINT

1. What are the differences between generalist palliative care and specialist palliative care?

Read the paper by Skilbeck and Payne (2003) (doi.org/10.1046/j.1365-2648.2003.02749.x) and the chapter written by Ryan and Johnston (2018).

2. Are there any clear differences in the approach over the span of 15 years?

THE SPECIALIST PALLIATIVE CARE TEAM

Bion and Coobs (2015) acknowledge the advances in intervention and treatment options in the critical care setting, and that many people with complex co-morbidities may have considered the option to not be admitted to a critical care environment for care. The value of advance care planning discussions allows the patient, their family and their healthcare providers to identify a ceiling of care, which would support decision-making and reduce the need for critical care admissions. The involvement of palliative care teams can complement the delivery of this aspect of care and also support the development of future care planning for those living with complex and life-limiting conditions.

There appears to be a lack of clarity and consensus about the best timeframe for the involvement and engagement of the specialist palliative care team in the delivery of care in the critical care setting. Matthews and Nelson (2017) (see Figure 16.5) identified that there are many similarities in the development of both critical care and palliative care delivery over the last 2 decades. A point of significance is the drive to acknowledge the value of palliative care intervention at any point in a person's **disease trajectory**; end of life care may be a part of this, but specialist palliative care services can also offer so much more. This lends itself to the concept of supportive care and that the specialist palliative care teams can provide input to patient care, even if the intention of the treatment is curative in nature.

In the UK in 2004, NICE provided a definition of supportive care that shares many similarities with the NICE (2004) and WHO (2019) views of palliative care; extending and emphasising the value of supportive care at any point in a person's illness and disease trajectory and also ensuring that there is equal emphasis on supportive care and treatment with curative intent. This should lead to the inclusion of palliative care for support and guidance for all as needed throughout the critical care admission. It is suggested that it may be useful to consider if a person is already known to palliative care services prior to their involvement and admission in the community setting.

It is also helpful to know that community and acute specialist palliative care services work in close proximity and that the palliative care team can be a useful source of information and guidance. Mercadante et al. (2019) propose two possible models for the integration of palliative care delivery in the critical care setting; the first being the 'integrative' approach, which is that the founding principles of palliative care are a part of day-to-day care delivery in the critical care setting. The second approach is the 'consultative' approach, where the palliative care team are invited into care delivery for their expertise and opinion.

Matthews and Nelson (2017) also acknowledge the need to future proof this aspect of care and linking this with the advances in care delivery, leading to important issues such as survivorship, mirroring the developments in cancer care delivery over recent years.

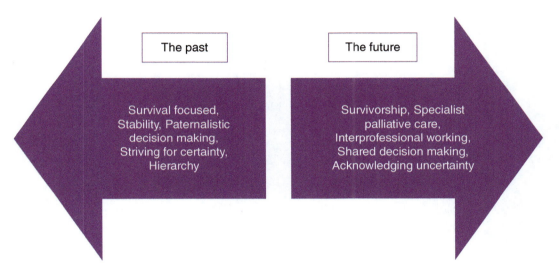

Figure 16.5 Changes in palliative care approaches

Source: Mathews and Nelson (2017); adapted and reprinted by kind permission of Springer Nature.

ACTIVITY 16.6: RESEARCH AND EVIDENCE-BASED PRACTICE

The role of the SPC team in the delivery of EoLC

Listen to this podcast from the Society of Critical Care Medicine – Enfield and Kollef discuss their study that looked at the value of early intervention from the specialist palliative care team in the critical care setting.

1. What key factors are identified in the study?

As you will have found from the last activity, Specialist palliative care teams can offer expert advice and opinion in a number of areas of complexity, linking with the identified ethos of palliative care defined by the World Health Organisation. Their care delivery is holistic in its approach across the physical, spiritual, emotional and social needs of the person and their family. Symptom control is a significant part of the role of the specialist palliative care team, with many people in the critical care setting experiencing a range of symptoms at the end of life and in the last days of life. Cosgrove et al. (2019) have identified this as a priority, with the acknowledgement of a number of key symptoms that may be experienced by patients at the end of their life in the critical care setting. These symptoms are not unique to critical care and are akin to those experienced by many people at the end of their life, regardless of the care setting. But the need to seek specialist support when they cannot be managed by the critical care team is vital to ensure comfort and dignity at the end of life and in the last days of life (Mercadante et al., 2018).

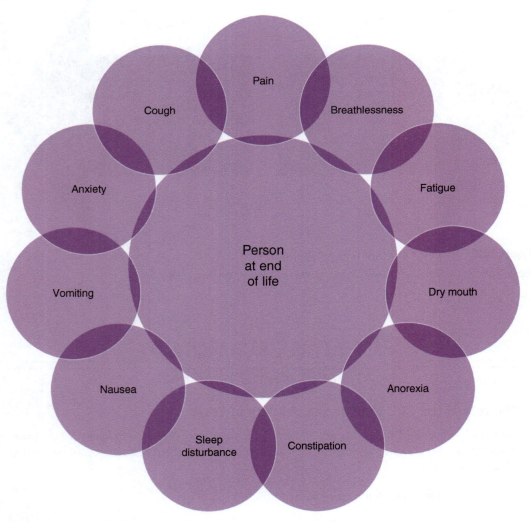

Figure 16.6   Symptoms that may be experienced by a person at the end of life

ACTIVITY 16.7: CASE STUDY

Peter is a 37-year-old man who was admitted to the critical care unit following a cardiac arrest whilst playing football with his friends. Before this event, Peter was a fit and active man who also enjoyed running and cycling regularly. He had no previous medical issues at all and this event has come as a huge shock to his family and friends.

Peter is married to Kelly; they have been together for 21 years and met at school. They have two children, Daniel is 8 and Olivia is 4. They are a very close family unit and both Peter's and Kelly's parents live very close by and play an active part in the family and in the provision of childcare. Kelly is a ward sister on an acute surgical ward in the hospital and Peter works as a manager at a local supermarket.

Peter has been on the critical care unit for 2 weeks and despite the support of inotropic drugs, ventilator support and renal support via filtration, he continues to deteriorate. Following multidisciplinary assessment and discussion this morning and discussion with his family, the decision has been made that there is no further treatment that can be considered to support Peter and that he is at the end of his life.

The team have discussed with Kelly that they will withdraw inotropic support over the course of the day, they will not continue with renal support, but as Peter is sedated and ventilated, they will look to his need for ventilator support and will ensure that Peter is assessed regularly for symptoms to ensure that these are effectively managed.

Kelly has expressed concern that Peter will be in pain and that he may experience discomfort at the end of his life. She has expressed that as a nurse, she has cared for many people at the end of their life and wants to ensure that his symptoms are well controlled. Kelly asks if it would be possible for her to be involved in some aspects of care for Peter.

1. How would the nurse support Kelly in this situation?
2. How would involvement of the hospital palliative care team support the nurse, team, Peter and Kelly in this situation?

SELF-CARE – ESSENTIAL FOR ONGOING CARE DELIVERY

Nurses working in the critical care setting deal with a number of challenging and often distressing situations; it is important for nurses to feel supported and to have an awareness of their own emotional health and wellbeing to ensure safe and effective care delivery; a point supported by the Nursing and Midwifery Council (2018) in The Code.

For nurses working in critical care there are a number of significant factors that may affect the emotional health and wellbeing of the nurse including:

- Intensity of relationship with patient and their family
- Complex ethical dilemmas and decision-making
- Withdrawal of treatments and interventions
- Time pressures
- Multiple interventions and treatments

There is evidence to suggest that there is an increased risk of emotional burnout for nurses in the critical care setting. A systematic review by Van Mol et al. (2015) identified 40 studies that had identified the risks of burnout in the critical care setting. The study suggests the need for ongoing research into this area as advances in treatments continue and the complexity of care needs increases, suggesting the need to ensure that support is available to nurses in order that they can maintain their emotional health and wellbeing.

Burnout can have a number of causes including the personality traits of the individual, control in a situation and work pressures. It is characterised by 'emotional exhaustion, depersonalization, and a sense of low personal accomplishment' (Kim Wong and Olusanya, 2017).

There are many interventions that could be considered in the critical care setting, with the importance of working as a team and supporting each other in addition to the opportunity for debrief within the team, following the death of a patient. The use of debrief has been suggested to offer nurses an opportunity to discuss the situation and to learn from their experiences (Kisorio and Langley, 2016).

THIS TOPIC
IS ALSO
COVERED IN
CHAPTER 1

It is important too that critical care nurses are aware of the support mechanisms that may be available to them in their own organisations, with many offering opportunities for counselling and debrief in addition to the Schwartz rounds in which complex cases are discussed in a supportive and reflective environment. It is suggested that engagement with their employing organisations is essential to ensure that the workforce feels supported and their voice is heard (Barker and Ford, 2018).

ACTIVITY 16.8: REFLECTIVE PRACTICE

Think back to your notes from Activity 16.1 at the opening of this chapter.

- What does end of life care mean to you?
- Have you cared for a person at the end of their life?
- Was this in a critical care setting or in another care setting?
- What differences do you think you may find in the delivery of end of life care in a critical care setting?

1. Reflect on your initial notes and consider your learning from this chapter. Do you have further learning needs?
2. How might you meet these learning needs through your own practice learning experiences?

Consider the further reading that is suggested in the 'go further' section at the end of the chapter.
There is no template answer to this activity as it is based on your own reflection.

In an ever-changing healthcare system, with developments and advances in treatment options and complexity in the healthcare needs of the population; one constant is the need to deliver good quality and dignified end of life care. Although we are looking to prognosticate and identify when it is believed a person is at the end of their life, it is not always possible to plan effectively for their needs or for these needs to be met. It is essential for us to consider that we do not just focus on the physical needs of the patient at the end of their life, but also the needs of their family and that we consider their holistic needs too (Bloomer, 2019). The implementation of palliative care as part of care delivered by all in the critical care setting, alongside specialist team input in areas of complexity can add significant value to the care of people at the end of their life and in the last days of their life.

In this chapter, we have identified some of the challenges in the delivery of end of life care in the critical care setting, we have considered the role of the multi-professional team and importantly the role of the nurse in the co-ordination of care delivery. We have considered the drive over recent years to move the focus of the delivery of care in the critical care setting and also the imperative importance of facilitating effective communication with all in a range of contexts to ensure that end of life care is person-centred at its heart. Finally, we have considered the impact of end of life care for the nurse and the need to ensure our own health and wellbeing in the delivery of quality care.

CHAPTER SUMMARY

This chapter has supported you to gain greater insight into the following topics:

- Defining end of life care
- How care in the last days of life is managed in the critical care setting
- The role of the multi-professional team in end of life care
- The need to ensure your own emotional health and wellbeing
- Palliative care in the critical care setting

GO FURTHER

Books

Dixon, J. (2018) 'Issues of referral to and accessing palliative care', in C. Walshe, N. Preston and B. Johnston (eds) *Palliative Care Nursing – Principles and Evidence for Practice* (3rd edition). London: McGraw Hill.

- If you want to develop further understanding of the differences between generalist and specialist palliative care and the role of the specialist palliative care team in the delivery of care; this book chapter provides detail and further context to help expand your understanding.

Costello, J. (ed) (2018) *Adult Palliative Care for Nursing, Health and Social Care*. London: Sage.

- If you want to gain greater insight into the needs of people living with a range of diseases and some of the current key issues in adult palliative care across health and social care provision, this book provides expert opinion and identifies current practice developments and challenges.

Russell, S., Coombs, M. and Loney, J. (2018) 'The last days and hours of life', in C. Walshe, N. Preston and B. Johnston (eds) *Palliative Care Nursing – Principles and Evidence for Practice* (3rd edition). London: McGraw Hill.

- If you want to extend your knowledge and understanding of the care of a person in the last days of their life and the role of the nurse in care delivery; this chapter provides a valuable overview of this important aspect of nursing care, with a holistic approach to the management of person and family centred care.

Journal articles

Mullick, A., Martin, J. and Sallnow, L. (2013) 'An introduction to advance care planning in practice', *BMJ*, 13: Article #347. doi.org/10.1136/bmj.f6064

- This article will help you to develop a further understanding of the legal issues associated with advance care planning and an overview of current approaches to advance care planning in the UK from a medical perspective, including some of the barriers and the facilitators to advance care planning.

Metaxa, V., Anagnostou, D., Vlachos, S., Arulkumaran, N., van Dusseldorp, I., Bensemmane, S., Aslakson, R., Davidson, J.E., Gerritsen, R., Hartog, C. and Curtis, R. (2019) 'Palliative care interventions in intensive care unit patients – A systematic review protocol', *Systematic Reviews*, 8: Article #148. doi.org/10.1186/s13643-019-1064-y

- This systematic review provides interesting consideration of how palliative care is facilitated in a range of critical cares settings across a range of countries.

Anderson, R.J., Bloch, S. Armstrong, M., Stone, P.C. and Low, J.T.S. (2019) 'Communication between healthcare professionals and relatives of patients approaching the end-of-life: A systematic review of qualitative evidence', *Palliative Medicine*, 33: 8. doi.org/ 10.1177/0269216319852007

- This systematic review engages with the qualitative evidence about communication between healthcare professionals and family members when a person is at the end of life. It provides some interesting insight into strategies utilised by healthcare professionals and how these may be enhanced.

Useful websites

www.eapcnet.eu/

- The European Association for Palliative Care is a valuable website that provides detail on current policy development and research in the field of palliative care. Here you can also access a range of resources including some national policies.

http://advancecareplan.org.uk/ (accessed November 13, 2020).

- Advance Care Plan is a resource for people living in England and Wales, which contains a range of valuable information about advance care planning and tools to support people to consider advance care plans.

https://goldstandardsframework.org.uk/ (accessed November 13, 2020).

- The Gold Standards Framework (GSF) is a useful website that provides insight and overview into the role of the framework in the delivery of excellent end of life care. The website provides information on the aims of GSF and how the national GSF centre provides support to healthcare professionals in their role.

REFERENCES

Adler, K., Schlieper, D., Kingden-Milles, D., Meier, S., Schallenburger, M., Sellman, T., Schwager, H., Schwartz, J. and Neukirchen, M. (2019) 'Will your patient benefit from palliative care? A multi exploratory survey about the acceptance of trigger factors for palliative care consultations among ICU physicians (letter)', *Intensive Care Medicine*, 45: 125–7 doi.org/10.1007/s00134-018-5461-9

Barker, R. and Ford, K. (2018) 'The Point of Care Foundation: The case for employee engagement in the NHS – Three case studies'. https://s16682.pcdn.co/wp-content/uploads/2018/09/Point_of_Care_Report_2018.pdf (accessed November 13, 2020).

Bion, J. and Coombs, M. (2018) 'Balancing care with comfort: Palliative care in critical care', *Palliative Medicine*, 29 (4): 288–90. doi.org/10.1177/0269216315574648

Bloomer, M. (2019) 'Palliative care provision in acute and critical care settings: What are the challenges?', *Palliative Medicine*, 33 (10): 1239–40. doi.org/10.1177/0269216319891789

Cosgrove, J., Baruah, R., Bassford, C., Blackwood, D., Pattison, N. and White, C. (2019) *Care at the End of Life: A Guide to Best Practice, Discussion and Decision-making in and around Critical Care.* London: The Faculty of Intensive Care Medicine. www.ficm.ac.uk/sites/default/files/ficm_care_end_of_life_0.pdf (accessed November 12, 2020).

Gamondi, C., Larkin, P. and Payne, S. (2013) 'Core competencies in palliative care: An EAPC White Paper on palliative care education – Part 1', *European Journal of Palliative Care*, 20 (2): 86–91.

Jang, S.K., Park, W.H., Kim, H., Chang, S.O. (2019) 'Exploring nurses' end-of life care for dying patients in the ICU using focus group interviews', *Intensive and Critical Care Nursing*, 52: 3–8. doi.org/10.1016/j.iccn.2018.09.007

Kim Wong, A.V. and Olusanya, O. (2017) 'Burnout and resilience in anaesthesia and intensive care medicine', *British Journal of Anaesthesia Education*, 17 (10): 334–40.

Kisorio, L.C. and Langley, G.C. (2016) 'Intensive care nurses' experiences of end-of-life care', *Intensive and Critical Care Nursing*, 33: 30–8. doi.org/10.1016/j.iccn.2015.11.002

Ma, J., Chi, S., Buettner, B., Pollard, K., Muir, M., Kolekar, C., Al-Hammadi, N., Ling, C., Kollef, M. and Dans, M. (2019) 'Early palliative care consultation in the medical ICU: A cluster randomized crossover trial', *Critical Care Medicine*, 47 (12): 1707–15. doi.org/10.1097/CCM.0000000000004016

Mathews, K.S. and Nelson, J.E. (2017) 'Palliative care in the ICU of 2050: Past is prologue', *Intensive Care Medicine*, 43 (12): 1850–2. doi.org/10.1007/s00134-017-4828-7

Mercadante, S., Gregoretti, C. and Cortegiani, A. (2018) 'Palliative care in intensive care units: Why, where, what, who, when, how?', *BMC Anesthesiology*, 18: Article #106. doi.org/10.1186/s12871-018-0574-9

National Institute for Health and Care Excellence (NICE) (2004) *Improving Supportive and Palliative Care for Adults with Cancer* (Cancer Service Guideline 4). London: NICE. Available from www.nice.org.uk/guidance/csg4 (accessed November 13, 2020).

National Palliative and End of Life Care Partnership (2015) *Ambitions for Palliative and End of Life Care: A National Framework for Local Action 2015–2020.* http://endoflifecareambitions.org.uk/wp-content/uploads/2015/09/Ambitions-for-Palliative-and-End-of-Life-Care.pdf (accessed November 13, 2020).

Nelson, J.E., Puntillo, K.A., Pronovost, P.J., Walker, A.S., McAdam, J.L., Ilaoa, D. and Penrod, J. (2010) 'In their own words: Patients and families define high-quality palliative care in the intensive care unit', *Critical Care Medicine*, 38 (3): 808–18. doi.org/10.1097/CCM.0b013e3181c5887c

NHS Digital (2019) *Hospital Admitted Patient Care Activity*. Available from: https://digital.nhs.uk/data-and-information/publications/statistical/hospital-admitted-patient-care-activity/2018-19 (accessed November 12, 2020).

North West Strategic Clinical Networks (2015) *North West End of Life Care Model.* https://www.nwcscnsenate.nhs.uk/files/2414/3280/1623/May_2015_Final_NW_eolc_model_and_good_practice_guide.pdf (accessed November 12, 2020).

Noyes, J., Mclaughlin, L., Morgan, K., Roberts, A., Moss, B., Stephens, M. and Walton, P. (2019) 'Process evaluation of specialist nurse implementation of a soft opt-out organ donation system in Wales', *BMC Health Service Research*, 19: Article #414. doi.org/10.1186/s12913-019-4266-z

Nursing and Midwifery Council (2018) *The Code – Professional Standards of Practice and Behaviour for Nurses, Midwives and Nursing Associates* . www.nmc.org.uk/globalassets/sitedocuments/nmc-publications/nmc-code.pdf (accessed November 13, 2020).

Ryan, K. and Johnston, B. (2018) 'Generalists and Specialist Palliative Care', in R. MacLeod and L. Van den Block (eds) *Textbook of Palliative Care*. Berlin: Springer. pp. 503–16.

Skilbeck, J. and Payne, S. (2003) 'Emotional support and the role of clinical nurse specialists in palliative care', *Journal of Advanced Nursing*, 43 (5): 521–30. doi.org/10.1046/j.1365-2648.2003.02749.x

Stokes, H., Vanderspank-Wright, B., Bourbonnais, F.F. and Wright, D.K. (2019) 'Meaningful experiences and end-of-life care in the intensive care unit: A qualitative study', *Intensive and Critical Care Nursing*, 53: 1–7. doi.org/10.1016/j.iccn.2019.03.010

The Choice in End of Life Care Programme Board (2015). *What's Important to Me: A Review of Choice in End of Life Care*. https://assets.publishing.service.gov.uk/government/uploads/system/uploads/attachment_data/file/407244/CHOICE_REVIEW_FINAL_for_web.pdf (accessed November 13, 2020).

Thomas, K., Armstrong Wilson, J., Gold Standards Framework Team (2011) *The GSF Prognostic Indicator Guidance*. www.goldstandardsframework.org.uk/cd-content/uploads/files/General%20Files/Prognostic%20Indicator%20Guidance%20October%202011.pdf (accessed November 12, 2020).

Todaro-Franceschi, V. (2013) 'Critical care nurses' perceptions of preparedness and ability to care for the dying and their professional quality of life', *Dimensions of Critical Care Nursing*, 32 (4): 184–90. doi.org/10.1097/DCC.0b013e31829980af

Van Mol, M.M.C., Kompanje, E.O., Benoit, D.D., Bakker, J. and Nijkamp, M.D. (2015) 'The prevalence of compassion fatigue and burnout among healthcare professionals in intensive care units: A systematic review', *PLoSONE*, 10 (8): e0136955. doi.org/10.1371/journal.pone.0136955

World Health Organization. (2013). *WHO Definition of Palliative Care*. http://www.who.int/cancer/palliative/definition/en (accessed January, 14 2021).

REHABILITATION AFTER CRITICAL ILLNESS

SALLY MOORE AND SAMANTHA FREEMAN

> "
> I thought being discharged from intensive care meant I was better. Months later when I was still struggling to get back to normal, I realised that had only been the start of my long recovery.
>
> **Raisa, 49, Critical Care Survivor**
> "

LEARNING OUTCOMES

When you have finished studying this chapter you will be able to understand:

- The importance of preparedness for discharge from critical care
- The importance of assessment of a person's rehabilitation needs
- The potential issue around physical recovery
- The psychological recovery following critical illness
- The ways we can support both the person and their family during their long-term recovery

INTRODUCTION

For those who survive a critical illness, recovery may be long and complex. Yet survival alone is not the only important outcome of a critical care stay (Jeitziner et al., 2015). Following a period of critical illness people may have not only physical changes to cope with but also emotional and cognitive problems as well (Olsen et al., 2017). The aim of the healthcare team is to ensure recovery is supported and people can regain as much of their ability to function as they had prior to their critical illness. When this is not possible, they need to be supported to adjust to any subsequent changes.

Therefore, the preparation and planning for recovery should start on admission to critical care (Evans, 2017). Utilising the knowledge and research available we can predict the complications and challenges of recovery and from the point of admission act in a way to prevent or reduce the incidence of these issues. In 2018 adjustments were made to the Pain, Agitation, and Delirium (PAD) guidelines to include rehabilitation/mobilization (Devlin et al., 2018). This document supports the notion of considering rehabilitation early in the person's critical care stay by reducing immobility.

As with many aspects of care delivery there is variation in services for people following critical care. Aftercare can range from follow up consultations or outpatient clinics to rehabilitation programmes (Mehlhorn et al., 2014). There are also charity support groups such as ICUsteps (www.icusteps.org/) that provide information and meetings where both the person who experienced critical illness and their loved ones can ask questions and share experiences. As well as service provision being variable across the UK, we also need to be mindful that people and their families will need different individualised aftercare.

In this chapter we will examine the challenges faced by a person recovering from a critical illness from a physical, psychological and social perspective. We will discuss how needs are assessed and what methods are used to deliver rehabilitation. We will also consider the broader impact of critical illness on the family and significant others.

We know that survivors of critical illness face increased **morbidity** (Gayat et al., 2008; Wittekamp 2010) and **mortality** for several years after their discharge from critical care (Cuthbertson and Wunsch, 2016; NICE, 2009a). There may also be permanent life changing effects and complications, and the failure to provide a robust rehabilitation plan for this group has been described as a 'major public health issue' (NICE, 2009a). Therefore, the pathway for each person during this less acute phase requires just as much care and attention from healthcare professionals as the person received whilst in the critical care unit.

WHAT'S THE EVIDENCE?

This so called 'major public health issue', that is a lack of a cohesive and consistent rehabilitation service for all critical illness survivors, should demand an equal sense of priority as the initial critical care **interventions**. The study below highlights the importance of a person-centred rehabilitation plan that seeks to humanise care whilst rebuilding autonomy.

Corner, E.J, Murray, E.J., and Brett, S.J. (2019) 'Qualitative, grounded theory exploration of patients' experience of early mobilisation, rehabilitation and recovery after critical illness', *BMJ Open*, 9: e026348. doi.org/10.1136/bmjopen-2018-026348

Comprehensive Critical Care (2000) demanded a structured assessment and plan for recovery after critical illness. This was expanded upon further in NICE clinical guideline 83 (Nice, 2009a). Then in 2017 NICE produced a document setting out the quality standards for rehabilitation after critical illness. The four quality statements can be seen in Table 17.1.

Table 17.1 Four quality statements

Quality statements
Statement 1 Adults in critical care at risk of morbidity have their rehabilitation goals agreed within 4 days of admission to critical care or before discharge from critical care, whichever is sooner.
Statement 2 Adults at risk of morbidity have a formal handover of care, including their agreed individualised structured rehabilitation programme, when they transfer from critical care to a general ward.
Statement 3 Adults who were in critical care and at risk of morbidity are given information based on their rehabilitation goals before they are discharged from hospital.
Statement 4 Adults who stayed in critical care for more than 4 days and were at risk of morbidity have a review 2 to 3 months after discharge from critical care.

Source: NICE, 2017. Reproduced under the NICE UK Open Content License. URL: www.nice.org.uk/Media/Default/About/Reusing-our-content/Open-content-licence/NICE-UK-Open-Content-Licence-.pdf.

All the above quality statements support early goal setting for rehabilitation, a structured approach to rehabilitation and a clear line of communication both with the person it affects and other health care teams. In the following activity you will be asked to consider these quality statements and the potential challenges that face the clinical team in ensuring the quality statements are acted upon.

ACTIVITY 17.1: CRITICAL THINKING

Consider the four quality statements set out by NICE in Table 17.1.

1. For each statement consider the challenges the clinical team may face when trying to ensure they are met.
2. Following this, consider ways in which we can overcome the challenges you have noted.

It is clear that a rehabilitation strategy or plan is crucial in optimising the recovery of the individual and that we should not be content for people to merely survive (NICE, 2009a). Implementation of an individualised structured rehabilitation programme is stated as pivotal in reducing length of stay (LOS), reducing readmission rates both to hospital and critical care, decreased use of primary care resources and improving the speed at which the person is returned to their previous levels of activity, or their best achievable condition.

The advent of rehabilitation and follow-up services occurred alongside the recognition of the importance of pre critical care admission events. This double-sided issue of examining what happens to people before and after their critical care admission is therefore a relatively new speciality with many research areas not yet thoroughly explored. This lack of underpinning evidence makes our practice challenging as what we are doing may feel intuitively right, but we need to strive to ensure our care is evidence-based. The longer-term mortality, morbidity, and quality of life in survivors of critical illness is a research priority.

The NICE Clinical Guideline 83 (2009a) refers to two domains of recovery: physical and non-physical. It goes on to expand these domains, which are also reflected in The Intensive Care Society's *Guidelines for the Provision of Intensive Care Services 2* (ICS) (2019), and they have been summarised in Table 17.2. This bundle of symptoms in the case of a critical care illness survivor is sometimes called 'Post ICU syndrome'. These challenges are in addition to, and will run alongside, their recovery from the illness that lead to their admission to a Level 3 area. NICE CG 83 (2009a) also warns us away from making assumptions about rehabilitation needs based on the features of the acute illness. All those who have experienced a critical illness should undergo an individual assessment of their needs; people who have had only short critical care admission may still require 'substantial help'.

ACTIVITY 17.2: REFLECTIVE PRACTICE AND TEAM WORKING

Before referring to Table 17.2:

1. Consider what physical and non-physical challenges may be faced by someone recovering from a critical illness. Then compare your thoughts to the challenges collated in provided in Table 17.2
2. Consider which members of the multi-disciplinary team are best placed to provide this

Table 17.2 Collated summary of physical and non-physical challenges

Physical	Non-Physical	
	Psychological	Social
Mobility	Anxiety, panic attacks	Financial
Fatigue	Depression	Employment
Nutrition	Recurrent nightmares	Housing
Swallowing	Intrusive memories	Breakdown of relationship
Communication	Poor memory	Loneliness/isolation
Polyneuropathy	Sleep disturbance	Loss of friendships
Myopathy	Stress	

Source: Adapted from ICS (2019); NICE (2017); NICE (2009).

The ICS (2019) and NICE (2009a) suggest 5 key times for rehabilitation and these times are used as a structure for the rest of the chapter whilst considering the areas suggested in GPICS2 as the main areas of attention for rehabilitation after critical illness.

ON ADMISSION TO CRITICAL CARE/DURING CRITICAL CARE STAY

As soon as a person is admitted to critical care clinicians should be thinking about their discharge. As with admissions to ward areas where common practice is to predict an expected date of discharge, the critical care MDT should be forward planning for each individual discharge to a lower level of care.

From the point of admission there are low level interventions that can be utilised to try to reduce the incidence of Post ICU Syndrome. Thinking about the old saying 'prevention is better than cure', routine and robust implementation of certain strategies can help reduce the incidence of post critical care morbidity.

The aim is to have the critically unwell person sedated and mechanically ventilated for the shortest amount of time possible (Evans, 2017; Marra, 2017). Orientation should be promoted at all times, even when the person is sedated. Pain should be managed and sleep promoted with a clear day and night routine, and reduced noise and intrusive lighting. Sleep aids should be employed for people who are awake. Interventions should be clustered where possible.

THIS TOPIC IS ALSO COVERED IN CHAPTER 15

The above strategies combined with early mobilisation will help to prevent **delirium**.

Early mobilisation has been shown to be beneficial in reducing physical and psychological morbidity after a critical illness (Adler, 2012; Arias-Fernandez, 2018). The exclusion criteria for early mobilisation is surprisingly small.

Certain events during a critical care admission can be indicative of post critical care morbidity, such as incidence of delirium, and begin to shape an individualised structured rehabilitation plan. Assessments should be performed within 4 days of admission or sooner if the person is to be discharged (ICS, 2019). If the short assessment highlights concern, then a longer more in-depth assessment should be performed. People admitted electively, especially those who have had the benefit of enhanced recovery programmes (Moore et al., 2017; Pedziwiatr et al., 2018), are less likely to require additional input from the interdisciplinary follow-up team but should still be assessed. Every person admitted to critical care should have a 'short clinical assessment' to identify those who could be at risk of psychological or physical morbidity after their critical care admission (NICE, 2009a). 'Relatively short [critical care] stays may still need substantial help' (NICE, 2009a), so though it is likely that shorter, less complicated or planned admissions will need less support with rehabilitation, we mustn't assume this.

ACTIVITY 17.3: RESEARCH AND EVIDENCE-BASED PRACTICE

Consider two different critical care admissions:

Farida is 61 and has a PMH of previous Myocardial infarction, insulin controlled T2DM and **hypertension**. Farida is admitted to a booked critical care bed after a planned laparotomy,

(Continued)

resection of bowel cancer and formation of a stoma. Farida was extubated in recovery and on admission to critical care the plan is for 24 hours of close monitoring, insulin sliding scale and usual ERAS+ care (Shida, 2017).

Freda is 61 and has a past medical history of a previous MI, insulin controlled T2DM and hypertension. Freda attended ED yesterday with abdominal pain and was found to have a bowel perforation. Freda was admitted to critical care as an unplanned admission after an emergency laparotomy, bowel resection and formation of a stoma. On admission Freda remains sedated, intubated and ventilated, is requiring cardiovascular support and is on an insulin sliding scale infusion.

1.   Without knowing the further events during both persons' admissions, reflect on the similarities and differences between Farida and Freda and suggest how their individualised rehabilitation plans may differ. Consider the recommendations for assessing and formalising these rehabilitation plans.

PHYSICAL ASSESSMENT

Immobility and a highly **catabolic** state in people with a critical illness can lead to muscle loss (Sharma et al., 2018). The effect of this can lead to reduced mobility and fatigue during recovery and poorer outcomes. To prevent this you, as the critical care nurse, will ensure with the **dietician** that nutrition and energy requirements are met. You will also, alongside the physiotherapist, perform passive movements, regular position changes and mobilise the person out of bed as early and as frequently as possible. Green et al. (2016) summarise the benefits of early mobilisation in critical care areas. All those experiencing critical illness should have early intervention with rehabilitation as this is considered beneficial in preserving or restoring physical function (Whelan, 2018). Repeated assessment and goal setting and outcome measures are integral to this intervention. The Chelsea Critical Care Physical assessment tool (CPAx) is one such tool (Corner, 2012). Addressing nutritional needs can be complicated but as already discussed above, this is crucial to survival and recovery. In critical care some people may continue to eat normally. Even if you are looking after someone who can eat normally you may need to support them with nausea and vomiting, poor appetite, taste changes and other issues which will lead them to have a less than ideal intake of food and drink. For this group you will need to closely monitor their intake with fluid balance and food charts. With your dietetic colleagues you will consider alternative ways to improve this. Supplements can be prescribed by dieticians or other prescribers. A 'little and often' approach may work well with family bringing specific items from home that the person has requested. Ensure the family are warned not to be offended when the usually much loved and requested meal is prepared and brought in for the person to ultimately 'just not fancy it'.

Others may need their nutrition delivering artificially either enterally, through their usual gastrointestinal tract, or parenterally, i.e. a specially prepared liquid feed given **intravenously** known as total parenteral nutrition (TPN). Both of these will require a dietetic assessment and prescription. Nutrition is discussed further in Chapter 10.

THIS TOPIC IS ALSO COVERED IN CHAPTER 10

Critical illness induced polyneuropathy and myopathy

Critical illness induced **polyneuropathy** and **myopathy** are long acknowledged complications that may be experienced by critically ill people (Hermans et al., 2008; Latronico et al., 2005). Thought to be caused by prolonged immobility, multiple organ failure, **sepsis**, Acute Respiratory Distress Syndrome and some medications, the precise mechanism is not fully understood. Polyneuropathies and myopathies lead to prolonged time on assisted ventilation, prolonging or preventing weaning from mechanical ventilation, increased critical care length of stay and increased hospital length of stay, with the fatigue and weakness taking up to a year to recover from.

Zhou (2014) found critical illness induced polyneuropathy and myopathy has a long-lasting impact with a 'compromised quality of life lasting for months to years' and is experienced by 25–45% of people admitted to critical care areas. This suggests the focus should be on prevention and multiple sources agree (Hermans et al., 2008; Lacomis, 2011) aggressive treatment of sepsis and multi-organ failure is the most effective measure. It is easy to see that this strategy will lead to reduced duration of immobility and time on ventilators, and reduced use of **sedation** and neuromuscular blockade. Other measures suggest limited use of steroids and tight hyperglycaemic and electrolyte control as effective approaches (Latronico, 2005).

THIS TOPIC IS ALSO COVERED IN CHAPTER 2, 5 AND 15

Once the muscular weakness (mostly seen in lower limbs and respiratory muscles), fatigue and altered peripheral sensation has been identified it is important to exclude other differential causes of weakness, such as Guillain Barré Syndrome and toxic, **metabolic** and nutritional neuropathies which may be correctable or require a different management strategy.

Communication

As we have discussed in previous chapters, communication is a big challenge for people with a critical illness. Inability to communicate effectively is an extremely frustrating experience for the people we are looking after and is partially responsible for psychological sequela. Addressing communication during the critical care admission can prevent issues further on during the person's experience.

Psychological impact of critical illness

THIS TOPIC IS ALSO COVERED IN CHAPTER 15

Acute psychological distress is a commonly seen and long recognised complication in people who have experienced a critical care admission (Benzer et al., 1983; Wade et al., 2012); supporting survivors of a critical illness through their psychological recovery is discussed in Chapter 15.

ACTIVITY 17.4: CASE STUDY

Winston, 73, was admitted to the critical care unit after an emergency repair of a ruptured Abdominal Aortic Aneurysm. Prior to this Winston was fit and well, other than medications for hypertension and hyperlipidaemia, and independent for the activities of daily living.

(Continued)

Winston was in critical care for three weeks and two days. During that time, he was intubated and ventilated, received inotropic support and renal support.

Winston needed a tracheostomy to facilitate weaning from the ventilator but was decannulated two days ago. He is being prepared for transfer to the ward.

Winston is clinically stable but has a nasogastric tube and is being fed via this as he failed a swallow assessment. Winston is currently being hoisted out of bed. He is also showing evidence of short-term memory problems and was CAM ICU +ve during his critical care admission.

1. What members of the multidisciplinary team will need to be involved in Winston's rehabilitation?
2. What will the aims and goals of the rehabilitation programme be?

Cognitive function

Those recovering from a critical illness have been recognised as 'high risk for long term cognitive impairment', this risk is further increased by the presence of delirium (Pandharipande et al., 2013). Assessing cognitive function should be performed throughout the rehabilitation and follow up pathway (NICE, 2009a) The socio-economic implications of altered cognition can be subtle and underestimated; thorough assessment recognition and goal setting is needed.

Diaries

In recent years the use of diaries has been advocated as an effective strategy for reducing psychological distress after a critical illness for both the person recovering from the illness and their loved ones (Backman and Walther, 2001; Costa et al., 2019; Jones, 2009; Jones et al., 2010;).The Intensive Care Society (ICS, 2019) suggests use of diaries is a way of 'capturing the experience' and facilitates reflection. Costa et al. (2019) refer to the diaries' ability to reduce memory gaps and contextualise events as the factors which improve psychological outcomes.

The diaries are usually completed contemporaneously by both clinicians and loved ones and may also contain photographs. They should be written in plain understandable lay terms avoiding jargon and contain a mixture of a record of progress for the critically ill person and sometimes a record of local national and world events (Aitken et al., 2013). Handing over the diaries should be done by a health care professional who can provide context and explanations to go with entries. Pattison (2019) describes how handing over the diaries needs to be done with forethought and support. Case notes are often required alongside the diaries to provide additional context. The appropriate level of detail should be assessed individually. Due to a lack of national guidelines for completing the diaries (Costa et al., 2019) the content can be varied and timing of when the diaries are offered can depend upon local practice.

ACTIVITY 17.5: CASE STUDY

Karen is 57 years old and has attended follow-up clinic after her 6-day admission to critical care with sepsis 3 months ago. Karen is recovering slowly and though she is improving in strength week by week is frustrated with the pace of her recovery. Karen has returned to work but is not sleeping well and feels her mood is low. Karen feels her family are overprotective and doesn't like how her family keep telling her how poorly she was. Karen asks to see her diaries.

1. What will be the benefits of Karen seeing her diaries?
2. How will the health care professional structure the diary feedback for Karen?
3. How should Karen be prepared for seeing pictures of herself, critically ill, that she may not have known existed?

ACTIVITY 17.6: REFLECTIVE PRACTICE

1. What do you perceive as the challenges in completing diaries?
2. What are your feelings about taking pictures of people who are not in a position to consent? How should these images be stored? Who should be able to see them? Consider general data protection regulations.
3. What do you think the response from the person in the pictures will be when they see them?

PREPARING FOR DISCHARGE FROM CRITICAL CARE

I'd looked after Alex a lot during her three weeks on critical care so I could tell how scared she was about going back to the ward. We had a good chat about it and the follow-up team came to see her before she went, and I even got a few of the ward staff to come and meet her and her family. That seemed to help with the discharge.

Amaarah, Staff Nurse

The transition from a Level 3 critical care environment to a lower level of care can be a time of complex challenges (Rosa et al., 2016). Preparing individuals for this change requires good communication to clarify what changes they will experience. It is reasonable to expect a period of readjustment to ward-based care from individuals who have had a critical care admission (NICE, 2009a). As far in advance as possible monitoring should be reduced and independence promoted. To allay any fears, discussing the move to the wards, how care is delivered and explaining the reduced nursing ratios whilst providing reassurance that the critical care discharge is happening because the person is recovering and ready for the 'step down' can help prepare the person to adjust. Common practice in the UK is for a critical care follow-up service to review these people on the wards and ensure rehabilitation progress is being made. These teams will ideally meet the person prior to their discharge to the ward and so can provide an element of continuity for their care.

Information giving at this point, and throughout all of the rehabilitation pathway, is well recognised as integral for progress (ICS, 2019), improving the person and their family participation and achievement of set rehabilitation goals.

Once the decision to discharge a person to a ward environment has been made, discharge should occur within 4 hours and as early as possible within the 'working day' (ICS, 2019). Out of hours discharges (those that do not occur between 07:00 and 21:59) should be avoided and are known to carry an increased risk of complication and readmissions to critical care (Vollam et al., 2018).

THIS TOPIC IS ALSO COVERED IN CHAPTER 3

Vollam et al. (2018) further recognised critical care readmission correlated with increased hospital length of stay, increased morbidity and mortality and that it could be suggested that a readmission to a critical care area within 48hrs is an indication of a premature discharge. From the perspective of the individual and their significant others a readmission would be a time of great stress and worry, likely leading to increased psychological distress. This should be considered and managed as part of the rehabilitation package.

Concerns regarding the recovery from the acute illness and the high risk of deterioration and readmission are central but in addition the nutrition, mobility, communication, cognitive function, mental health and social situation will be examined and discussed. Referral to the appropriate teams and implementation of strategies to address acknowledged needs will form part of the individualised rehabilitation plan. This individualised plan should have been initiated prior to discharge from the critical care area. Those discharged from critical care areas often will require ongoing input from members of the interdisciplinary team such as physiotherapy, dieticians, **speech and language therapists** and psychologists alongside the clinical team with overall responsibility, sometimes referred to as the parent team.

The role of critical care follow-up teams, as we have previously discussed, is a relatively new speciality. NICE CG 83 (2009a) describes a key principle of care as having a health care professional coordinating the rehabilitation care pathway and ensuring continuity of care. This is usually the critical care follow-up nurse or can be any member of the interdisciplinary team. Ward staff will often require support in caring for these individuals from the follow-up team due to their complex needs. Ward staff may be required to care for individuals with invasive lines or other equipment. Support from follow-up services can facilitate discharges to lower levels of care by creating the continuity and providing the expert support needed. In their Cochrane review of five studies Schofield-Robinson et al. (2018) found little difference in outcomes for those who received standard care rather than support from a follow-up service due to insufficient evidence available to determine effectiveness. Variety in the component parts of the follow up models made comparisons difficult. Nonetheless, provision of **follow-up** services within the UK continue to be recommended in national guidelines (NICE, 2009a, 2017; ICS 2019).

Spirituality is easily overlooked. As part of routine admission questions, the spiritual needs of the person should be enquired about and possible options to meet these needs should be explored throughout the hospital stay. Hospital-based chaplaincy is usually accessible, or faith leaders from the community who are willing to come in to visit. Based on the requirements of the individual, access to spiritual support should be facilitated in an effort to recognise and rehabilitate the whole person. Being able to engage with their faith again will be a key point of recovery for a spiritual person. Providing spiritual care is an area where the individual's family can be involved and Abuatiq (2015) suggests in a case report that persons who have their spiritual needs addressed have reduced levels of psychological distress and that this is crucial to an effective recovery.

During stay on ward

Adapting to a lower level of care, moving from a critical care unit to a ward is often a difficult time. The change in nurse to patient ratios means people may wait longer for assistance, interventions and medications. Preparation and reassurance will go some way to allaying these concerns along with input from the follow-up or rehabilitation team. It is essential at this point that the person and their loved ones are supplied with the correct information, tools and strategies to help themselves through their recovery. The importance of information-giving at all points through a person's critical illness has been a cited as central to rehabilitation (ICS, 2019).

The work already started on the critical care unit, especially by physiotherapists supporting early mobilisation and prevention of deconditioning, continues whilst on the ward. Close working with the person to ensure they understand the value of mobilising, eating and drinking, optimising memory and cognitive function is crucial. The rehabilitation package should continue to be individualised with clear goals set and be regularly reviewed.

This is an opportunity to repeat the psychological assessment tools and support the individual as dictated by their score or as felt appropriate after discussion. Low key interventions such as talking to the person about their critical care experience and normalising as appropriate can be helpful. Knowing when to refer on to more specialist intervention from a psychologist should be part of the pathway.

Preparing for discharge from hospital home or to community care

Again, preparation for the next step is required and involves the interdisciplinary team considering referrals for services and equipment that may be needed for a safe and successful discharge from hospital. This assessment should continue to be individualised and **holistic**. Goals should continue to be set with full consideration of the baseline functional status the individual is aiming for. Including loved ones in these plans will be helpful.

2-3 months after critical care discharge

GPICS 2 (ICS, 2019), NICE CG 83 (2009a) and NICE quality standard 158 (2017) recommend those who have experienced a critical care admission of greater than 4 days or those people with recognised complications of a critical illness be invited to a follow-up clinic around 2-3 months after discharge from hospital. Subsequent outpatient follow up visits may also be needed at 6 and 12 months.

As before, the physical, psychological and social wellbeing of the person is assessed and compared to previously set rehabilitation goals to ensure progress is being made. Ideally this is done by a **multi-professional team** led by an **intensivist**. Ongoing access or referral to other team members should be facilitated through this clinic. Psychological assessment tools can be revisited and interventions as dictated by scores put in place. A medication review may be needed.

ACTIVITY 17.7: CRITICAL THINKING

'Correlation is not causation'.

When evaluating research consider the difference between causation and correlation.
   In a Dutch retrospective cohort study van Beusekom et al. (2019) looked at the risk of developing new chronic health conditions for ICU survivors. Findings indicated an increase in chronic conditions after a critical illness, but also noted a higher level of chronic conditions in the group before their critical illness.

(Continued)

1. Has the episode of critical illness caused the person to be at increased risk of developing a chronic illness? Or is this a positive correlation and the fact they had pre-existing chronic conditions the cause?
2. Do you agree with the main results and conclusions of this article?

SOCIAL, FINANCIAL AND RELATIONSHIPS IMPACT OF CRITICAL ILLNESS

The fact that this has been left for the last few paragraphs of the chapter is not an indication that this topic is of low importance. The ongoing long-term socio-economic and relationship implications of critical illness persist for some people long after their immediate recovery from the acute illness (Davidson, 2017). The needs of this group are diverse (McPeake at al., 2019).

It is important that you are aware of possible socio-economic issues that may be encountered and are able to discuss them, perhaps to recognise or forewarn, or to signpost to support services should they be needed.

Financial worries are often of immediate concern when someone is unable to work. A social work referral may be needed in addition to ensuring your critical care unit has literature available which may direct a person or their friends and family to access financial support. Help and guidance through the benefits system could well be required.

A knock-on effect may be housing worries: it may be that a person can no longer afford their house, or it may become apparent that the current residence will not be suitable for the person when they leave the hospital. Adaptations may be needed, or a completely different form of housing could be indicated.

Keeping employment and returning to work may be difficult. Mobility, fatigue and cognitive function may stop a person from returning to their usual job; perhaps reduced hours or a phased return would help. Again, support agencies will be needed to ensure the person is aware of their rights as an employee and what reasonable adjustments they can expect from their employer.

Relationship dynamics can change after someone has experienced a critical illness and Davidson and Netzer (2017) talk of 'role strain' and impact upon 'family integrity' for both the person and their loved ones. A partner may become a carer and having witnessed their loved one going through a critical illness they may become overprotective and cautious. Altered roles at home can impact intimate relationships. Libido may be reduced due to fatigue and altered body image. Fear can also cause couples to be wary about resuming sexual relationships. Embarrassment can prevent people asking for help with returning to a healthy sex life.

There is also evidence to indicate that the significant others of a person who has been critically ill may experience acute to long term psychological distress (Azoulay et al., 2005). This study found incidence of severe PTSD correlated with increased risk of anxiety and depression. These family members often act as informal carers, especially after the person leaves the critical care area and is heading towards home. The benefit for the critically ill person of these informal carers is recognised and therefore leads to an obvious need to support these family members to ensure their burden is reduced and that they are able to provide this support (Davidson and Netzer, 2017). Diaries, as discussed above, may contribute to this. Ideally psychological support would expand to include family as needed, but from a resource and funding perspective this may not be feasible. This is where lay support groups and forums may have value.

ACTIVITY 17.8: THEORY STOP POINT

'The large investments made during intensive care are only sustained when continued support is in place following discharge' (ICS, 2019)

Research of the long-term implications of critical illness upon both the survivor and their loved ones is a relatively new area of study.

1.   What do you think the value of this research is?
2.   What are the common research methods used for studies in this area?
3.   Is the money invested in critical care worth it? After the large financial investment in caring for the critically ill what do you think about the comparable lack of resources for the rehabilitation phase of the individual's recovery?
4.   Are we failing by not ensuring optimal recovery for this vulnerable group with inadequate provision of rehabilitation services?
5.   How would more research into this specialist area affect the service provision?

CHAPTER SUMMARY

This chapter has supported your understanding of:

*   The important concept that preparing for discharge from a critical care area begins on admission
*   Recovery as recovering from a critical illness can be a lengthy and complex process, which requires a holistic approach including the person's physical, psychological and social wellbeing
*   The multi professional team who will have a central role in co-ordinating rehabilitation
*   The tools available for psychological assessment
*   Your awareness of services you may need to signpost a person towards for additional support for both the person and their loved ones

GO FURTHER

As a critical care nurse, you should be aware of the resources available to aid recovery. Familiarise yourself with the organisations below and understand when you might need to direct someone to them.

1.   Can you find any other support groups or forums?
2.   Does your department facilitate any groups?

You should be clear that you are only signposting towards possible support agencies and are not endorsing any services external to the NHS.

Books

Awdish, R. (2017) *In Shock: My Journey from Death to Recovery and the Redemptive Power of Hope*. London: St. Martin's Press.

• An autobiography from a doctor sharing her experience of a critical illness.

Bauby, J.-D. (2008) *The Diving Bell and the Butterfly*. London: HarperCollins.

• This poignant memoir from a French journalist dictated through blinking after a catastrophic brain stem stroke gives insight into the frustration of not being able to communicate.

Watson, C. (2020) *The Courage to Care: A Call for Compassion*. London: Chatto and Windus.

• An anthology of stories about compassionate nursing.

Journal articles

Held, N. and Moss, M. (2019) 'Optimizing post-intensive care unit rehabilitation', *Turkish Thoracic Journal*, 20 (2) 147–52. www.ncbi.nlm.nih.gov/pmc/articles/PMC6453631/ (accessed November 13, 2020).

• This paper provides a summary of literature reviewing post ICU rehabilitation strategies.

McPeake, J., Mikkelsen, M.E., Quasim, T., Hibbert, E., Cannon, P., Shaw, M., Ankori, J., Iwashyna, T.J. and Haines, K.J. (2019) 'Return to employment after critical illness and its association with psychosocial outcomes: A systematic review and meta-analysis', *Journal of the American Thoracic Society*, 16 (10). www.atsjournals.org/doi/abs/10.1513/AnnalsATS.201903-248OC (accessed November 13, 2020).

• This article is about returning to work (or not).

Wintermann, G.B., Rosendahl, J., Weidner, K., Strauß, B., Hinz, A. and Petrowski, K. (2018) 'Self-reported fatigue following intensive care of chronically critically ill patients: A prospective cohort study', *Journal of Intensive Care*, 6 (27). www.ncbi.nlm.nih.gov/pmc/articles/PMC5930426 (accessed November 13, 2020).

• Fatigue after critical illness is an often-reported, long-lasting complaint. This prospective cohort study reviews the data around self-reported fatigue.

Useful websites

www.criticalcarerecovery.com

• An NHS resource for individuals, families, carers and professionals.

www.icusteps.org (accessed November 13, 2020).

• This is a charitable organisation which provides support for people and their families during rehabilitation after critical illness.

https://dipexcharity.org (accessed November 13, 2020).

• A charitable multimedia approach to sharing qualitative research around illness.

www.healthtalk.org (accessed November 13, 2020).

- The website for an informal network of health care providers who are interested in use of diaries for critically ill people on the intensive care unit.

www.icu-diary.org (accessed November 13, 2020).

- A diary that is written for those admitted to the ICU completed during their time of sedation and ventilation. It is written by relatives, nurses and others. The person can read their diary afterwards and is able to understand better what has happened to them.

Podcasts

Walking home from the ICU. https://podcasts.apple.com/us/podcast/walking-home-from-the-icu/
    id1497431005

- A series of podcasts from North American clinicians and critical care survivors about rehabilitation, recovery and their critical illness experience.
- Aitken, L. (2019) 'Helping patients to recover psychological health after critical illness', Continuous Critical Care Nurse podcast, August 7. https://podtail.com/en/podcast/med reach-critical-care-nursing/prof-leanne-aitken-helping-patients-to-recover-psy/

A fast paced yet thorough guide through the available research regarding psychological recovery after critical care.

REFERENCES

Abuatiq, A. (2015) 'Spiritual care for critical care patients', *International Journal of Nursing and Clinical Practices*, 2: 128. doi.org/10.15344/2394-4978/2015/128

Adler, J. and Malone, D. (2012) 'Early mobilization in the Intensive Care Unit: A systematic review', *Cardiopulmonary Physical Therapy Journal*, 25 (1): 5–13.

Aitken, L., Rattray, J., Hull, A., Kenardy, J.A., Le Brocque, R., and Ullman. A.J. (2013) 'The use of diaries in psychological recovery from intensive care', *Critical Care*, 17: 253. doi.org/10.1186/cc13164

Arias-Fernandez, P., Romero-Martin, M., Gomez-Salgado, J. and Fernandez-Garcia, D. (2018) 'Rehabilitation and early mobilization in the critical patient: Systematic review', *Journal of Physical Therapy Science*, 30 (9): 1193–201.

Audit Commission (ed.) (1999) *Critical to Success*. London: Audit Commission for Local Authorities and the National Health Service in England and Wales. http://www.wales.nhs.uk/sites3/documents/768/CriticalToSuccess.pdf (accessed November 13, 2020).

Azoulay, E., Pochard, F., Kentish-Barnes, N., Chevret, S., Aboab, J., Adrie, C., [...] and Schlemmer, B. (2005) 'Risk of post traumatic stress symptoms in family members of intensive care unit patients', *American Journal of Respiratory and Critical Care Medicine*, 171 (9): 987–94.

Bäckman, C.G. and Walther, S.M., (2001) 'Use of a personal diary written on the ICU during critical illness', *Intensive Care Medicine*, 27: 426–9.

Benzer, H., Baker, S. and McDaniel. C. (1983) 'Psychological sequel of intensive care', *International Anaesthetic Clinics*, 21: 169–78.

Corner, E.J., Wood, H., Englebretsen, C., Thomas, A., Grant, R.L., Nikoletou, D. and Soni. N. (2012) 'The Chelsea Critical Care Physical Assessment Tool (CPAx): Validation of an innovative new tool to measure physical morbidity in the general adult critical care population – An observational proof-of-concept pilot study', *Physiotherapy*. doi.org/10.1016/J.physio.2012.01.003

Costa, A.V., Padfield, O., Elliott, S. and Hayden, P. (2019) 'Improving patient diary use in intensive care: A quality improvement report', *Journal of the Intensive Care Society*. doi. org/10.1177/1751143719885295

Cuthbertson, B.H., and Wunsch, H. (2016) 'Long-term outcomes after critical illness: The best predictor of the future is the past', *American journal of Respiratory and Critical Care Medicine*, 194 (2). doi.org/10.1164/rccm.201602-0257ED

Davidson, J.E. and Netzer, G. (2017) 'Family response to critical illness', in J.O. Bienvenu, C. Jones and R.O. Hopkins (eds) *Psychological and Cognitive Impact of Critical Illness*. Oxford: Oxford University Press. pp. 191–211.

Department of Health (ed.) (2000) *Comprehensive Critical Care: A Review of Adult Critical Care Services*. London: Department of Health. http://webarchive.nationalarchives.gov.uk/20130107105354/http://www.dh.gov.uk/prod_consum_dh/groups/dh_digitalassets/@dh/@en/documents/digitalasset/dh_4082872.pdf (accessed November 13, 2020).

Devlin, J.W., Skrobik, Y., Gélinas, C., Needham, D.M., Slooter, A.J.C., Pandharipande, P.P., [...] and Alhazzani, W. (2018) 'Clinical practice guidelines for the prevention and management of pain, agitation/sedation, delirium, immobility, and sleep disruption in adult patients in the ICU', *Critical Care Medicine*, 46 (9): e825-73. doi.org/10.1097/CCM.0000000000003299

Evans, S., Senaratne, D.H.S. and Waldman, C. (2017) 'Continuing rehabilitation after intensive care unit discharge: Opportunities for technology and innovation', *ICU Management and Practice*, 17 (3): 178–80.

Gayat, E., Cariou, A., Deye, N., Vieillard-Baron, A., Jaber, S., Damoisel, C. [...] and Mebazaa. A. (2018) 'Determinants of long term outcome in ICU survivors: Results from the FROG ICU study', *Critical Care*, 22: Article #8.

Green, M., Marzano, V., Leditschke, I. A., Mitchell, I., and Bissett, B. (2016) 'Mobilization of intensive care patients: A multidisciplinary practical guide for clinicians'. *Journal of Multidisciplinary Healthcare*, 9: 247–56.

Hatch, R., Young, D., Barber, V., Griffiths, J., Harrison, D.A. and Watkinson, P. (2018) 'Anxiety, depression and post traumatic stress disorder after critical illness: A UK-wide prospective cohort study', *Critical Care*, 22: Article #310. doi.org/10.1186/s13054-018-2223-6

Hermans, G., De Jonghe, B., Bruyninckx, F., and Van Den Berghe, G. (2008) 'Clinical review: Critical illness polyneuropathy and myopathy', *Critical Care*, 12 (6): 238.

Intensive Care Society (ICS) (2019) *Guidelines for the Provision of Intensive Care Services* (2nd edition). London: ICS. Available from https://www.ics.ac.uk/ICS/ICS/GuidelinesAndStandards/GPICS_2nd_Edition.aspx (accessed November 13, 2020).

Jeitziner, M.M., Hamers, J.P., Bürgin, R., Hantikainen, V. and Zwakhalen, S.M. (2015) 'Long-term consequences of pain, anxiety and agitation for critically ill older patients after an intensive care unit stay', *Journal of Clinical Nursing*, 24 (17–18): 2419–28. doi.org/10.1111/jocn.12801

Jones, C., (2009) 'Introducing photo diaries for ICU patients', *Journal of the Intensive Care Society*, 10: 183–5.

Jones, C. Bäckman. C., Capuzzo. M., Egerod, I., Flaatten, H., Granja, C., Rylander, C. and Griffiths, R.D. (2010) 'Intensive care diaries reduce new onset post-traumatic stress disorder following critical illness: A randomised, controlled trial', *Critical Care*, 14 (5): R168.

Lacomis, D. (2011) 'Neuromuscular disorders in critically ill patients: Review and update', *Journal of Clinical Neuromuscular Disorders*, 12 (4): 197–218.

Latronico, N., Shehu, I. and Seghelini, E. (2005) 'Neuromuscular sequelae of critical illness', *Current Opinion in Critical Care*, 11: 381–90.

Marra, A., Wesley, E. and Pandharipande. P.P. (2017) 'The ABCDEF bundle in critical care', *Critical Care Clinics*, 33 (2): 225–43.

Mckinley, S., Aitken, L.M., Alison, J.A., King, M., Leslie, G., Burmeister, E. and Elliot, D. (2012) 'Sleep and other factors associated with mental health and psychological distress after intensive care for critical illness', *Intensive Care Medicine*, 38: 627–33. doi.org/10.1007/s00134-012-2477-4

McPeake, J.M., Henderson, P., Darroch, G., Iwashyna, T. J., McTavish, P., Robinson, C. and Quasim, T. (2019) 'Social and economic problems of ICU survivors identified by a structured social welfare consultation', *Critical Care*, 23: Article #153. doi.org/10.1186/s13054-019-2442-5

Mehlhorn, J., Freytag, A., Schmidt, K., Brunkhorst, F.M., Graf, J., Troitzsch, U., Schlattmann, P., Wensing, M., Gensichen, J., 'Rehabilitation interventions for postintensive care syndrome', *Critical Care Medicine*, 42 (5): 1263–71 doi: 10.1097/CCM.0000000000000148

Moore, J., Conway, D., Thomas, N., Cummings, D. and Atkinson, D. (2017) 'Impact of a peri-operative quality improvement programme on postoperative pulmonary complications', *Anaesthesia*, 72 (3). doi.org/10.1111/anae.13763

National Institute for Health and Clinical Excellence (NICE) (2006) *Nutrition Support for Adults: Oral Nutrition Support, Enteral Tube Feeding and Parenteral Nutrition* (Clinical Guideline 32). London: NICE. Available from www.nice.org.uk/guidance/cg32 (accessed November 13, 2020).

National Institute for Health and Care Excellence (NICE) (2007) *Acutely Ill Patients in Hospital: Recognition of and Response to Acute Illness in Adults in Hospital* (Clinical Guideline 50). London: NICE. Available from www.nice.org.uk/guidance/cg50 (accessed November 13, 2020).

National Institute for Health and Care Excellence (NICE) (2009a) *Rehabilitation after Critical Illness in Adults* (CG 83). London: NICE. Available from www.nice.org.uk/guidance/cg83 (accessed November 13, 2020).

National Institute for Health and Clinical Excellence (NICE) (2009b) *Depression in Adults: Recognition and Management* (Clinical Guideline 90). London: NICE. Available from www.nice.org.uk/guidance/cg90 (accessed November 13, 2020).

National Institute for Health and Clinical Excellence (NICE) (2011) *Generalised Anxiety Disorder and Panic Disorder in Adults: Management (Clinical Guideline 113)*. London: NICE. Available from www.nice.org.uk/guidance/cg113 (accessed November 13, 2020).

National Institute for Health and Care Excellence (NICE) (2017) *Rehabilitation After Critical Illness in Adults* (Quality Standard 158). London: NICE. Available from www.nice.org.uk/guidance/qs158 (accessed November 13, 2020).

National Institute for Health and Clinical Excellence (NICE) (2018) *Post-traumatic Stress Disorder*. NICE Guideline 116. London: NICE. Available from https://www.nice.org.uk/guidance/ng116 (accessed November 13, 2020).

National Patient Safety Agency (NPSA) (2007) *Recognising and Responding to Early Signs of Deterioration in Hospitalised Patients*. London: NPSA.

National Patient Safety Agency (NPSA) (2009) *Framework of Competencies for Recognising and Responding to Acutely Ill Patients in Hospital*. London: NPS.

Olsen, K.D., Nester, M., Hansen, B.S. (2017) 'Evaluating the past to improve the future – A qualitative study of ICU patients' experiences', *Intensive and Critical Care Nursing*, 43: 61–7. doi.org/10.1016/j.iccn.2017.06.008

Page, P., Simpson, A. and Reynolds. L. (2019) 'Bearing witness and being bounded: The experiences of nurses in adult critical care in relationship to the survivorship needs of patients and families', *Journal of Clinical Nursing*, 17 (17–18). doi.org/10.1111/jocn.14887

Pandharipande, P.P., Girard, T.D., Jackson, J.C., Morandi, A., Thompson, J.L., Pun. B.T. [...] and Ely, E.W. (2013) 'Long term cognitive impairment after critical illness', *New England Journal of Medicine*, 369 (14): 1306–16.

Pattison, N., O'Gara, G., Lucas, C., Gull, K., Thomas, K. and Dolan, S. (2019) 'Filling the gaps: A mixed-methods study exploring the use of patient diaries in the critical care unit', *Intensive and Critical Care Nursing*, 51: 27–34. doi.org/10.1016/j.iccn.2018.10.005

Pędziwiatr, M., Mavrikis, J., Witowski, J., Adamos, A., Major, P., Nowakowski, M. and Budzyński, A. (2018) 'Current status of enhanced recovery after surgery (ERAS) protocol in gastrointestinal surgery', *Medical Oncology*, 35: Article #95. doi.org/10.1007/s12032-018-1153-0

Pilcher, D.V., Duke, G.J., George, C., Bailey, M.J. and Hart. G. (2007) 'After hours discharges from intensive care increases the risk of readmission and death', *Anaesthesia and Intensive Care*, 35 (4): 477–85.

Resuscitation Council UK (RCUK) (2020) *ReSPECT*. https://resus.org.uk/respect/ (accessed November 13, 2020).

Righy, C., Rosa, R.G., Amancio da Silva, R.T., Kochann, R., Migliavaca, C.B., Robinson, C.C., Teche, S.P., Teixeira, C., Bozza, F.A. and Falavigna. M. (2019) 'Prevalence of post-traumatic stress disorder symptoms in adult critical care survivors: A systematic review and meta-analysis', *Critical Care*, 23: Article #13. doi.org/10.1186/s13054-019-2489-3

Rosa, R.G., Maccari, J.G., Cremonese, R.V., Tonietto, T.F., Cremonese, R.V. and Teixera. C. (2016) 'The impact of critical care transition programs on outcomes after intensive care unit (ICU) discharge: Can we get there from here?', *Journal of Thoracic Disease*, 8 (7): 1374–76. doi.org/10.21037/jtd.2016.05.30

Schofield-Robinson, O.J., Lewis, S.R., Smith, A.F., McPeake, J. and Alderson, P. (2018) 'Follow-up services for improving long term outcomes in intensive care unit survivors', *Cochrane Systematic Review*. doi.org/10.1002/14651858.CD012701.pub2

Sharma, K., Mogensen, K.M. and Robinson, M.K. (2018) 'Pathophysiology of critical illness and role of nutrition', *Nutrition in Clinical Practice*, 34 (1): 12–22. doi.org/10.1002/ncp.10232

Shida, D., Tagawa, K., Inada, K., Nasu, K., Seyama, Y., Maeshiro, T., Miyamoto, S., Inoue, S. and Umekita, N. (2017) 'Modified enhanced recovery after surgery (ERAS) protocols for parient with obstructive colorectal cancer', *BMC Surgery*, 17: Article #18. doi.org/10.1186/s12893-017-0213-2

van Beusekom, I., Bakhshi-Raiez, F., van der Schaf, M., Busschers W. B., de Keizer, N., Dongelmans, D. (2019) 'ICU survivors have a substantially higher risk of developing new chronic conditions compared to a population-based control group', *Critical Care Medicine*, 47 (3): 324–30. doi.org/10.1097/CCM.0000000000003576

Vollam, S., Dutton, S., Lamb, S., Petrinic, T., Young, J.D. and Watkinson, P. (2018) 'Out of hours discharges from intensive care, in hospital mortality and intensive care readmission rates: A systematic review and meta-analysis', *Intensive Care Medicine*, 44 (7): 1115–29. doi.org/10.1007/s00134-018-5245-2

Wade, D.M., Hankins, M., Smyth, D.A., Rhone, E.E., Howell, D.C.J., Mythen, M.G. and Weinman. J.A. (2015) 'Detecting acute distress and risk of future psychological morbidity in critically ill patients: Validation of the intensive care psychological assessment tool. Critical Care', 18: Article #519. doi.org/10.1186/s13054-014-0519-8

Wade, D.M., Howell, D.C., Weinaman, J.A., Hardy, R.J., Mythen, M.G., Brewin, C.R., Borja-Beluda, S., Matejowsky, C.F. and Raine. R.A. (2012) 'Investigating risk factors for psychological morbidity three months after intensive care: A prospective cohort study', *Critical Care*, 16: R192.

Wade, D.M., Mouncey, P.R., Richards-Belle, A., Wulff, J., Harrison, D.A., Sadique, M.Z. [...] and Rowan, K.M. (2019) 'Effect of a nurse-led preventive psychological intervention on symptoms of posttraumatic stress disorder among critically ill patients: A randomized clinical trial', *JAMA*, 321 (7): 665–75. doi.org/10.1001/jama.2019.0073

Whelan, M., Van Aswegen, H. and Corner, E. (2018) 'Impact of the Chelsea Critical Care Physical assessment tool on clinical outcomes of surgical and trauma patients in an intensive care unit: An experimental study', *South African Journal of Physiotherapy*, 74 (1): a450. doi.org/10.4102/sajp. v74i1.450

Wittekamp, B.H.J., Van Zanten, A.R.H. and Tjan, D.H.T. (2010) 'Intensive care aftermath: Morbidity and disabilities after critical illness in adults', *Netherlands Journal of Critical Care*, 4 (1): 16–21.

Zhou, C., Wu, L., Ni, F., Ji, W., Wu, J. and Zhang, H. (2014) 'Critical illness polyneuropathy and myopathy: A systematic review', *Neural Regeneration Research* 9(1): 101–10. doi: 10.4103/1673-5374.125337

APPENDIX

CHAPTER 1 ANSWERS TO ACTIVITIES

Answers to Activity 1.1: Critical Thinking

1. To support you making a judgment you can use critical appraisal tools. You may look at how the research was conducted, who it was conducted by and how it was funded. Depending on the type of research methodology used you may look at the sample of participants, how they were selected and do they accurately represent the target population. There are a number of ways a piece of evidence can be biased and the Critical Appraisal Skill Programme (https://casp-uk.net/)will help you identify these.

2. Types of evidence you may have listed:

   - Randomised controlled trials
   - Qualitative research
   - Quantitative research
   - Mixed methods research
   - Literature review
   - Systematic reviews
   - Case studies
   - Clinical expertise
   - National guidelines
   - Local policy
   - Media
   - Patient views

Answers to Activity 1.2: Research and Evidence-based Practice

1. Some of the challenges faced when implementing the sepsis care bundle could be:

   - Lack of resources/staff
   - Staff knowledge and skills
   - Powerless to escalate within the team due to team culture
   - Lack of leadership support for junior staff
   - It could also be the lack of understanding that all the elements need to be delivered together
   - There can be limited evidence base surrounding some of the individual elements in a bundle. Measuring effectiveness can be hampered by the delivery with the other elements.

2. To overcome these barriers possibly:

- Raise awareness within the department – posters, emails, reminders and audits
- Structured education programme
- Stronger leadership to lead by example and to improve both culture and retention of staff

Answers to Activity 1.3: Theory Stop Point

1. What do you think the barriers are when trying to implement a care bundle in a practice area?

- Acceptance of the care bundle either as a bundle or of one individual element
- Compliance with delivering the care bundle across the team
- Time to embed change in practice
- Knowledge and understanding of the team regarding the importance or impact of the care bundle

2. What could be the negatives of using care bundles?

You may not know which element of the care bundle is having the most positive or negative effect as all are delivered together

3. How do you think the effectiveness of care bundles is assessed?

Audits of compliance in delivery against a relevant outcome such as the reduction in ventilator acquired pneumonia when the VAP bundle is adhered to.

Answer to Activity 1.4: Critical Thinking

1. When watching the video you may have come up with different answers to the questions posed which is fine, but you need to be conscious that your opinion can be influenced by others through what they say and how they behave.
2. Your perception is affected by three factors:

- Your past experiences: You might act on information based on experiences, someone you have previously cared for with a similar condition and the knowledge gained.
- Your expectations: You may interpret information in such a way that it confirms the expected action you plan to take. You also may pay more attention to the information that fits your expectations.
- Filters: You may unconsciously 'filter out' some information and disregard it.

Answer to Activity 1.6: Critical Thinking

1. • This may have been due to the power imbalance between the nurse and the other members of the team.
   • She may not have been assertive enough in her suggestion. In stressful, highly critical events it can be difficult to hear, focus and communicate with all team members.
2. Using a structured commutation tool may be helpful, not doubting herself and reiterating her point, if this does not work then escalating the issue and speaking with more senior staff to support her.

Answer to Activity 1.8: Case Study

3. Other strategies you can try:

- Assessment and management of all the factors: is she in pain, hungry, thirsty, needing the toilet.
- Consideration of the environment, dim light, move to see a window if possible, remove as much technology as is safe, reduce the alarm noises.
- Encourage, if appropriate, family involvement in care. Ask the family if she has any music she would find calming. Ask the family to read or speak to her, offering reassurance. Hold her hand.
- Constant reorientation to place and date and time.
- Promotion of sleep.

Answers to Activity 1.11: Critical Thinking

2. Some barriers to effective teamwork:

- Lack of trust across the team
- Lack of clear leadership
- Lack of a shared goal or vision
- Lack confidence in your own ability
- Traditional professional cultures or hierarchy

3. How would you overcome these?

- Choosing the right people in the team (where possible)
- Work towards developing an atmosphere of trust
- Being clear about roles and responsibility as well having a clear, common goal
- Encourage communication – debrief and constructive feedback
- Team building needs time!

CHAPTER 2 ANSWERS TO ACTIVITIES

Answer to Activity 2.1: Case Study

1. We have made the assumption that the person can write in English and has a reasonable level of reading and writing ability
2. Some issues may be:

- The person may be a non-English speaker or writer
- They may have an impaired grip due to muscle weakness, increased oedema in their hands or as part of their illness
- Lines and drip may hinder movement or make the person anxious to move

Answer to Activity 2.2: Reflective Practice

1. The app could aid communication without the need for the person to write
2. An issue in practice is the availability of a device which the app can be downloaded on, and cleaning of this device in between uses.

Answer to Activity 2.3: Critical Thinking

1. As this is a discussion or reflective activity there is no correct answer, you may want to consider the tool and how easy it is to use. Also, is the assessment consistent across the staff when used?

Answer to Activity 2.4: Theory Stop Point

1. There is lack of consistency due to the need of sedation to be tailored to the individual's needs additionally some variation is due to prescriber preference
2. In addition to the two points above there may be licencing law differences in certain countries, poor availability of the medication and the cost of certain sedatives

Answer to Activity 2.5: Theory Stop Point

1. What can help is:

   - Differentiate between night and day, access to window, dim lights in the evening
   - An evening routine to signal that it is evening
   - Study in the day and some activity
   - Reduction of noise at night time

Answer to Activity 2.7: Critical Thinking

1. As a minimum you need to involve:

   - The person
   - Physiotherapist
   - Nurse
   - Doctor

Answer to Activity 2.8: Case Study

1. Communication in challenging situations can be distressing. It is important that you have space for your own emotions. There are some strategies to help you consider all the elements of communication; one is called SPIKES
   It stands for:

   - **S**etting
   - **P**erception
   - **I**nvitation
   - **K**nowledge
   - **E**motions
   - **S**trategy

Just think about each of the above before you communicate with the family. The main thing is to remain calm.

2. Explain to the family why this is happening and that it is temporary. Suggest ways in which they can structure the visit and try to engage Michelle. Bring in items from home such as a photograph and maybe play Michelle's favourite music. It might help to read to her. Let them know they can take a break from visiting or see if there are other family members who they can share the visits with.

Answers to Activity 2.10: Reflection

1. There can be a perception that family visits can upset the critically ill person. There also may be a view that family visits get 'in the way' of the nurse caring for the person. There may also be restrictions due to infection control reasons, but this is not the norm.
2. There can be some tensions in families during visiting, it can put stress and pressure on the family to visit. It can also be difficult or costly to keep visiting. The critically ill person may not always want visitors there all the time.

CHAPTER 3 ANSWERS TO ACTIVITIES

Answers to Activity 3.1: Critical Thinking

Planned admissions to critical care areas have a much greater chance of surviving to hospital discharge. This cohort will be in better health throughout the process and will have benefited from optimisation before their admission.

Those with a planned admission to critical care have a better out as they can prepare for admission. For example, they can give up smoking or lose weight. Their procedure is also planned and therefore is less likely to have negative complications. They may wake up with some disorientation, but they will have more awareness of their circumstances and are more likely to be cooperative with the weaning from the ventilator. All of these factors can result in a shorter stay and fewer complications as a result of critical illness.

Answers to Activity 3.2: Research and Evidence-based Practice

1. Research results and findings will be used to guide the writing of documents. Application of these documents will differ depending on whether it is a policy, a formal mandatory document, or a guideline, a non-mandatory recommendation.
2. Communication cascades can be formal or informal. You may find emails, newsletters, and communication boards a good source of information. Communication may be built into the structure of your working day. You may only find out about a change in practice when a colleague comments 'did you know...?' or perhaps gives you feedback on an element of your practice.

   Mandated services and targets are often from the government level via NHS England to the hospital, which will cascade through the organisation to you. This may be attached to a financial penalty or reward.

   Practice-based educators, mandatory training, and local resources such as the intranet library of documents are available to ensure you and your practice are up to date.

Answer to Activity 3.3: Theory Stop Point

1. To overcome barriers to implementing change by considering the following:

   - People change when they *see a need*
   - People will change when they *know how*
   - People change when they are *actively involved*
   - People *need support* during the process
   - People change when they *feel secure*
   - People are not always rational, new knowledge alone is not enough
   - People change their attitudes slowly

Answer to Activity 3.4: Research and Evidence-based Practice

1. You may find a nurse-led critical care outreach team, or a multi-disciplinary rapid response team or medical emergency team. Their remit and structure will be varied. Consider spending some time with the team as part of your development.

   Not all teams cover 24 hours a day 7 days a week.

   Some hospitals do not have interventional emergency teams (apart from cardiac arrest teams) and rely on a ward-based response system.

   Quantitative research on the value of these teams is equivocal. Qualitative research is more supportive of the existence of these teams. Talk to your colleagues and ask what their opinion of these teams is.

   Critics feel these teams can deskill ward doctors and nurses. Supporters highlight the sharing of skills and knowledge as a core function and benefit of such teams.

Answers to Activity 3.7: Case Study

1. Whilst Carol's respiratory rate is normal, she has an increased work of breathing. A normal breathing pattern and rhythm is barely noticeable. Carol appears to be working hard to breathe; this is a clear subjective assessment that Carol isn't as well as she was previously.

   Not all people that deteriorate will have a raised early warning score. As a qualified nurse, you will be observant of subtle changes in Carol's condition that may indicate Carol is deteriorating. New confusion is a recent addition to the National Early Warning Score 2 and can be a sign of sepsis. Along with a known source of infection and your assessment that Carol doesn't look as well you have fulfilled the criteria for starting the sepsis bundle.

2. You will inform the nurse in charge and the medical team looking after Carol. You can also discuss your assessment with the Critical Care Outreach Team.

   Communication should be delivered in a structured format and conclude with recommendations or a plan. This is especially relevant when needing to complete a time-specific intervention where you may need additional skills.

Answers to Activity 3.8: Critical Thinking

Q1&2 are about your personal experience.

3. The SBAR tool aids communication, however there needs to be a culture change for all health care providers to adopt and sustain structured communication formats.

Answers to Activity 3.9: Case Study

1. Julia's hypotension and tachycardia are likely to be related to chemotherapy-induced nausea and vomiting. Additionally, as she has been receiving chemotherapy, Julia may be neutropenic and at risk of infection and sepsis. Hypotension and tachycardia can also lead to an Acute Kidney Injury.

    Julia meets the criteria for the sepsis bundle and this should be commenced.

    Oxygen should be delivered to keep saturations within Julia's normal range.

    Julia needs to have her blood taken, including Lactate and Blood cultures.

2. Intravenous access should be established, and IV fluids commenced. IV antibiotics will need to be prescribed and given.

    Commence a strict fluid balance chart. This should be reviewed hourly.

    Consider a urinary catheter to facilitate this. If Julia is not passing 0.5ml/kg/hr the medical staff should be informed. Julia is 67kg, therefore 0.5 x 67 = 33.5mls of urine per hour is the target.

    You should record Julia's observations as per the local policy for the EWS.

    If Julia is neutropenic consider if a side room is needed and available.

Answer to Activity 3.10: Case Study

1. It appears that Andrew has multi-organ failure in addition to a poor functional baseline. Would it be in Andrews's best interest to subject him to the interventions likely with a critical care admission? Is Andrew likely to survive a critical care admission and cope with the aftereffects of critical illness and rehabilitation afterward?

    Does Andrew have the capacity to discuss these issues, and can you involve Andrew's significant others in this discussion?

    This may be time to decide Andrew would not be for escalation to Level 2 or Level 3 care, but ward level care can continue. Or this may be time to consider Andrew's comfort and symptom control is the priority and to discontinue active treatment of his organ failure.

    These are difficult discussions best performed by trained clinicians with full involvement of Andrew and the multi-disciplinary team in any decision-making.

Answer to Activity 3.11: Case Study

What preparations are required for this transfer?

Answer

1. Firstly, it must be discussed and agreed that the benefit of transferring David outweighs any risks inherent in his transfer. Next, stabilise David's condition as far as possible prior to moving him:

Airway: David is currently maintaining his airway but as he is only responding to pain this puts him at a point when he may not be able to continue to protect his own airway. Airway adjuncts such as a nasopharyngeal or oropharyngeal can be considered. David can be nursed in a lateral position. Alternatively, intubation with a cuffed oral **endotracheal tube** (COETT) may be considered to establish a definitive airway. In this scenario monitoring of end tidal CO2 is essential for a transfer; this is a best practice method of monitoring the position of the COETT. Displacement of a COETT during transfer is not an uncommon adverse event.

Breathing: David is already on the maximum amount of Oxygen possible. His respiratory rate (RR) is low. Consider the possible causes of this and whether they can be treated. For example, if David has recently had any medications which can suppress the RR, such as opioids or sedatives, can this be reversed? The reversal agent for opioids is Naloxone and for sedatives it is Flumazenil.

Cardiovascular: David's blood pressure is low. You could consider commencing IV fluids to support this. It is essential David has a least 2 reliable points of IV access for the transfer. These should be established prior to the move.

It is likely David is being incontinent of urine due to his low level of consciousness. You need to accurately monitor David's fluid balance and protect his skin integrity. This could be done with a urinary catheter or use of incontinence pads, which could be weighed for fluid balance purposes.

Disability: The biggest risk due to the low level of consciousness is an unprotected airway as already discussed.

David has been having regular seizures; have his anti-epileptic medications been optimised to prevent further seizures? It is also essential to ensure David's environment does not present any danger to him were he to have any further seizures.

David's blood sugar is low and should be corrected prior to transfer. Capillary blood glucose of less than 4 mmol/L needs correcting.

2. Equipment

You will need: A monitor with minimum:

- Three lead electrocardiograph display.
- Saturations
- Blood pressure, set on a regular cycle
- RR
- EtCO2 if intubated.

The monitor needs to have a full battery and consider if spare batteries are needed.

Oxygen cylinders will quickly run out if you are delivering 15L/min via a non rebreathe mask. Ensure you have enough oxygen and then take a spare as well.

David has intravenous fluids running, consider if a volumetric pump is needed to continue running this. A drip stand on the bed and a pressure bag may be sufficient.

The critical care transfer bag will be required. This is a standardised bag, which contains whatever you may require to manage an emergency during the transfer.

3. Staff

    Do you have enough people and are they correctly trained people for this transfer?

    *   A porter to push the bed
    *   An experienced critical care nurse with transfer training
    *   An experienced critical care doctor with transfer training

4. Communication

    Ensure all the team members are familiar with each other and their roles.

    Discuss where you are going, which route is the safest and least congested and consider safe havens along the way should you need to stop and perform any interventions.

    Using the transfer checklist as a team, talk through an assessment of David and consider what scenarios may present during the transfer and how you would manage them. For example:

    'If he has a further fit, we will give more Lorazepam. It is made up ready and labelled. We have flushes with us, and we will use the free cannula in his right Antecubital fossa'.

    'Ok, I'll just quickly flush that cannula before we go and make sure it's patent'.

    This level of communication helps focus the team to clearly manage any adverse events. It opens communication, gives opportunity for all team members to participate and may prevent adverse events. An open two-way communication is essential.

    Before setting off with David you will speak to the CT scan department and make sure they are ready for him. You do not want to be waiting in a corridor or other unsafe area with someone who is critically ill.

    You will also speak to the critical care unit and ensure they will be ready to accept David when you leave the scan department.

    At the end of the transfer attempt to debrief with your colleagues, even if this is a quick informal sign off to say it was uneventful. Should there have been an adverse event this should be documented, the incident reported and a more in-depth debrief may be required.

CHAPTER 4 ANSWERS TO ACTIVITIES

Answers to Activity 4.1: Critical thinking

These factors could make an individual more vulnerable to HCAI:

1. Age
2. Long term conditions
3. Immunosuppression
4. Impaired cognition
5. The use of invasive devices
6. Surgery
7. The use of antibiotics
8. The use of corticosteroids
9. Organisational factors, such as poor staffing levels, low bed stock, insufficient single rooms, poor access to equipment, poor standards of cleanliness

11. Cultural factors such as lack of leadership, inadequate knowledge and skills, lack of accountability, poor motivation and compliance with policies.

Answers to Activity 4.2: Reflective Practice

1. Bacteria can be found on the skin, the upper respiratory tract, the gut, the nose, the throat, in the mouth, in the vagina.
2. The human body has an innate immune system that provides a number of anatomical barriers that prevent bacteria creating abnormal colonisations or moving into sterile areas. Examples include

    - Skin – Sweat
    - Gastrointestinal tract – peristalsis, gastric acid, gut flora
    - Nasopharynx – mucus, saliva
    - Eyes – tears

3. Any treatment that disrupts these barriers could promote an abnormal colonisation, so for example

    - Any general surgery that breaks the skin
    - An invasive device that punctures the skin
    - A device that moves from a contaminated area to a sterile area, e.g. ET Tube, urinary catheter.
    - Antibiotics that disrupt bowel flora

Answers to Activity 4.4: Reflective Practice

1. These figures may surprise you as they seem very low when compared to the 90%+ hand hygiene compliance figures that are routinely publicised by Trusts. Perhaps the reason for this is the way Trusts often measure and produce audit data does not have the same level of scrutiny that peer reviewed research papers have.
4. The difference in figures might have a number of different explanations. It might be that trust auditors lack the experience and/or time to collect authentic data. It may be they are concerned about the implications of reporting low levels of compliance.

Answers to Activity 4.6: Critical Thinking

Hand hygiene is often seen as an habitual practice that is learnt at a young age and triggered by an emotional feeling of dirtiness, not the removal of transient micro-organisms. In other words, people are programmed from a young age to wash their hands when they feel dirty. As such contact with body fluids makes people feel dirty and it brings out an instinct to wash hands. It is the need for personal protection that drives this behaviour. Contact with a 'clean' environment or social contact, for example taking someone's blood pressure, does not activate the same response. Omissions of hand hygiene are typically seen after these types of 'clean' activities.

Answers to Activity 4.7: Case Study

1. Your practice assessor might have said this because many people have a habitual preference for soap and water over AHR. The researcher tells us that soap and water makes people feel cleaner. How people think about things is an important component of how they use evidence-based practice.

2. If people continually favour soap and water over alcohol hand rub this is likely to have a negative impact on their overall compliance. HCWs are already time poor and soap and water takes considerably more time than hand rub. Skin may also be damaged through overuse of soap and water and this also has a detrimental impact on compliance.

3. It can be difficult to challenge colleagues but as a student nurse it is important that you have the courage to speak up. Perhaps you could share with your practice assessor some of the things you have learnt about AHR. Bring her attention to the World Health Organisation guidelines, or discuss with her the Trusts policy which will state times when hand rub should be used.

Answers to Activity 4.10: Case study

The ultimate aim for Suzanne is to enhance practice by enabling changes in practice. Change can be uncertain and uncomfortable and because of this will often fail. If Suzanne managed this project by following the principles of a change management model like ADKAR, the process may be eased.

A – Awareness

Announce the change, explain why it is needed, give colleagues a chance to ask questions and make suggestions.

D – Desire

Gauge reactions, if colleagues are resistant or indifferent, address their concerns. Identify champions to support you.

K – Knowledge

Address any gaps in knowledge and/or skills. Produce enabling resources like flowcharts, checklists, posters etc.

A – Ability

Run a small pilot scheme to highlight any problems, monitor performance, give feedback, set goals, adjust as necessary.

R – Reinforcement

Monitor the change over time, give positive feedback, encouragement, are there rewards you can give?

CHAPTER 5 ANSWERS TO ACTIVITIES

Answers to Activity 5.1: Reflective Practice

Consider the roles of key anatomical structure involved in respiration.

1. What are the names and key function? Nose, pharynx (throat), larynx (voice box), trachea (windpipe), bronchi and two lungs.

2. Consider what barriers may occur in the respiratory tree that can impede gaseous exchange. Loss of muscle control of the upper airway; trauma; swelling; occlusion/blockage from secretions or foreign body.

3. Can you list some of the common causes of air, blood, pus or chyme entering the pleural cavity? Open pneumothorax as a result of penetration of the chest wall; closed pneumothorax as a result of rupture of the respiratory tree; haemothorax are a result of trauma or sheering forces; empyema as a result of infection, trauma or tumour; chylothorax as a result of trauma to the lymphatic system in the chest cavity.

Answers to Activity 5.2: Case Study

1. What is causing Harold's respiration rate to increase?

   Respiratory acidosis or if there is evidence of carbon dioxide retention, a low oxygen level, hypoxic drive.

2. What type of respiratory failure is Harold likely to be experiencing? Type 2 respiratory failure – hypoxia with a raised pCO_2 (hypercapnia).

Answers to Activity 5.3: Reflective Practice

Both the insertion of an ETT or a tracheostomy bypasses the normal physiology of the person's upper airway.

1. Consider what natural defences the insertion of the airway affects. Cough reflex, swallow reflex and nasal hairs and cilia in the upper airway, all of which contribute to the removal of bacteria and other debris. It also bypasses the process that humidifies the air entering the lungs.
2. Consider how the bypassing of these defences may affect the person. Sputum retention. Increase in risk of infection of the lungs.
3. Artificial humidification. Bronchial toilet to remove secretions and maintain airway patency. Regular change of position to help with drainage of the secretions into the upper airways in preparation for suctioning.

Answers to Activity 5.4: Reflective Practice

1. Given the potential risks of the procedure, why do you think it would be in the person's best interest to have a tracheostomy inserted? Write this down in a list.

   To enable the person to be woken up more quickly. To help to wean from artificial ventilation.

   To help with communication and to commence an oral diet if tolerated.

   To help with the clearing of secretions.

   Where there is a loss of control of the airway to protect from aspiration and help with breathing.

Answers to Activity 5.5: Reflective Practice

1. Consider which members of the multidisciplinary team are required to establish artificial ventilation.

   Senior doctor with experience in advanced and difficult airway management.

Experienced nurse or anaesthetic technician or paramedic.

Technician to prepare the ventilator

Circulating practitioner to support as necessary.

Where a tracheostomy is inserted, as well as the above, a second doctor experienced in bronchos-copy and a theatre scrub nurse to assist the doctor inserting the tube.

2. Consider why it is necessary to have a dedicated department, i.e. intensive care, to look after these patients.

    Consider the following...

    Ensuring security of the airway related sedation levels.

    Constant observation of the ventilator for life-threatening complications.

    Immediate access to experienced staff who can intervene in emergency situations and support more junior staff.

    Ready access to point of sample blood testing equipment such as blood gas analysers.

    Ready access to bedside suction devices.

    Bedside availability of backup oxygen and temporary ventilation equipment in the event of ventilator failure.

Answers to Activity 5.7: Critical Thinking

1. How does positive pressure ventilation adversely affect the lungs?

    Barotrauma

    Bronchospasm

    Shearing of the mucosal membranes through air shuttling in and out of the airway.

    Damage to the cilia

    Increase in lung secretions resulting in atelectasis

    Loss of cough reflex and retention of sputum.

    Laryngeal nerve damage

2. What issues can you think of that can arise from the use of sedation, paralysing agents to facilitate positive pressure ventilation?

    All the above plus...

    Disorientation leading to psychosis and delirium

    Loss of muscle mass through immobility

    Joint stiffness

Answers to Activity 5.8: Case Study

1. What type of respiratory failure does Sandra have?

    Type 1. Hypoxia with no prior lung disease.

2. How would you persuade Sandra to consent to this treatment plan?

   Advise her on the advantages of supporting her breathing and allowing her to rest.

   Advise her on the detailed control and support the ITU can offer her oxygenation.

   Support her that she will never be left without someone by her side.

3. What resources do you need to prepare prior to Sandra's admission to your ACCU?

   Ventilation/oxygen sources

   Suction

   Necessary and adequate staff from all necessary disciplines.

   Monitoring equipment

4. Which members of the multidisciplinary team are required to support Sandra?

   Nurses

   Doctors

   Physiotherapists

   Dieticians

   Radiographers

   Medical technicians

   Speech and language therapists to judge swallow reflex in the event of a tracheostomy

   Laboratory staff

   Haematologists

   Biochemists

   Microbiologists

   Radiologists

Answers to Activity 5.10: Theory Stop Point

1. Consider the procedure outlined above and list the equipment you think you would need to decannulate a person.

   Dressing pack

   Gauze and two transparent semi-permeable dressings such as Tegaderm™ or Opsite™

   Sterile normal saline

   Gloves, apron and protective eye wear

   Appropriately sized tracheostomy tube and one a size smaller (available not opened)

   Facemask or nasal specs if patient requiring oxygen

   Microbiological swab

   Tracheal dilators

Functioning suction unit and appropriate sized suction catheters

Stethoscope

Resuscitation equipment

2. What assessment would you carry out before and after this procedure?

Prior to procedure

The patient is able to maintain adequate gas exchange self-ventilating +/- supplemental oxygen. Occasionally patients may require non invasive ventilation (NIV) post decannulation for the management of chronic conditions such as obstructive sleep apnoea (OSA) or chronic obstructive pulmonary disease (COPD).

There are no signs of deteriorating bronchopulmonary infection or excessive pulmonary secretions.

The patient has a stable lung status with oxygen therapy less than 40%.

The initial reason for the insertion of the tracheostomy has been resolved and/or been considered (e.g. upper airway obstruction, cranial nerve palsy).

The patient is cardiovascularly stable.

After the procedure

Increased work of breathing

Inability to clear secretions

Damage to the trachea including stenosis

Tracheomalacia and granuloma

Stridor

Change in voice quality

Increase in work of breathing

An emergency tracheostomy kit should be kept nearby the person for 24 hours post decannulation in case of emergency.

CHAPTER 6 ANSWERS TO ACTIVITIES

Answers to Activity 6.2: Reflective Practice

1. Cardiovascular focused assessment of the person's skin, face, neck, and peripheries would be to look and touch the person. Do they have pink and moist mucous membranes? Are their peripheries warm to touch and their usual colour? Do they have bilateral, strong regular pulses? Is their capillary refill time <2 seconds?
2. Abnormality could be dry mucous membranes suggesting dehydration, evidence of cyanosis. Any lumps or swelling which could be signs of deep vein thrombosis. Signs of oedema. Pulse that is weak irregular, absent, or bounding

Answers to Activity 6.3: Case Study

1. Your first concern would be to stabilise and improve Gerry's cardiovascular status as this is compromised due to hypovolaemia.
2. Additional assessments would include capillary refill time, arterial blood gas for Hb and oxygenation, temperature, assessment of wound drains.
3. The surgeon is required for emergency review. The first factor to be considered is whether the hypovolemic shock has resulted from haemorrhage or fluid losses, as this will dictate treatment. When aetiology of hypovolemic shock has been determined, replacement of blood or fluid loss should be carried out as soon as possible to minimize tissue ischemia. Nursing care focuses on assisting with treatment targeted at the cause of the shock and restoring intravascular volume. Retrieve the packed red blood cells, are they prescribed? Plan for transfusion.

Answers to Activity 6.4: Reflective Practice

1. Optimise the person's Starling's curve through improving filling pressures to improve cardiac output. Caution should be exercised to prevent overloading.
2. Once fluid filling has been established if the improvement in the person's condition is inadequate then further assessment should be completed and suitable medication may be considered such as drugs to improve cardiac output and/or manipulate vascular tone.

Answer to Activity 6.5: Theory Stop Point

Living with an LVAD –

- Lack of sleep
- Reduced physical activity
- Stress and fear
- 'To live a normal life' and be able to socialise
- Intelligence to be able to manage the device at home
- Fear for the future, and living in constant hope for a transplant that may never come
- Psychological impact of continually waiting for a heart transplant
- Fear of technology failure

Answers to Activity 6.6: Case Study

1. The below might be causing Brenda's symptoms:

   Whilst there are many similarities in symptoms, women can present with different symptoms of acute coronary syndrome compared to men. These symptoms are often overlooked or misinterpreted. Women can complain of pain between the shoulder blades, nausea and vomiting and shortness of breath. Brenda's symptoms are suspicious of acute coronary syndrome and this should be excluded.

2. This quality standard from NICE will advise on the different investigations required and different treatment strategies depending on the findings.

   www.nice.org.uk/guidance/qs68/documents/acute-coronary-syndromes-including-myocardial-infarction-briefing-paper2

CHAPTER 7 ANSWERS TO ACTIVITIES

Answers to Activity 7.1: Theory Stop Point

Review your knowledge about the control of blood pressure in relation to cardiac output, especially stroke volume, and vascular tone.

1. Think about what conditions may apply to create a drop in cardiac output and blood pressure.

    a) Lack of circulating volume
    b) Lack of pump (i.e. cardiac muscle tone/function)

        a. This can be broken down into a broken electrical system in the heart

            and/or

        b. Poor myocardial function from damage or ischaemia.

    c) Lack of vascular tone leading to pooling of blood in the circulation resulting a poor venous return

2. Then, consider why sepsis may be overlooked when monitoring patients.

    a) Sepsis can be overlooked as a reduction in blood pressure is a late indicator of sepsis.
    b) A reduction in cardiac output can be as a result of the issues mentioned above but can be attributed to other conditions such as dehydration or cardiac problems.

Answers to Activity 7.2: Case Study

1. What are Massum's risk factors for sepsis?

    - Diabetic (impaired immune system)
    - Breach of skin integrity (leg ulcer)

2. What might alert you to investigate Massum's condition in more detail?

    - Breathlessness
    - Mental vagueness
    - Associated risk factors

3. What observations would you take?

    - Respiration rate for a full minute
    - Oxygen saturation
    - Blood pressure
    - Pulse rate for a full minute
    - Consciousness level
    - Temperature (tympanic)

4. Who would you contact for further support or advice?

    - In the community you could contact (depending on your findings)
        o General practitioner
        o Hospital referral
        o Emergency ambulance

5. What strategy or method might you use whilst communicating with other healthcare professionals?

    - SBAR

Answers to Activity 7.3: Case Study

1. Do you think this is sepsis? If so why?

    - >75 years old (risk factor)
    - NEWS2 score = 7
    - Possible new altered mental state (high risk factor)
    - Recent trauma
    - Tachypnoeic (moderate to high risk factor)
    - Tachycardic (moderate to high risk factor)

2. Do you think this is not sepsis? If so why?

    - Tachycardia could be due to confusion and pain (excluded by use of analgesics)
    - Confusion – from the original incident

3. Based on your considerations, what would you do next?

On balance, Billy has a number of risk factors for developing sepsis that are greater than the reasons for no sepsis. I would strongly recommend urgent senior medical review using SBAR and commence sepsis 6 strategy. Early intervention will stop deterioration and further serious complications.

Answers to Activity 7.4: Research and Evidence-based Practice

1. Consider the enduring influence of the death of a class mate on Peter the anaesthetist's mental health, Jill's delay in recovery and the physical and mental impact on Jaco.

You can see that Peter, now middle aged, clearly recalls the events of the loss of his friend when he was at school. This has impacted on his life in a good way in that it took him into medicine. However, he lives with the memory of the loss every day and he continually asks, 'what if…'. Jill and Jaco have experienced the condition and the words they use to recall the events appear to show a serious psychological impact on them which they live with every day: depression, PTSD, anxiety, emotional triggers such as sounds and so on.

2. Review the symptoms the victims recall and consider how many people, including yourself, may have had these symptoms that can cause sepsis and death. Also review the rapid timeframe of the progression of the condition.

In Peter's case, his teenage friend felt unwell on a Friday afternoon with a headache and she died on Sunday afternoon, less than 48 hours later. Jill was at home when she felt unwell and had she delayed 3 hours she would have been unlikely to survive. Jaco had flu like symptoms towards the end of a working day, felt achy and shivery, went to A&E and collapsed. These stories illustrate how quickly the condition can progress and how severe it can become.

Answer to Activity 7.5: Reflective Practice

1. Actions to consider:

    a. Reflection in action (at the time it is happening)

Patients in intensive care often show very subtle signs of deterioration. However, there may be many causes for these changes. In the back of every nurse's mind should be the possibility of a developing sepsis. In intensive care it is easy to monitor for changes that would indicate sepsis through ready access to equipment to monitor blood levels such as blood pH and lactate.

b.   Reflection on action (after the event)

Many times this writer has had to recall his actions following a particularly challenging shift of work. Each time I have considered the events and learned something which I have added to my knowledge and experience and implemented in future practice.

CHAPTER 8 ANSWERS TO ACTIVITIES

Answer to Activity 8.1: Critical Thinking

High levels of potassium in the blood stream is known as hyperkalaemia. The effects of hyperkalaemia on the body include bradycardia/weak pulse, irregular heartbeat, muscle cramps/weakness and irritability. Slowly rising levels of potassium, often associated with chronic kidney disease, can be tolerated by the body but abrupt changes can be fatal.

Answers to Activity 8.2: Case study

1.   Normal renal function

- Sodium   3.5 – 5.0 mmol/L
- Potassium   135 – 145 mmol/L
- Creatinine   50 – 110 umol/L
- Urea   2.5 – 7 mmol/L

2.   A minimum expected hourly urine output in critical care: 0.5 mls/kg/ hour. Therefore, if an adult weighed 70 kgs, the minimum expected hourly urine output would be 35 mls/hour.

3.   A Vascath is a flexible tube that is often inserted into the subclavian, jugular or femoral vein.

Answer to Activity 8.3: Reflective Practice

This is very much dependent on the extent of the renal failure and eGFR result. For example, if a person you are caring for has an eGFR of 30mls/min, their stage of Chronic Kidney Disease would be Stage 3b. An eGFR > 90 mls/min is considered normal. It is important to understand the CKD classification to fully assess and understand the severity of disease process for people in your care.

Answer to Activity 8.4: Critical Thinking

Your care should always be aligned to local hospital policy and procedure. Knowing how to safely don (put on) and doff (take off) the personal protective equipment (PPE) is an important nursing skill. Always seek guidance and support from specialist services to help mitigate risk of cross-infection and take time to plan care delivery safely. Typical forms of PPE include theatre gowns, gloves, aprons, face masks and visors.

Answer to Activity 8.5: Research and Evidence-based Practice

Hepatitis D is also known as the Delta Hepatitis and is a liver infection caused by the Hepatitis D Virus (HDV). Hepatitis D only occurs in people who are also infected with the Hepatitis B virus. Hepatitis D is rare in most developed countries but common in Mediterranean counties, sub-Saharan Africa, the Middle East and South America. It is spread from the infected blood or body fluid entering the body of someone who is not infected.

Hepatitis E is a liver disease that is caused by the Hepatitis E Virus (HEV). It is mainly spread by the oral-faecal route due to contaminated water or food supplies. Person-to-person infection is uncommon. The HEV is widespread in South East Asia, India, Central Africa and Central America.

Answers to Activity 8.6: Case study

1. Bilirubin is an orange-yellow chemical made during the breakdown of red blood cells. Bilirubin passes through the liver for excretion from the body.
2. The reference range for serum bilirubin is 1 – 17 μmol/L
3. Ascites is a build-up of fluid in the abdomen. Liver disease is the most common cause for ascites though it can be caused by cancer and heart failure. The build-up of fluid occurs between two layers that make up the peritoneum. Ascites is usually painful, and symptoms can include nausea, loss of appetite, tiredness and breathlessness.

CHAPTER 9 ANSWERS TO ACTIVITIES

Answers to Activity 9.1: Critical Thinking

3. Priorities of care:

- Emergency and safety checks.
- Check rates of infusions and when they are due to run out. Prepare replacement infusions promptly.
- Consider pressure area care especially as the patient has been prone.
- Are any allergies recorded?
- What is the person's resuscitation status? Consider this in the context of her being in the prone position
- Past medical history, helps inform the team of the person's functional baseline/performance status before admission.
- Any advance directives in place.
- Do they have family and, how are they?
- You could ask if Joyce is unstable during any interventions such as repositioning or syringe changes.
- What are Joyce's other blood results apart from her arterial gases?
- When did Joyce last have her bowels opened?

Priorities:

Immediate safety checks and syringe replenishment should remain a priority but given the deterioration over the last 24 hours, a clear plan from the medical team is also needed. You can approach the medical team and ensure they know how unstable Joyce is and that an early review is a priority. It is also important to ensure your colleagues and nurse in charge are aware.

It appears proning has improved Joyce's oxygenation from 8.9 to 9.8 KPa, and saturations improved from 90 to 95%

Joyce is in a positive fluid balance, which may be due to Sepsis, Heart failure or an Acute Kidney injury. The resulting generalised oedema is seen with the 'leaking' skin.

Abbreviations used

PEEP	Positive End Expiratory Pressure and is the pressure applied by the ventilator at the end of each breath to ensure that the alveoli are not so prone to collapse.
I:E Ratio	Inspiratory: Expiratory ratio refers to the ratio of inspiratory time: expiratory time
vT	Tidal volume, it is measured in millilitres and is the volume of air displaced between inhalation and exhalation
IBW	Ideal Body Weight
AF	Atrial Fibrillation
MAP	Mean Arterial Pressure
RASS	Richmond Agitation-Sedation Scale is a medical scale used to measure the agitation or sedation level of a person
pH	This is the measure of acidity or alkalinity of a substance and ranges from 1 to 14, 1 being the most acid and 14 the most alkaline. Water is 7 and classed as neutral. Blood normal range is 7.35 to 7.45
pCO_2	Partial pressure of carbon dioxide dissolved in arterial blood and should normally be between 4.5kPa to 6.1kPa
pO_2	Partial pressure of oxygen dissolved in arterial blood and should normally be greater than 10kPa
HCO_3	Bicarbonate
sO_2	Oxygen saturation
kPa	Kilopascal. This is the unit of measure used for the partial pressure

8.   The implications of her fluid balance

Though it appears Joyce is well hydrated as she is oedematous and has a positive fluid balance, it may be that due to capillary leakage, part of the mechanism of sepsis, the fluid is in her tissues and leaving her intravascularly depleted. Prior to commencing cardiovascular support it should have been considered if Joyce had been adequately fluid resuscitated. Monitoring CVP and venous saturations will indicate whether or not Joyce needs additional fluids as well as the Noradrenaline infusion to support her blood pressure. Joyce's blood pressure is being supported with an intravenous inotrope; alongside this you must ensure Joyce continues to receive appropriate fluids. Additional haemodynamic monitoring may be required to guide this.

Answers to Activity 9.2: Reflective Practice

Your priority should certainly still be Joyce but good communication with her loved ones is also important. It's possible you could afford a couple of minutes away from the bedside to let Joyce's family know the time frame for them being allowed in or to speak to someone for an update. If you do leave the bed area, you must let a colleague know that the patient will be unattended.

You may find you do have adequate knowledge to speak with families; importantly though you must recognise when you do not know an answer. Generally families will appreciate you saying this rather than giving them incorrect information. You can follow this up with an attempt to get the correct information or by ensuring that the correct member of the MDT speaks with them.

Seeing a relative in an unusual position, such as proned, can be distressing. Without using jargon, it would be ideal to prepare Joyce's family for this, however they also need to understand that the need to prone Joyce is worrying for the team and occurred because her oxygen needs have been extremely high. It may not be appropriate for yourself as a junior team member to communicate the severity of the situation.

4. Positives and negatives of open visiting

Positive for person and relatives	Positive for staff	Negative for person and relatives	Negative for staff
Calmed/comforted	Caring for a calmer person may be more stable, able to deliver nursing interventions	Visitor may tire them	Can interrupt nursing interventions
Family kept up to date	Can get background information/history	Not all visitors may be welcome	Staff may feel intimidated by some relatives
Open visiting allows families to work around other commitments they may have	Promotes person-centred nursing as you can get to know the family and the person you are caring for.	Relatives may feel they have to stay all the time, can become exhausted	Large groups of visitors can be disruptive. It can be time-consuming to manage their questions and needs, taking time away from caring for the critically ill person

Answers to Activity 9.3: Critical Thinking

1. The main medications we are concerned about here are inotropes
2. Syringe changes are a point of care which may cause the patient to become unstable. There will be policies and protocols in place to ensure this and other procedures are done in the safest possible way. Best practice would be to adhere to these local guidelines when completing a procedure. In the case of infusions, which are providing cardiovascular support these are often 'piggybacked', that is, the new infusion commenced prior to the old infusion ending. This is due to the fact many of these drugs have a short half-life and even the shortest period without the medication in progress will lead to cardiovascular instability.

Answers to Activity 9.5: Reflective Practice

1. Do you feel you understand the physiology behind why Joyce's skin is damp and what the cause is?

    Sepsis can cause cardiovascular collapse through vasodilation and capillary leakage. Fluid will leak from the circulating volume into surrounding tissues. Tissue has a finite ability to hold excess fluid and when this has been exceeded, some leakage from the skin may be noted. This will be worse if the skin is damaged or broken in any areas.

2. Consider how you would explain this to Joyce's son. What communication approaches could help you?

When communicating with loved ones it is best to start by clarifying what they already know and understand. Using this as a starting point you will confirm with them what further information they require and ensure you give this at an appropriate level. Avoid jargon and answer queries honestly. Be prepared to repeat information and check back with them that they have understood and their questions have been answered. Observe Joyce's son for non-verbal cues that may direct your conversation with him.

There are advanced communication skills courses available which you could consider attending. Often a model for communication can help, see below for the SPIKES Model.

Answers to Activity 9.6: Reflective Practice

1. Possible MDT members:

   - Nurses
   - Doctors
   - Physiotherapist
   - Dietician
   - Occupational therapists

2. - Is Joyce stable enough to be moved?
   - Timing of the move; are any other interventions about to happen/needed to be completed first?
   - What else is happening on the critical care unit?
   - Is anything else acute occurring, how busy are your colleagues?
   - A minimum of 5 staff will be required including an airway-trained person.
   - Do you have all your equipment ready and available?
   - Have family been informed?

Joyce's face is likely to be swollen and this is upsetting for family. Turning Joyce over may lead to a period of instability or deterioration; it may be useful to prepare the family for that.

The turning team should discuss possible scenarios and have a plan ready. E.g. if Joyce was to immediately de-saturate would the team prone her again?

Answers to Activity 9.7: Critical Thinking

1. What tools are used in your clinical area to help reduce the risk of pressure ulcers?

Standards for pressure area care vary between critical care units. Risk assessment tools, such as the Waterlow score or the Braden and Norton scales, are often used to stratify risk and form the basis of pressure area care for patients. However, the reliability of these scales and scoring systems is debated when used in critical care, meaning prevention and management are usually based on the bedside nurse's clinical judgement and the preferences of the individual.

Some tools you may come across in ACCUs that aim to reduce the risk of a patient acquiring a pressure sore include:

- Pressure relieving equipment such as mattresses; fixators for medical devices including catheters, drains and tubes; and equipment which aims to offload pressure points such as heel-lift boots

- Repositioning schedules (ideal frequency is again widely debated in the literature)
- Skin care products such as barrier creams
- Continence management with urinary catheters and bowel management systems where indicated

Many other aspects of high-quality nursing care also indirectly promote skin health and reduce risk of skin damage. This includes things such as:

- Sedation holds
- Adequate nutrition and hydration
- Delirium and pain management
- Weaning of drugs such as inotropes and vasopressors when able

2. Based on your own experiences, think generally about the potential advantages and disadvantages of repositioning critically ill patients

Nurses can often feel worried and conflicted about repositioning patients, especially when they are on lots of organ support or unstable. The risks and benefits of repositioning a particular patient need to be considered before each planned maneuver.

Advantages	Disadvantages
Promotion of patient comfort	Risk of device dislodgement including artificial airway and central venous catheters
Reduces the risk of skin becoming damaged and pressure sores developing	Potential deterioration in patient condition, especially if they are on a high amount of organ support or are unstable
Allows provision of personal care	May cause discomfort or pain and require increased use of sedatives
Gives opportunity for skin assessment	Disrupts sleep and may therefore increase risk of delirium
Sitting out of bed or in 'chair' positions promotes use of abdominal muscles and may reduce the risk of pneumonia	Musculoskeletal injuries to staff
Some positions, such as prone positioning, may improve oxygenation	Time consuming
Facilitates physiotherapy and rehabilitation	Requires a minimum of 4 nurses to perform safely

- Scoring systems to assess risk
- Documentation of regular position changes/skin inspection
- Pressure-relieving mattresses and cushions
- Endotracheal Tube holder
- Urinary Catheter tube holder.
- Naso-gastric tube holder.
- Heel protector boots.
- Pressure-relieving dressings
- Appropriate absorbent pads
- Correct manual handling equipment to prevent friction.

Answers to Activity 9.8: Critical Thinking

1. Write down what your initial action plan might be following the discovery of Joyce's pressure damage.

After discovering pressure damage, it is important to relieve pressure from the area as much as possible. In this case, tube ties had caused the damage, so these could be repositioned away from the damaged skin, or if this were not possible, dressings could be applied to act as a physical barrier. Some units use special pressure relieving devices to position ET tubes securely in a way that does not cause pressure damage, so this might be something to consider. A lot of these devices cannot be used, however, when a patient is in prone position. The wounds might need to be cleaned, and barrier creams or ointments could be applied to the surrounding skin. In Joyce's case, good mouth and lip care would also be essential given the location of the pressure sores. Communication with Joyce's relatives about her acquiring a pressure sore would also need to be considered.

*   Use appropriate tools to prevent further damage.
*   Document including pictures and photographs.
*   Include in handover to colleagues
*   Incident report as per local policy

2. What MDT members would need to be involved?

Local practices for the management of pressure ulcers would need to be adhered to. Escalation to the senior nurse on duty and the medical team caring for Joyce would also be good practice.

*   Senior Nurses
*   Tissue Viability Nurse Specialist
*   Medical illustrations – might be indicated to make it easier to monitor wound healing
*   Physiotherapy – ensure pressure damage isn't exacerbated during treatment and that appropriate moving and handling equipment is utilised
*   Dietician – wound healing may require additional nutritional considerations

3. What would you need to document?

It would be useful to complete a wound care plan, including full details of the size and appearance of the wound, in addition to any initial actions taken so that nurses looking after Joyce on future shifts know what has happened. An incident report might need to be completed depending on local policy and practice.

Discuss your ideas with a colleague and take a look at our care plan.

Answers to Activity 9.10: Critical Thinking and Reflective Practice

When communicating with a patient or their loved ones it may help to follow a conceptual framework or model such as SPIKES.

This stands for:

*   Setting
*   Perception
*   Invitation
*   Knowledge

- Emotions
- Strategy

(Baile et al., 2000)

Initially assess the other parties' understanding of what you are going to discuss, this can also help you to moderate your input at the correct level for them.

- Avoid using jargon
- Clarify their comprehension of what they've been told
- Ensure they don't have any other questions
- Summarise

It does not always have to be this formally structured but having a framework in mind may help.

Answers to Activity 9.11: Critical Thinking

1. Family updates and discussions should ideally be led by the intensive care consultant with the bedside nurse also present. The family members most important to Joyce should be present. Some may choose not to participate, and this should be respected. The lead clinician can, again, be managing the discussion with a structure in mind but this does not have to be communicated with the family. It's important to meet the family's agenda in this conversation as well as the agenda of the medical team. Setting out a rigid structure for the conversation may prevent the family from feeling they are being listened to.

2. Questions Joyce's family may ask could be extremely varied.

   They may want specifics regarding therapies and treatments or may want more 'bigger picture' information.

   They may request advice about contacting other family members who are far away or on holiday.

   They may request prognostication or a second opinion.

   Clinical teams will often not have all the answers for these families.

   This list of questions is far from exhaustive.

3. A family discussion such as this is an opportunity for the team to ascertain from the family what Joyce's wishes may be in this situation. Whilst Joyce is unable to communicate her wishes, her family are in the best position to ensure we understand what Joyce would want.

   It's important the family do not feel any burden of decision-making and that the information they provide is assessed alongside the clinical picture for the consultant to make a decision regarding ongoing care. In absence of a person's capacity and an advanced directive of power of attorney for health the consultant is the only person with decision-making responsibilities.

Answers to Activity 9.12: Critical Thinking

Using a structured model for handover should alleviate any concerns you may have and ensure it is thoroughly done.

If you didn't feel confident about handing over regarding Joyce, you could ask Jane to observe you and feedback. You could also request feedback from the nurse you've handed over to.

CHAPTER 10 ANSWERS TO ACTIVITIES

Answers to Activity 10.1: Critical Thinking

1. Some advantages of using the MUST:

   - It is a nationally recognised and validated tool that many healthcare institutes are familiar with using
   - Assists in the identification of persons at risk of malnutrition that may have been missed by relying only on their general condition
   - Provides an action plan for low to high risk categories

2. Some disadvantages of using the MUST:

   - It takes time to complete and may not be completed accurately by everyone
   - It is not always easy to measure and weigh people experiencing critical illness accurately due to issues such as not having the necessary equipment, cardiovascular instability of the person or the person may have had rapid weight gain due to intravenous fluid administration.
   - The person experiencing critical illness may not be able to give you information regarding their weight 3-6 months previous.

Answer to Activity 10.2: Critical Thinking

1. People receiving nutritional support in the ACCU should have the route, risks, benefits and goals of their nutritional support reassessed regularly. This monitoring should be done by health professionals with the relevant skills. The NICE protocol for nutritional, anthropometric and clinical monitoring of nutritional support should be referred to when monitoring those receiving nutritional support in hospital. It is advisable to involve a dietician or other trained health professional to perform this.

Laboratory monitoring is also required, particularly in those receiving parenteral nutrition and might include:

- Sodium
- Potassium
- Urea
- Creatinine
- Glucose
- Magnesium
- Phosphate
- Liver function tests including International Normalised Ratio (INR)
- Calcium
- Albumin
- C-reactive protein
- Zinc
- Copper

- Full blood count including MCV
- Iron, ferritin
- Folate, B12

Answers to Activity 10.3: Theory Stop Point

What do you think are some of the potential advantages and disadvantages of each of the swallow tests detailed in Table 10.1?

Test	Advantages	Disadvantages
Swallow tests involving water and food	• Uses substances that the person will be swallowing in real-life • No special equipment required • Reasonably simple and inexpensive to perform • Test results are typically provided immediately • Can identify if there are certain food or liquids that need to be avoided • Can identify any positions that the person can move into that might assist swallowing	• Water can be difficult to swallow for people with dysphasia • There is a slight risk of aspiration • Only gives an indication of swallow function at the moment in time when the test is being carried out • Ensuring the thickness of the food is altered accordingly • Must be carried out by a trained specialist • Relies on the observations of the operator being reliable • Requires the person undergoing the test to be able to understand and follow instructions
Evans Blue Dye Test	• Minimal specialist equipment required • Does not require specialist training to perform • Simple and inexpensive to perform	• Results are not available for 48 hours • Does not consider that the person may aspirate on larger volumes of a substance or different consistencies • There is controversy regarding the accuracy of this method

FibreopticEndoscopicEvaluation of Swallowing (FEES)	• Tests results are typically available immediately after the test
	• The results are usually very accurate
	• Uses substances that the person will be swallowing in real-life
	• Can identify a specific part of the swallow where there is an issue so treatment can be established to target the specific issue
	• Can identify if there are certain food or liquids that need to be avoided
	• Can identify any positions that the person can move into that might assist swallowing
		• A FEES can be uncomfortable for the person undergoing the procedure
		• Risks include:
		   ○ Nosebleed
		   ○ Vomiting
		   ○ Laryngospasm
		   ○ Aspiration
		• A trained specialist is required to perform the test
		• The person undergoing the FEES must be able to understand and follow instructions
		• The test only gives an indication of swallow function at the moment in time when the test is being carried out.

Answers to Activity 10.4: Reflective Practice

1. Having dietary restrictions may leave you feeling frustrated and angry. You may be worried that you will never be able to eat again or that you may permanently require a nasogastric tube or other method to give you food. Being fed teaspoons may leave you feeling undignified and a hinderance to people. It might stop you asking for food and drink even though you are hungry or thirsty due to embarrassment or not wanting to be a nuisance.

2. The texture of pureed food may be offputting, especially if several foods are pureed together. Having to eat pureed food may remove your dignity especially if you are depending on someone else to feed you.

3. Staff members drinking cups of tea or eating biscuits may not concern you. However, these may be some of the things that you are craving, and this again might leave you feeling angry and frustrated. It might spoil your relationship with some staff members as you believe them to be inconsiderate and uncaring for eating and drinking in front of you.

Answers to Activity 10.5: Case Study

1. There are several possible reasons that might have resulted in Amara aspirating on her evening meal:

It is not unusual for people on the ACCU to experience generalised weakness and tiredness when they are recovering. Amara was assessed by the SLT in the morning, it might be that she was more rested at this time and as the day progressed, she became fatigued, resulting in a weakened swallow in the evening. It is also important to consider the position that Amara was in when she had the swallow test and whether this was replicated when Amara was eating in the evening. Typically, the optimal position for a person when they are eating is sat upright, ideally in a chair, with their chin flexed slightly forward. Another reason that Amara might have had difficulty swallowing her evening meal is that the consistency of the meal may not have been optimal for her to swallow.

2. Amara will need to be assessed and monitored for any ill effects of aspiration, for example, aspiration pneumonia.

As discussed at the beginning of the chapter, adequate nutrition plays a vital role in the maintenance, functioning and healing of every system within the body. It is important that Amara receives adequate nutrition whilst she is unable to take diet orally, this might be through another route such as a nasogastric tube.

Amara will require further review and assessment by the SLT. It is important that the SLT accurately documents the consistency of any diet and fluids that are to be given orally to Amara as well as educating Amara and those caring for her about how to swallow safely and optimal positioning for eating and drinking.

The nurse will need to ensure that when Amara is assessed as safe to take oral diet and fluids again that she is optimally positioned to safely swallow and that the consistency of any oral intake meets the requirements prescribed by the SLT. It is important that the nurse continues to ensure Amara is adequately monitored for any symptoms of aspiration both during and after oral intake.

Amara might be anxious when she receives oral intake in the future. It is important that the MDT reassure and educate Amara and address her concerns to facilitate her to receive adequate oral intake as part of her recovery and rehabilitation.

Answers to Activity 10.6: Critical Thinking

1. Checks to confirm initial placement of tube:

   pH testing is the first line test method. Once the NGT has been inserted, gastric contents should be aspirated via the NGT. The aspirate is then dripped on pH testing strips. Please note that only strips that are CE marked and manufactured to test human gastric aspirate should be used. If the pH is between 1 and 5.5 and there is no clinical concern, it is usually considered safe to feed.

   If you are unable to obtain a gastric aspirate or if the aspirate is outside the pH range (this could be for reasons such as the misplacement of the tube or due to medications that the person is taking) an X-ray to confirm placement should be performed. The X-ray must only be interpreted by someone who is assessed as competent to do so. NG feeding must only take place once the competent person who has interpreted the X-ray documents that it is safe to do so.

   Once initial tube placement has been confirmed, it may be useful to measure the length of the external tube in case this is needed to assist with the confirmation of placement when performing repeat checks.

2. Repeat checks after initial correct placement has been confirmed:

   It is possible for a tube that was correctly placed initially to move from the stomach into the oesophagus or lungs leading to aspiration which could prove to be fatal. For this reason, it is important to check the position of an inserted NG at regular intervals including before administering each feed or medication and at least once daily. It is important that you check your local guidelines to establish how regularly NGT position needs to be checked in your clinical area.

   It is recognised that continuous feeding via the NGT and acid reducing medication can increase the pH of stomach contents resulting in aspirates that are not within the 'safe' feeding pH range of 1–5.5. It is not safe to expose these individuals to X-rays daily. In circumstances where initial placement has been confirmed and there is no reason to suspect tube displacement the only practical method of assessing whether the tube remains correctly placed is to measure the external length of the tube. You must check the external length of the tube remains the same as it was when documented on insertion and the fixation tapes have not moved or become loose before administering anything down the NGT.

   If you have reason to believe the tube might have become displaced, for example, the person has been pulling at the NGT, coughing, retching or vomiting or there are signs of respiratory deterioration, it is important to check the back of the person's throat. If the tube is coiled in the mouth you will need to remove this. If the tube isn't coiled but you are not certain that the tube is in the correct position, an X-ray to confirm position would be indicated.

   Source: NPSA (2011).

Answers to Activity 10.7: Case Study

1. What events do you believe led to the death of Ahmad?

   The first thing to consider before inserting any enteral feeding tube is to assess whether it is safe and the right decision for the person. A nutritional risk assessment had been performed that identified EN would benefit Ahmad. However, NGT insertion is rarely an emergency procedure and in this case study, it would have been safer for the NGT to be inserted during the day when there are more trained staff available rather than overnight. The insertion of an NGT can be a difficult procedure in some people, and the insertion can be further complicated in the unconscious person due to their inability to swallow. The ST6 in the scenario was called to another potential emergency whilst inserting the NGT. This may have distracted them from the insertion and affected their situational awareness.

The FY2 might not have been adequately trained to perform any checks that may be needed to confirm correct placement of the tube and may have had misplaced confidence in their ability. The FY2 did not document that the tube was in the correct position and that it was safe to start feeding. This would leave Mark in a vulnerable position if the FY2 denied that they had told Mark the NGT was safe to use.

The event took place at night and it is not uncommon for staff to experience sleep deprivation when working night shifts. Sleep deprivation can affect performance and there is a direct relationship between sleep deprivation and medical errors.

2. What interventions might have prevented the death of Ahmad?

As stated above, sleep deprivation is a known causal factor in medical and nursing errors. Waiting to insert and confirm the position of the NGT during the day would have been safer.

It is possible that the staff involved in inserting and caring for the NGT were not fully aware of the risks associated with NGT feeding. Educating staff in the safe use of NGTs is essential.

It is not clear that the FY2 was competent to confirm the position of the NGT. Whenever delegating a task, it is important to ensure you delegate to a competently trained person. The FY2 did not complete the documentation to state that it was 'safe to commence feeding'. Perhaps if the FY2 had been prompted to document the confirmation of the tube this may have triggered them to interpret the X-ray more carefully or recognise their lack of competence in this area.

Answers to Activity 10.8: Critical Thinking

1. High GRVs can result in the person experiencing critical illness receiving interruptions in nutrition. Monitoring GRVs can potentially lead to the overdiagnosis of feeding intolerance, possibly leading to the unnecessary reduction or stopping of EN causing or exacerbating malnutrition in this already vulnerable category of individuals.
2. In 2 of the studies presented by Wang et al., (2019) not monitoring GRV was shown to increase the overall cumulative calorie intake of individuals receiving EN. Additionally, not monitoring GRV was shown to reduce the use of prokinetic medication. However, there is concern that not monitoring GRV leads to increased vomiting, which is distressing for the affected individual. Vomiting also raises concerns regarding the risks of the person aspirating and the theoretical risk of causing ventilator acquired pneumonia, although no evidence of this was found in the review.
3. The authors recognise that their review has several limitations and that further research is needed to provide an evidence-base for the monitoring of GRVs.

CHAPTER 11 ANSWERS TO ACTIVITIES

Answers to Activity 11.2: Case Study

1. You could consider a brief bedside neurological assessment (ACVPU) but this is a crude measure. The assessment tool of choice would be using the Glasgow Coma Scale (GCS) and examining pupil size and response.
2. It is likely that Tina is experiencing concussion from the assault and head injury. Patients with classical concussion may experience post traumatic amnesia, confusion/disorientation, dizziness and memory loss.

Answer to Activity 11.3: Critical Thinking

1. It is possible to donate the following tissue

    - cornea
    - sclera (white of the eye)
    - heart valves
    - skin
    - bone
    - tendons
    - amniotic tissue (following birth)

Answers to Activity 11.4: Case Study

1. Critical Care Units and Emergency Departments can refer a potential organ donor to the Organ Donation and Transplantation (ODT) Duty Office Hub on 03000 20 30 40. Potential donors are screened and then referred to the appropriate regional organ donation teams.
2. As pressure rises in the brain due to injury, critical structures including the brainstem are compressed. There is limited room for swelling because the brain is housed within an inflexible container (the skull). As pressure rises, brain tissue is pushed through the foramen magnum onto the spinal cord.
3. Typically, each critical care unit will have an organ donation resource box and organ donation link nurse. These will often have the phone number of the Organ Donor Register, so a healthcare professional is able check the Register.
4. Collaborative working is always advised. Plan the discussion amongst the multidisciplinary critical care team. Include the specialist nurse – Organ Donation in this planning and in discussion with the family. The discussion should be offered in a private room, free from distraction.

Answer to Activity 11.5: Theory Stop Point

1. Autoimmune disorders that sometimes result in critical care admission include myasthenia gravis, Guillain–Barré syndrome, systemic lupus erythematosus, rheumatoid arthritis and systemic vasculitis.

CHAPTER 12 ANSWERS TO ACTIVITIES

Answers to Activity 12.1: Critical Thinking

1. The most important function of the skin is to act as a barrier between the person and the external environment. Any breach of this barrier can lead to water and heat loss and infection.

Thermoregulation can be affected in several ways, including loss of skin and fluid through injuries such as burns. Septic shock often has symptoms such as oedema and sweating that cause prolonged exposure to moisture and result in skin damage. Diarrhoea and urine can also damage the skin through moisture damage and due to the enzymes present in faeces.

It is common for the person being cared for in the ACCU to have wounds and/or invasive devices such as central lines in place. These breach the skin's protective barrier and increase the risk of an already vulnerable person developing an infection.

The critically ill person's consciousness level may be reduced, either by medication or illness. This can reduce the person's sensory perception of pain associated with tissue damage and can also make them unable to change position or communicate that they are experiencing pain related to tissue damage. Medications such as inotropes reduce blood flow to the skin which can cause necrosis and increase a person's risk of other skin disorders such as pressure injuries. Other medications such as antibiotics may cause diarrhoea.

2. Addressing hygiene is essential when caring for the critically ill person due to the risk of increased exposure to moisture and the increased risk of infection caused by critical illness and the presence of invasive devices. It is important that you perform a thorough skin assessment of the critically ill patient to help you to plan nursing care that will not only manage the current skin condition of the person but also help to reduce the risk of any deterioration in skin condition from occurring. Once you have performed a comprehensive skin assessment, an evidence-based plan needs to be implemented that addresses any current or potential issues that you have identified in the assessment. It may be necessary to refer the critically ill person to other specialists such as a tissue viability nurse specialist, dietician, dermatologist or surgeon. The critically ill person's skin must be assessed regularly and the plan must be reviewed to assess its effectiveness and changes made as appropriate.

3. Barriers to performing interventions might include the severity of illness experienced by the critically ill person. For example, some patients may become haemodynamically unstable when being repositioned. Devices such as cardiac monitors and renal filter machines can also pose barriers to repositioning patients as the position of the person receiving monitoring and treatment through these devices can affect the devices' ability to work effectively. Staffing numbers can create a barrier. Most critically ill people will require at least 3 people to reposition and provide hygiene care to them. This can be very difficult in areas that are understaffed and/or have a high level of dependency, for example if several patients are experiencing diarrhoea or undergoing procedures. Other barriers may be that the person experiencing critical illness declines to be cleaned or repositioned. In cases such as this it is important to identify why this might be: is the person experiencing a lot of pain, are they embarrassed? You must then try to work with the person to resolve the issue and be aware that in some cases the person may not have the capacity to decline care, but this must be formally assessed.

Sometimes, it may be difficult to provide care due to visitors being present. You must communicate with visitors regarding the importance of carrying out interventions. On occasion it may be possible to involve relatives and carers in caring for the critically ill person, for example, a person with a learning disability may feel more at ease if their carer is present when being repositioned or given a bed bath. However, this must be assessed on a case by case basis and lay people delivering care must be shown how to provide the care to your institution's standard and must always be supervised.

Answers to Activity 12.2: Critical Reflection

1. Sometimes you might identify that risk assessments are incomplete, contain inaccurate or wrong information or are not completed as regularly as instructed by the care plan or local policy. It is important that you ensure you complete this documentation as accurately as possible to assist in the critically ill person you are caring for in receiving the best possible treatment.

2. The potential risks to the patient of the skin risk assessment not being completed accurately include deterioration in their skin condition. This can lead to unnecessary pain and discomfort as well as leading to scars that can negatively affect their body image and serve as a constant reminder of their stay in ACCU, potentially increasing the risk for the person to experience psychological difficulties after discharge. Deterioration of the skin can lead to both skin and systemic infection making the vulnerable, critically ill person even more unwell and increasing their ACCU and hospital length of stay. Another consequence of not completing risk assessments accurately is that it may lead to the person receiving unnecessary interventions, this can interrupt their rest and sleep and lead to needless breaches of their privacy and dignity.

3. Some of the potential risks to the nurse of not completing the skin risk assessment accurately are: If the affected person's skin deteriorates, this will increase workload for the nurse and organisational costs in the long-term due to requirement for additional interventions such as dressing changes and pressure relieving devices. Also, if accurate, regular assessments are not performed and it is not recognised that the person's skin condition has improved, the nurse may be performing unnecessary tasks that will further increase workload. Inaccurate or incomplete assessment that results in the deterioration of the critically ill person may lead to formal complaints being issued. This can lead to costs in litigation and damage to the reputation of the organisation and staff involved in caring for the affected person, particularly if the allegations are found to be true.

Answer to Activity 12.3: Theory Stop Point

The nursing process is a useful, systematic tool that can help you to plan and implement care. When supporting people experiencing critical illness to maintain healthy skin you might think about the following:

Assess

Your area will have its own tool that it uses for skin assessment. The assessment might include the following:

*   Body mass index
*   Age
*   Sex
*   Mobility
*   Nutritional state
*   Illness
*   Whether the person is continent or not
*   Oedema
*   Skin temperature
*   Moisture – is the skin dry/oily/wet
*   Skin turgor

- Skin integrity – any breaks in the skin
- Pain
- Skin colour and discolouration

Plan

From your assessment a goal must be developed, and your plan should identify interventions that will assist in achieving this goal. The person experiencing critical illness might have a pre-existing skin condition, for example eczema or psoriasis and although this may not be the priority of health professionals when managing critical illness, it is important that skin conditions are managed appropriately and, where possible, deterioration of the condition is prevented.

Pre-existing skin conditions can affect people in several ways. People with skin conditions can be affected psychologically if they consider their condition to be unsightly; conditions such as eczema and psoriasis can cause pain and irritation and can also lead to infection if not managed correctly. If the person you are caring for has a pre-existing skin condition, it is advisable to discuss with either the affected person or someone who knows them about their skin care regime and what treatments the person uses as well as any cleansers etc. that should be avoided.

If the person experiencing critical illness has any other skin problems, for example wounds, your plan should include interventions that will encourage healing and prevent deterioration. This might include implementing a regular turning regime, the use of pressure relieving devices, nutritional support, tending to the hygiene needs of the person regularly, continence management, identifying the appropriate dressing and referral to a specialist in tissue viability.

Your assessment may have identified that the person does not have any skin related issues; if this is the case, your plan needs to be comprised of interventions that will prevent any deterioration in the condition of their skin. This will include interventions such as nutritional support, pressure relieving devices, appropriate hygiene care and possibly continence management.

Your plan should be person-centred and evidence-based. You will need to clearly document the plan to ensure it can be followed by other health professionals caring for the person in your absence. Your plan should also include a time frame for the evaluation of the interventions you have identified.

Implementation

Once a plan has been developed it is time to implement the plan. During this phase of the nursing process it is important that the implementation of the plan is documented, so adherence to the plan and its effectiveness can be evaluated.

Evaluation

Your evaluation should explore whether your plan has been effective. This will include looking at whether the plan was implemented appropriately and whether the interventions have achieved or are achieving the goal identified in the planning phase of the process.

From this evaluation you will start the nursing process again and identify whether the plan needs to be modified or whether it is effectively achieving the goal you identified and should continue to be followed unchanged.

Answer to Activity 12.4: Case Study

1. The first step in caring for Joseph is the completion of an assessment of his skin and wound with the assessment tool that is utilised within your area of work. From the assessment an evidence-based plan needs to be developed and implemented. The plan will include caring for Joseph's hygiene needs. This will include how often Joseph should be cleaned and what products will be used to clean and protect his skin. Joseph should also be assessed for his suitability for an indwelling catheter or a convene if he does not already have one in place and the use of a faecal pouch or insertion of a faecal management system. A thorough pain assessment should be performed, and adequate analgesia prescribed and administered to relieve any pain or discomfort experienced by Joseph.

A medication review may identify medications that cause diarrhoea or corrosive faeces that can be stopped or changed to medications without these side-effects. An anti-diarrhoeal such as loperamide hydrochloride may be added to Joseph's current medication regime if the benefits are perceived to outweigh the risks. Consultation with the dietician will also be useful, especially if Joseph is being fed enterally, as a feed that reduces the side-effect of diarrhoea may be recommended. It is also important to consider Joseph's increased risk of developing a pressure injury due to his MASD and ensure adequate pressure relieving measures are commenced, such as the regular repositioning of Joseph and the use of relevant pressure relieving devices.

Answers to Activity 12.5: Case Study

1. As Priscilla has already developed a pressure injury, she is at a high risk of developing further injuries. Therefore, Priscilla will require regular skin assessments and a plan of care to prevent further deterioration in her skin integrity. The initial assessment should include the assessment and documentation of the category of injury (i.e. Category 2) using a validated pressure injury categorisation tool (NICE, 2014). The location of the injury as well as its size and shape and the condition of the wound bed needs to be assessed. Malodour, heat and excessive or purulent exudate may be signs of infections and should, along with wounds that are not healing, trigger the review of a specialist such as a tissue viability nurse. The amount and consistency of any exudate should be documented. As well as assessing the wound itself it is important to pay attention to the integrity of surrounding skin as this is potentially at risk of deterioration.

2. NICE, (2014) recommend that for Category 2, 3 and 4 pressure injuries a dressing that promotes a warm, moist healing environment is used. You will also need to consider the position of the pressure injury as this may affect such things as the shape of the dressing you choose or the adhesiveness of the dressing. Pain tolerance and the amount of exudate present will also impact on dressing choice (NICE, 2014); wounds with large volumes of exudate will require a more absorbent dressing.

3. For anyone with or at risk of developing a pressure injury it is important to consider methods to redistribute the pressure that can cause pressure injuries. This may include regular repositioning of the person or pressure redistributing devices such as an alternating air pressure mattress; these mattresses have air cells that inflate and deflate alternately to relieve pressure on the body. Regular repositioning of Priscilla, avoiding positions that place pressure on her sacrum, may help with healing and prevent further deterioration of her pressure injury as well as providing some relief from any pain she might be experiencing.

Priscilla's pain should be assessed, and adequate pain relief prescribed and administered to ensure she is comfortable and that her pain is not preventing her from mobilising which could potentially lead to further pressure damage and non-coherence with treatment.

Priscilla may benefit from education regarding her pressure injury and strategies that she can use to offload pressure from vulnerable areas, such as her heels, if she is well enough and has the strength to do this.

Another important factor to consider is Priscilla's nutritional status. Early referral to a dietician will help to ensure Priscilla is receiving the correct diet to facilitate wound healing and prevent further skin deterioration.

Answer to Activity 12.7: Critical Thinking

1. The National Burn Care Referral Guidance (2012) recommends that the following individuals should be referred to a specialist burn care service:

   - Any adults with burns covering 3% or more of their TBSA and children with burns covering 2% or more of TBSA
   - Anyone with full thickness burns
   - Anyone with a burn affecting the entire circumference of their body (circumferential burn), for example a finger, toe, leg or torso.
   - Any individuals who have burns that do not heal within 2 weeks of the injury
   - Anyone with a burn that is believed to be caused by a non-accidental injury

The guidance also recommends the following reasons for prompt discussion with a consultant in a specialist burn centre:

   - Burns to hands, feet, genitals, or perineum
   - Chemical, electrical and friction burns
   - Any cold injury
   - Any unwell child or any child who has a high temperature and a burn
   - If there are any concerns about the burns injuries and co-morbidities that might affect the treatment or healing of the wound

CHAPTER 13 ANSWERS TO ACTIVITIES

Answers to Activity 13.1: Critical Thinking

Is there anything else you need to ask the night shift nurse before they leave?

   The structure of the SBAR is designed to ensure that critical information is identified and shared. A clinical handover should always have structure. Some nurses make notes as they receive handover and it is essential to explore anything you are uncertain about prior to the night shift nurse leaving duty. Additionally, there should be robust clinical documentation of events for you to access which could answer some questions prior to your own care delivery.

3. From what has been handed over so far, do you have concerns about Declan's ventilation and blood pressure?

Normal blood pressure for an adult is 120/80 mmHg. Declan's blood pressure is 101/72 mmHg which is a cause for concern. Importantly, his MAP is 59 mmHg which means poor perfusion of oxygen and nutrients to his central organs. Declan needs an urgent medical review of his respiratory and circulatory systems.

4. What is the significance and implication of a cervical vertebral fracture and high cervical cord injury for the patient?

People who suffer high cervical cord injury can experience respiratory impairment. Sometimes, signals from the brain which normally control inspiration and expiration can no longer pass the cervical cord injury. This can lead to an apnoeic state and people with such injuries are often intubated and/or have a tracheostomy to support their breathing.

Answers to Activity 13.3: Reflective Practice

Reflect on the situation above and consider your first concerns.

1. How will you record the physiological observation and what do each of the values mean?

These observations should always be performed under direct supervision of your practice assessor. It takes time to fully understand ventilation terminology, so be sure to seek guidance and support. The observations are collated on an 'ICU' or 'critical care observation chart'. These track changes in respiratory status and haemodynamic stability so need to be completed accurately.

2. How are you going to plan to update the family and which words are you going to use to describe his high cervical cord injury?

It is important to plan for such sensitive discussions. Usually this would be a team approach with the consultant leading the discussion. Sometimes it is helpful to show scan pictures and images to family/relatives to help them understand the injury. The task of breaking bad or significant news to a family is a challenging nursing duty. However, you can plan for this event and it does become a little easier with experience. Relatives must be offered privacy during these conversations and allow time to address their inner turmoil. Furthermore, health professionals must avoid technical jargon when explaining the injury. Instead use words and phrases that are easily accessible to distressed relatives.

3. Can you list all members of the MDT that would be involved in Declan's care at this point?

The team might include a consultant intensivist, critical care nurse, radiologist, pharmacist, care support workers, dietician, clerical staff, physiotherapist, and specialist nurses [list not exhaustive].

4. Although Declan's partner states she is the next of kin, you establish they are not married and do not have a civil partnership, so who is his next of kin?

It is important to establish who is the legal next of kin at the earliest opportunity. Avoid assumptions and gather facts. These conversations are sometimes challenging but the communication skills of the nurse are significant here. If tensions rise, steer the conversation back to the care of Declan. This, sometimes, allows families to focus. It is necessary to ask who each family member is and what their relationship to the person in your care is. People often express wishes for who their next of kin is but, due to Declan's critical illness, his autonomy has been relinquished and this is not possible.

5. Can information be released to the press about Declan's condition and how would you manage such a phone call?

High profile cases of people admitted to critical care can often attract media attention and interest. Sometimes the police need to contact the unit to obtain updates and exchange important information, but a password system is often instigated. The media can purport to be concerned family members to extract information. All aspects of Declan's care are confidential, and you must not release any information. Always seek guidance and support about such telephone calls.

Answers to Activity 13.4: Critical Thinking

1. Each team member brings their own unique talents gained through specialist education programmes. Consequently, they possess unique skills to input into the person's treatment ultimately improving their care.
2. Contribution to the person's care typically occurs during formal rounds where the person's status and care plan is reviewed using a structured systematic approach, drawing on the experiences and knowledge of each team member.

Answers to Activity 13.5: Critical Thinking

1. What could be causing Declan's blood pressure to fall?

There is often significant blood loss following long bone (femur) and pelvic fractures. These might require urgent surgical intervention. In the short term, Declan's haemodynamic stability is the priority and he may require a blood transfusion if bleeding is suspected.

2. Which inotropic therapies could be considered to improve his blood pressure?

The use of a noradrenaline infusion via a central catheter is appropriate but this should only be commenced following a medical review and subsequent signed prescription.

3. Why is achieving a MAP of 60 – 70 mmHg significant?

Maintaining an adequate blood pressure is essential to ensure the flow of oxygen and nutrient rich blood cells to central organs. If the MAP falls below 60mmHg, cardiac output diminishes which can lead to tissue hypoxia and ischaemia.

Answers to Activity 13.6: Critical Reflection

1. What strategy are you going to develop to explain Declan's injury to him once he is fully conscious?

This will undoubtedly be a difficult nursing duty and time should be taken to prepare for the discussion. The lead clinician will attempt to ascertain Declan's understanding of his injuries prior to explaining the full extent and prognosis. The discussion must be a team approach and carefully planned. The use of scans and images might be helpful to allow Declan to understand his injuries. Clinical information must be shared slowly and sensitively with a clear plan of care on what will happen next.

2. What other services offer long term care and support for patients with high cervical cord injuries?

It is vital to gather expert advice prior to discussing Declan's injuries with him. There are regional spinal injury centres across the UK that offer guidance and support on specialist spinal care services. Typically, the consultant intensivist, working in partnership with other medical teams, makes a referral to these specialist centres to explore long term care options.

CHAPTER 14 ANSWERS TO ACTIVITIES

Answers to Activity 14.1: Reflective Practice

1. Routine postnatal care

   History taking

   Observations

   Breast care

   Wound care

   Vaginal Loss

   Bladder and bowel function

2. Debrief

   Time to adjust

   Clear communication

   Bonding and attachment with baby

3. Midwives

   Obstetricians

   Anaesthetists

   Physiotherapists

   Neonatal teams

   Breast feeding support

Answers to Activity 14.2: Critical Thinking

1. **Mild hypertension**: Systolic BP 140–149 mmHg, Diastolic BP 90–99 mmHg

   Moderate Hypertension: Systolic BP 150–159 mmHg, Diastolic BP 100–109 mmHg

   Severe hypertension: Systolic BP ≥160 mmHg, Diastolic BP ≥110mmHg.

   Chronic hypertension: Hypertension present before 20 weeks' gestation or if the woman is taking antihypertensive medication before pregnancy. It can be primary or secondary in aetiology.

Gestational Hypertension: New hypertension presenting after 20 weeks without significant proteinuria.

Pre-eclampsia: New hypertension presenting after 20 weeks with significant proteinuria.

Severe pre-eclampsia: Pre-eclampsia with severe hypertension and/or symptoms, and/or biochemical and/or haematological impairment.

Eclampsia: Convulsive condition associated with pre-eclampsia

Source: NICE, 2019.

2. Take a full clinical history:

    Signs and symptoms of preclampsia include severe headache, problems with vision , e.g. blurring or flashing lights, severe pain just below the ribs, vomiting and sudden swelling of the face, hands or feet.

    Perform blood pressure reading. Repeat to confirm accuracy of reading (see above for parameters).

    Perform dipstick proteinuria testing. If dipstick screening is positive (1+ or more) seek medical advice from the obstetrician.

    Perform blood tests, measure full blood count, liver function and renal function.

    Seek medical advice.

Answers to Activity 14.3: Case Study

1. Take a full history to ascertain why she Imogen feels unwell/perform risk assessment.

    Perform basic observations.

    Escalate/ask for help/refer to senior team

    Document events

2. Risk of sepsis due to forceps delivery, invasive procedure (manual removal of placenta) and blood transfusion.
3. Antenatal considerations: care of unborn foetus, regular foetal monitoring, regular midwifery/ obstetric review, consider MDT discussion around timing and mode of delivery.

Answers to Activity 14.5: Case Study

1. Communication: ask Doha how she feels, ask about the baby

    Offer debrief

    Consult with midwives

    Analgesia requirements

    Feeding support

2. Breast engorgement

Lochia (vaginal loss) assessment

Offer to check perineal sutures, give ice packs

Check urine output

3. Midwives

Obstetricians

Breast feeding support worker.

Answers to Activity 14.6: Reflective Practice

1. Look at the different parameters on each chart in your clinical setting. They are different for women and babies. For example, a normal respiratory rate for a woman is 10–20 breaths per minute. The normal respiratory rate for a healthy baby is 30–60 breaths per minute.
2. This will be dependent upon your own clinical experience. A MEWS chart will help you identify trends and changes in the maternal condition and prompt you to escalate any concerns.
3. Identifying the correct, most suitable chart available for the situation.

   Practitioners may become reliant on the numbers rather than the overall clinical picture.

   Access to training.

   This list may be different depending on your own clinical experience.

Answers to Activity 14.7: Reflective Practice

1. Attachment and bonding will be severely disrupted.

   Baby will be cared for by partner or grandparents or in some cases maternity staff or foster parents.
2. Good documentation.

   Keep a diary for Mum which contains all relevant information e.g. baby's feeds, how much, how long etc.

   Take photographs and videos of first few days.

   Encourage relatives to visit with baby.

   Contact midwives to help support skin to skin with baby.
3. Partners, relatives, grandparents and midwives and neonatal staff.

Answers to Activity 14.8: Reflective Practice

1. Communication

   Offer condolences

   Encourage discussion about the baby

Facilitate time with the baby where possible

Leaflets and information giving.

2. Don't be frightened

Be honest about your own feelings

It is ok to step away

Seek support from your colleagues

3. Don't be afraid to show your feelings.

Some of you might be frightened of seeing a stillborn baby

Talk with your supervisors

Don't worry if you don't know what to say to bereaved parents

4. Practice supervisors and assessors

Peers, colleagues, friends

Answers to Activity 14.9: Reflective Practice

1. Maternal experience of critical care:
   - Ineffective communication
   - Distress at the environment
   - Sensations of loss
   - Guilt and lack of role fulfilment associated with the inability to bond with or feed their baby
   - Lack of control and loss of dignity
   - Long-term physical and psychological trauma

2. Good communication
   - Referral to appropriate support services, e.g. health visitors
   - Arrange debrief for clinicians to go through the maternal records and discuss events with the mother
   - Continuity of carer to reassure the woman and her family

CHAPTER 15 ANSWERS TO ACTIVITIES

Answer to Activity 15.1: Reflective Practice

1. This is a reflective activity so there are no right or wrong answers. However, you may consider wanting to wear your own clothes, access to your telephone, your family visiting. You may find music relaxing, wanting to watch the television or read a book. You may want to know the time and date by having a clock nearby or be able to see out of a window.

Answers to Activity 15.2: Critical Thinking

1. The positives are that this provided a structured assessment of the person to ensure accurate diagnoses and quicker treatment. The team can also assess treatment effectiveness over time.

2. The disadvantages of delirium screening could be:

A false-positive screening, although rare with either the CAM-ICU or the ICDSC, may result in unnecessary pharmacologic or nonpharmacologic treatment. The nurse may be concerned about labeling a person with a diagnosis.

3. To support the effectiveness of the team, regular and evidence-based education and support are needed. Perform regular audits of practice to identify if an assessment is carried out and what the subsequent actions were. This can also identify any gaps in the team's knowledge and feedback into the education provision.

Answer to Activity 15.3: Theory Stop Point

1. The limitation of this study is that the study was carried out in a single centre in one country. We do not fully know the difference in sedation practice, staffing numbers, pain management approaches, and physical restraint use between this country and our own so we need to be cautious when considering the study's findings and our practice.
2. The tool may have been implemented hospital wide, so the department was limited in their choice. This may also have been personal preference or custom and practice.

Answers to Activity 15.4: Critical Thinking

1. Causes of agitation could be:

   - Pain
   - Thirst or hunger
   - Discomfort
   - Fear and anxiety
   - Needing to go to the toilet
   - Confusion as to time, place, date

2. Addressing the underlying causes of agitation is key to its management so working through the list like the one above or the one you created would be a good strategy.

Answer to Activity 15.5: Reflective Practice and Critical Thinking

1. As this is a reflective activity, there are no right or wrong answers. This is a challenging ethical debate, one better discussed rather than written. I propose that the difference between holding a person for comfort and holding to control their movement lies in the amount of force exerted and the intention of the member of staff. The issue of consent should always be considered along with mental capacity, but in people receiving treatment in critical care units, waking from sedation, consent is a complex area.

Answers to Activity 15.6: Case Study

1. A risk of limiting daytime routine is the inability to establish and improved sleep pattern. Allowing a person to 'sleep' also prevents rehabilitation and movement; it increases the risk of infection and pressure damage. As the wake/sleep cycle is not correct the person will continue to be agitated at night, possibly receiving medication that could have been avoided.

2. An assessment to establish if Refaat is experiencing delirium would enable the team to appropriately manage his recovery.

3. The allowance and support of visiting can increase stimulus and help with structuring the person's day. Watching television together or reading a book or newspaper to them can help, as well as updating them on what is happening in the family or their friendship group. Letting the family know that delirium is transient and not to be worried if Rafaat doesn't seem himself at the moment. Letting them know the importance of re-orientation. Allowing them time to express any concerns they may have and offering support.

Answers to Activity 15.7: Critical Thinking

1. Depression may develop post critical care for several reasons, but you may have in your list:

   - Loss of control
   - A significant change in health status
   - Change of body image
   - Unable to communicate effectively
   - Unable to eat and drink
   - Loss of free will
   - Lack of connection with loved ones
   - Reduction of income or loss of employment due to illness
   - Loss of opportunities such as starting university or new employment

Answers to Activity 15.8: Theory Stop Point

1. Poor handover of information between departments, disjointed service transferring between hospital and community healthcare services. Poor access to follow-up services. Lack of speciality services for post critical care rehabilitation

2. Shared access by all services to the person health care records. Funding specialty rehabilitation services for those who have experienced critical illness.

Answers to Activity 15.9: Reflective Practice and Critical Thinking

1. This will be a personal view

2. People who may not be able to access this resource are those who have limited or no access to the internet, those who may be homeless, those who do not speak or read English. The resource could also be a paper copy, offered in different languages and accessible formats (large print, braille). There could be an audio recording made available.

Answers to Activity 15.10: Case Study

1. He should have had an assessment for PTSD-like symptoms whilst he was still in the hospital. If there was an early indication he was at risk of psychological trauma, low-level interventions may have been used at that point. However, the timing of the follow-up visit is crucial. PTSD-like symptoms have to persist for more than 6–8 weeks before any therapeutic interventions would be offered (National Institute of Mental Health, 2020).

2. Other symptoms he may exhibit and would be asked about during the follow-up visit are:

   - Heightened awareness/irritability
   - Feeling jumpy
   - Intrusive thoughts/memories
   - Feeling he is reliving events
   - Churning stomach
   - Racing pulse
   - Anger (especially outbursts)
   - Poor concentration span

3. In addition to Dala's psychological needs, the family may need some psychological support. They may also need financial support and support with childcare.
4. Referral to a psychologist or to Improving Access to Psychological Therapies (IAPT) services would be beneficial, as well as a social worker or family liaison team.

CHAPTER 16 ANSWERS TO ACTIVITIES

Answer to Activity 16.2: Research and Evidence-Based Practice

1. All three tools presented by the Cosgrove et al. (2019) support decision making for critical care healthcare professionals in often complex situations. The tools should not be used in isolation, but in conjunction with the wider content of the document, in addition to the importance of multi-professional teamworking, effective assessment and clinical judgement to inform decision-making processes that will impact on the delivery of care at the end of life.

   The tools encourage critical care practitioners to maintain focus and clarity in end of life care situations, not just in dealing with ethical and clinical dilemas, but in ensuring that all aspects of care delivery at the end of life are considered. Central to all of this is communication and seeking to ensure that dignity and comfort are a priority.

   The tools in isolation don't facilitate communication, but they do identify the importance of communication and of assessment to support communication between the patient, their family and the entire healthcare professional team involved in the delivery of care.

Answers to Activity 16.3: Case Study

1. In this situation, it is important that the nurse works as part of the multi-professional team, with a central role in continuous care delivery both to Elizabeth and to her family.
2. You may have considered here that **communication** is a main priority for the nurse, with Elizabeth and her family and with the team. In addition, the nurse will also prioritise the **management of any symptoms** that Elizabeth may experience, ensuring that they escalate any concerns about this to the medical team so that Elizabeth is comfortable and as effectively symptom controlled as possible. If symptoms are problematic, the nurse may wish to consider the input of the specialist palliative care team for advice and support. The nurse may also consider **spiritual support** for Elizabeth and her family and seek the input of the chaplaincy team, if this is important to Elizabeth and her family.
3. **Communication** is key in this situation and the nurse will need to ensure that Elizabeth's family are aware of the situation and ensure that they understand the information provided to them by the

medical team; the nurse would also be a part of that conversation. There are many factors that will need to be considered for Elizabeth's family, including the needs of her husband Reginald and the 3 young grandchildren that Elizabeth cares for. **Input from the bereavement service** in the hospital would be a useful source of support here; in some acute trusts bereavement teams provide support to families as a person deteriorates and is approaching death. They can provide resources to support families, including guidance on how to speak to children about death and resources, such as books, that can help families to talk together. The bereavement teams will also support the family in the initial bereavement period alongside the critical care team. The nurse may also wish to discuss with Elizabeth's family if Reginald will need additional support and if a **social worker** may be helpful.

The nurse will also ensure that Elizabeth's family are supported to be with her as much as they want to, and that they have **access to facilities** that will help with their comfort, including a rest room (if this is available).

4. The nurse **may feel sad** that Elizabeth is deteriorating and that she is going to die; they may feel that they could have done more to help with her condition and **disappointed** that the interventions that they have utilised have not been successful. The nurse may have been caring for Elizabeth and her family throughout the length of her admission to the critical care setting; in this time, they will have spent time with Elizabeth and her family and feel that they have developed a **therapeutic relationship** with them.

The nurse may manage their own emotions by allowing opportunity to discuss these with a colleague; other colleagues may also be feeling sad about the situation. It is valuable for colleagues to talk to each other and to debrief following the death of a person in their care. The team may also offer clinical supervision and the nurse may wish to engage with this to discuss their experience. The nurse may have activities outside of work that they engage with to support their emotional health such as running, yoga or spending time with their family and friends.

Answer to Activity 16.4: Reflective Practice

1. Your response to this question will vary based on your own personal experience in practice.

However, effective multi-professional working can be facilitated by:

a. Developed multi-professional team meetings
b. Team members understanding and appreciating the valuable contribution that each of them offers to the delivery of care
c. The use of group-based reflective discussion, e.g. clinical supervision
d. Clear and effective documentation via a shared system, e.g. electronic patient records

Answers to Activity 16.5: Theory Stop Point

1. Comparison between generalist and specialist palliative care; based on the work of Skilbeck and Payne (2003)

Generalist Palliative Care	Specialist Palliative Care
Provided by usual team of healthcare professionals	Provided by specialist palliative care team or hospice care provider
Identified as having low to moderate complexity of care need	Identified as having moderate to high complexity of care need

2. Ryan and Johnson (2018) in their chapter identify that there needs to be clarity between the level of complexity and the outline of the roles for those who provide generalist and specialist palliative care as indicated by Skilbeck and Payne (2003); but there are emerging models in the delivery of palliative care. As we move towards a model of shared care and away from palliative care being just about care at the very end of life, there is a real drive to integrate how generalist and specialist palliative care practitioners work together, with an ethos of collaboration, team working and coordination. The role of the specialist palliative care practitioner is to work alongside the main team, to educate and to support.

Answer to Activity 16.6: Research and Evidence-Based Practice

1. In their work, Enfield and Kollef identified that early introduction of palliative care in the critical care setting led to:

    - Less days on ventilator
    - Advance care planning discussions
    - Greater access to hospice care provision
    - Ease of intervention of specialist palliative care into the critical care unit

Answers to Activity 16.7: Case Study

1. Effective communication and the development of a therapeutic relationship is key in this situation. It will be a very difficult situation for Kelly as she has knowledge and experience in her role as a nurse and she is facing the loss of her husband. The nurse will need to work in partnership with Kelly and identify if and how she would like to support his care; this may involve giving support with personal care such as mouth care or supporting Peter's hygiene needs. The nurse will need to check regularly with Kelly how she continues to feel about supporting his care and will need to feel supported by the team to engage with this in partnership with the nursing team.

    The nurse can also talk to Kelly about the resources that will be available to her to support her children at this time and may wish to consider the involvement of the bereavement team, in order to ensure that Kelly has all of the information and support that she needs to support her children. It is essential that the nurse provides reassurance to Kelly and that effective assessment guides symptom management with close liaison with the wider multi-professional team.

2. In this situation, the specialist palliative care team can provide additional support to Peter, Kelly and their family; they can also provide expert advice to the team caring for Peter and Kelly in order to ensure that the team effectively manages any symptoms that Peter may experience. The specialist palliative care team can also provide further enhanced holistic assessment to ensure that any concerns that Kelly may have are managed appropriately and provide guidance to the team caring for Peter and Kelly in any key priorities. The specialist palliative care team will complement the main care team and provide an additional and valuable source of support and guidance for all involved; this is of particular relevance in this situation due to the many physical, social and psychological complexities that may be present.

CHAPTER 17 ANSWERS TO ACTIVITIES

Answers to Activity 17.1: Critical Thinking

Consider the four quality statements set out by NICE in the box above.

1. For each statement consider the challenges the clinical team may face when trying to ensure they are met.
2. Following this, consider ways in which we can overcome the challenges you have noted.

Statement 1 Adults in critical care at risk of morbidity have their rehabilitation goals agreed within 4 days of admission to critical care or before discharge from critical care, whichever is sooner.

1. All those in critical care are at risk of increased morbidity and should have their rehabilitation goals assessed. This assessment may be perceived as low priority within the ever-expanding work-load for critical care unit staff leading to it not being completed.
2. Processes need to be in place to ensure this assessment is built into the care of the whole person. Increased education for critical care staff will help ensure good understanding of the value of the assessment.

Statement 2 Adults at risk of morbidity have a formal handover of care, including their agreed individualised structured rehabilitation programme, when they transfer from critical care to a general ward.

1. Again, this includes all those discharged from a higher level of care to a lower level of care. Input is required from relevant members of the interdisciplinary team; the document needs to be accessible and easily amended by all team members and then easily accessed by the team responsible for ongoing care.
2. Follow-up teams will utilise this plan to structure interventions and set goals. Educating all those involved in the care of these individuals should ensure they understand the value of the programme and encourage adherence to the plan.

Statement 3 Adults who were in critical care and at risk of morbidity are given information based on their rehabilitation goals before they are discharged from hospital.

1. Information-giving is commonly recognised as integral to good recovery from any episode of ill health. The communication needs of the group will be diverse and require different media, formats and languages to be considered.
2. The critical care and follow-up teams should have information packs which can be tailored to meet individual requirements. This may need to be supplied in more than one medium (e.g. large print, braille, audio, translation), but definitely needs to be in some form that can be referred back to on subsequent occasions as retention of information can be challenging for people after a critical illness.

Statement 4 Adults who stayed in critical care for more than 4 days and were at risk of morbidity have a review 2 to 3 months after discharge from critical care.

1. Highlighting and consistently capturing which individuals meet this criterion of increased risk and providing a robust MDT pathway to the 2–3-month review.

2. Mechanisms need to be in place to highlight the people who fall into this category and meet the criteria for a follow outpatient appointment. Appropriately trained staff, usually a multi-disciplinary team, should be available to deliver the outpatient clinic. This requires time, funding and space.

(National Institute of Health and Care Excellence, 2017)

These four quality statements should be the central structure of a clear rehabilitation pathway for all those discharged from a critical care area. Delivery of the rehabilitation pathway depends upon education and training of staff and appropriate resources.

Answer to Activity 17.2: Reflective Practice and Team Working

1.

Physical	Interdisciplinary team member
Mobility	Physiotherapist Nurse
Fatigue	Nurse
Nutrition	Dietician Speech and Language Therapist Nurse
Swallowing	Speech and Language Therapist
Communication	Speech and Language Therapist Nurse Doctors
Polyneuropathy	Physiotherapist Nurse Doctors
Myopathy	Physiotherapist Nurse Doctors

Non-Physical	
Psychological	**Interdisciplinary team member**
Anxiety, panic attacks	Nurse Psychologist
Depression	Nurse Psychologist
Recurrent nightmares	Nurse Psychologist
Intrusive memories	Nurse Psychologist
Poor memory	Nurse Psychologist
Sleep disturbance	Nurse Psychologist
Stress	Nurse Psychologist

Social	Interdisciplinary team member
Financial	Social Worker
Employment	Social Worker DWP
Housing	Social Worker DWP
Breakdown of relationship	Family Nurse Psychologist

Social	Interdisciplinary team member
Loneliness/isolation	Family Nurse Psychologist
Loss of friendships	Family Nurse Psychologist

(Adapted from ICS, 2019; NICE, 2009; NICE, 2017)

Answers to Activity 17.3: Research and Evidence-based practice

Consider two different critical care admissions

1.

Farida	Freda	Rehabilitation plan
Planned admission: will have received pre op assessment, information about procedure and attended Surgery School. May have been to visit the critical care unit prior to admission. Expecting to wake on the Critical Care unit, family prepared that will need a short admission to Level 2 care after the operation.	Urgent admission-limited pre-operativeinformation.Unknown post-operative course.	We need to acknowledge these differences will likely lead to very different rehabilitation trajectories. Farida will receive short rehabilitation assessment prior to discharge. Freda will have comprehensive rehabilitation assessment within four days of her admission.
Planned Stoma	Stoma formed during emergency surgery	Farida will have been counselled regarding stoma preoperatively discussing need, location and care post op. Freda will need to address these issues as appropriate afterwards, a more psychologically challenging situation.
Woken in recovery, admitted to CCU once extubated	Longer duration of intubation	Screen for Post Intensive Care Syndrome, Freda is at much greater risk of physical and psychological sequalae, but both will need assessing. Must not assume Farida will not have any rehabilitation needs after her admission.
Farida will be expecting care as per Surgery School (ERAS+)	Concepts of early mobilisation and pulmonary rehabilitation will be introduced as appropriate	Farida will be expecting these activities, they will be a new concept for Freda.
Whilst recovering from surgery will continue under the care of Oncology team, likely through this will have access to psychological support	Surgical team less likely to have access to ongoing psychological support.	Need to ensure both receive psychological support as needed.

Answers to Activity 17.4: Case Study

1. What members of the multidisciplinary team will need to be involved in Winston's rehabilitation?

    Dietician: to prescribe nasogastric feed and provide guidance with weaning from enteral feed to an oral route.

Speech and Language therapist: monitoring swallow, provide guidance for reintroducing oral feeding and drinking. Ensure speech and communication is adequate and assist with this if not.

Physiotherapist: improve mobility, build strength and stamina. Promote pulmonary rehabilitation.

Occupational therapist: assess functional status and memory, treat, support and guide as needed.

Follow-up nurse: often pivotal role in liaising with MDT. Provides continuity and support for the person and their loved one during the transition from critical care to the ward. Support psychological recovery and initiate low key interventions to assist with this, refer to psychologist as needed depending on psychological assessment tool scores, or subjective assessment.

2. What will the aims and goals of the rehabilitation programme be?

The broad goal is to return Winston to as near his baseline function as possible. This will be broken down into smaller measurable and achievable goals within each specific area.

For example, the initial plan might be for Winston to:

Hoist out of bed twice a day and sit in his chair for 1 hour each time.

Puree diet and teaspoons of thickened fluids

Maintain strict food chart for dietician to review

IPAT score 6 on discharge from CCU, repeat in one week.

Refer to Occupational Therapy for assessment of memory and cognitive function.

Minimum weekly visit from follow-up team

Monitor delirium, wean quetiapine if delirium is settling.

Goals will constantly be reassessed and rewritten.

Answers to Activity 17.5: Case Study

1. What will be the benefits of Karen seeing her diaries?

Research indicates access to critical care diaries helps with psychological recovery from a critical illness. Seeing her diaries may help Karen to understand why her family are so protective and why her recovery is slow.

2. How will the health care professional structure the diary feedback for Karen?

It is important to provide a safe quiet space for Karen to see her diaries. Someone should be on hand to read with her, helping to explain or give context. Karen may not wish to go through it all in one sitting. Karen should be advised that it may make her feel upset or distressed and that this is a normal reaction.

3. How should Karen be prepared for seeing pictures of herself, critically ill, that she may not have known existed?

The existence of the photos should be introduced gently to Karen and she should be reassured they are stored securely, and that it is her personal choice as to whether she will see them or not.

Answers to Activity 17.6: Reflective Practice

1. Completing the diary may be seen as low priority by staff busy looking after someone critically ill. Staff may feel unsure about what to include and how to phrase things. It can be difficult to avoid jargon. Is the diary electronic or paper and where should it be stored? Family and friends may be encouraged to keep a diary as well, should this be separate?

2. It may feel wrong to take pictures without the consent of the person. Local policy should be available to guide this practice. Refer to GDPR regarding storage of a digital image.

3. The person should be prepared for seeing the images and may need psychological support from a psychologist to do this. Clinical context will likely be needed from the follow-up team.

Answers to Activity 17.7: Critical Thinking

1. The article suggests that there is an increased incidence of new chronic conditions in people after a critical illness compared to a population control group. However, there is also an increase in new chronic conditions in people with pre-existing chronic conditions post critical illness compared to other critical illness survivors who did not have pre-existing chronic health conditions. The control group was also found to experience the same increased incidence of new conditions in those who had pre-existing conditions.

   Also, critical illness survivors without pre-existing conditions were at increased risk of developing chronic conditions, and those in the population control group who had pre-existing chronic conditions were more likely to develop further chronic conditions.
   The development, or not, of new chronic conditions appears to be multi-factoral.

2. The article concludes with the recommendation that survivors of a critical illness are at greater risk of developing new chronic conditions. This is further increased in those who had pre-existing chronic conditions. This should inform and shape the follow-up service delivered to this group.

Answers to Activity 17.8: Theory Stop Point

1. Research is a strong driver in ensuring we provide effective and cost-effective interventions in healthcare. It informs practice and improves outcomes.

2. Both qualitative and quantitative research is used in this area; however, there has been an increase in mixed methodology research. The use of mixed methodology is a deliberate choice to add value above that which could be achieved by a single study approach This approach can capture both the measurable effect of treatment and the person's experience of that treatment.

3. Whether or not the cost of critical care can be justified is a complex moral, ethical and philosophical debate. How we measure the value of survivorship is subjective. If we simply measure the value in time, rehabilitation costs seem unnecessary. If, however, we measure quality of life for our critical illness survivors, rehabilitation costs must carry equal weight.

4. NICE (CG 83) describes the failure to provide a robust rehabilitation plan after critical illness as a 'major public health issue'.

5. Further research could guide clinicians in utilising their finite resources in the most effective areas.

GLOSSARY

Accessory Organs   Organs that are not part of the digestive tract but have a digestive function.

Aerobic   Presence of oxygen

Afterload   The resistance within the circulation against which the heart has to pump to eject blood

Alimentary Canal   The long tube of organs, comprising the oesophagus, stomach and intestines that runs from the mouth to the anus.

Analgesia   An analgesic is any member of the group of drugs used to achieve analgesia, relief from pain.

Antenatal   Before birth, during or related to pregnancy.

Anti D   Immunoglobulin neutralises any RhD positive antigens that may have entered the mother's blood during pregnancy. If the antigens have been neutralised, the mother's blood does not produce antibodies.

Antibiotic Stewardship   Programmes and interventions that aim to optimise the use of antibiotics.

Antigen   Something that stimulates production of antibodies

Antimicrobial Resistance   The development by a disease-causing microbe, through mutation or gene transfer, to survive exposure to an antimicrobial agent that was previously an effective treatment.

Antipsychotics   A class of medication primarily used to manage psychosis and a range of other psychotic disorders.

Arrhythmia   Abnormal cardiac rhythm

Artery Forceps   These are surgical clamps that are used to compress an artery to stem bleeding

Aspiration   Food entering the trachea or lungs.

Aspiration Pneumonia   A lung infection caused by material from the mouth or stomach entering the lungs.

Atrial Fibrillation (AF)   A heart condition that causes irregular and abnormally fast heart rate.

Autoimmune Disorders   Disorders that cause the immune system to produce antibodies that attack normal body tissues.

Balloon Tamponade   An obstetric balloon inflated in the uterus to apply pressure to the bleeding vessels from the placental site.

Bile A yellow/green liquid produced and secreted by the liver comprising bile salts, cholesterol and fat soluble hormones.

Bilirubin The product of the breakdown of haemoglobin.

Brainstem A critical structure located in the distal part of the brain which is composed of the midbrain, pons and medulla oblongata. Together, these structures control breathing, blood pressure and the relay of impulses from the brain to the body and vice versa.

Brainstem Death The permanent loss of brain stem function including breathing and consciousness; this is an irreversible event.

C-Spine The Cervical Spine, often referred to as the neck, is the upper portion of the spinal vertebrae. These vertebrae connect the spine to the skull

Caesarean section Surgical procedure to deliver a baby through the abdomen.

Cardiopulmonary Bypass Cardiopulmonary bypass is a technique in which a machine temporarily takes over the function of the heart and lungs during surgery, maintaining the circulation of blood and the oxygen content of the patient's body.

Cardiotocography (CTG) Machine used to continuously record the heartbeat of the fetus and the contractions of the woman's uterus during labour.

Care Bundles Bundles contain three to five evidence-informed practices to be delivered collectively and consistently with the aim of improving the person's outcome.

Care in the Last Days of Life Care provided to a person who is in the last days of life and identified as deteriorating and approaching death; with care also extending to their family carers. Care can be provided in a range of settings and often requires input from a range of professionals from the multi-professional team.

Catabolic Breaking down larger molecules into small ones. It is what happens when you digest food and the molecules break down in the body for use as energy. Large, complex molecules in the body are broken down into smaller, simple ones.

Cerebral Perfusion Pressure (CPP) The amount of pressure needed to maintain blood flow to the brain. CPP is regulated by two balanced opposing forces: Mean Arterial Pressure, the driving force that pushes blood into the brain, and Intracranial Pressure, the force that keeps blood out.

Chain/circle of Infection A process that describes cross infection through a chain of interrelated events. This begins when an agent leaves its reservoir or host through a portal of exit, and is conveyed by some mode of transmission, then enters through an appropriate portal of entry to infect a susceptible host.

Cholesterol A fatty substance made in the liver and found in animal sources of food.

Cilia Hair-like projections within the main airways

Coagulation Blood clotting

Cognitive bias/unconscious bias these are biases that we have that are influenced by our background, our experiences, and any social stereotypes we may choose to believe.

Collagen A protein that is the main component of connective tissue.

Connective Tissue   Tissue that performs the functions of binding and supporting.

Continuum   A coherent whole characterized as a collection, sequence, or progression of values or elements varying by minute degrees.

Delirium   Abrupt change in the brain that causes mental confusion and emotional disruption. It makes it difficult to think, remember, sleep, pay attention, and more. It is usually temporary and can often be treated effectively.

Depression   Depression is a low mood that lasts for weeks or months and affects your daily life. The symptoms can range from mild and short term to severe and enduring.

Detoxification   Removal of toxic substances.

Diarrhoea   The passage of 3 or more loose or liquid stools in 1 day.

Dietician   A specialist trained to assess, diagnose and treat diet and nutritional problems.

Disease Trajectory   The duration and pattern of a specific disease process.

Diuretic   A medication taken to increase the excretion of water through urination.

Dysphagia   Difficulty swallowing.

Embolism   Occlusion of a blood vessel by a fragment such as from a thrombus or other undissolved material, e.g. fat, gas, tissue fragments.

Endotracheal Tube   A flexible plastic tube that is put in the mouth and then down into the trachea

Epidemiology   Study of the distribution of health-related events in a given population

Equivocal   Not clear one way of the other, uncertain, ambiguous.

Ergometrine   A medication used to cause contractions of the uterus to prevent or treat excessive bleeding after childbirth.

Erythema   Reddening of the skin typically caused by increased blood flow to the capillaries resulting from skin damage.

Exacerbation   An episode of worsening symptoms.

Fatigue   Extreme tiredness resulting from physical or mental activity or due to illness.

Follow-up   A multi-disciplinary service addressing the needs of critical care survivors.

Gallstones   These are small stones that form in the gallbladder, a small organ found near the liver.

Haemodynamic   Relating to the heart and circulation

Healthcare Associated Infection (HCAI)   An infection occurring in a patient during the process of care in a hospital or other health care facility which was not present or incubating at the time of admission.

Hepatitis   this is a term used to describe inflammation of the liver.

Holistic Care   Person-centred and total care needs that considers not just physical health, but also psychological, spiritual, social health and associated care needs.

Homeostasis   Homeostasis is the state of steady internal, physical, and chemical conditions maintained by living systems.

Hypercholesterolaemia Elevated levels of (usually low density) cholesterol in the blood.

Hypertension High blood pressure.

Hypotension Low blood pressure

Hypovolaemia Low volume of blood

Incontinence The inability to voluntarily control urination and defaecation.

Inflammation/Inflammatory Response The body's response to injury resulting in redness, heat and swelling, designed to move white blood cells to the affected area.

Inhalation Injury Damage to the respiratory tract or lungs caused by inhalation of heat, smoke or chemicals.

Inotropes/inotropic agents Medicines that change cardiac contractility.

Instrumental Deliveries Births assisted with the use of instruments such as forceps or ventouse (suction).

Intensivist A doctor specialising in Intensive Care.

Interstitium This is a fluid filled space that exists between structural barriers. These could be between cell walls, the layers of the skins and internal organs.

Intervention Treatments and actions that are performed to help the critically ill person reach their goals.

Intracranial Pressure The pressure within the craniospinal compartment, a closed system that comprises a fixed volume of neural tissue, blood, and cerebrospinal fluid.

Intrapartum Refers to the period of time when a woman is in labour and lasts until the delivery of the placenta.

Intravenous Inside a vein.

Invasive Device A medical device introduced into the body, either through a break in the skin or a naturally occurring opening.

Ischaemia Lack of oxygen supply arising either through lack of blood supply or lack of oxygen in the blood.

Ischaemic Stroke A stroke caused by a reduction in the amount of oxygen reaching the brain.

Laryngeal Masks A medical device that keeps a patient's airway open during anaesthesia or unconsciousness. It is a type of supraglottic airway device.

Liver Function Tests Groups of blood tests that measure the enzymatic status of the liver, protein and bilirubin levels which provide information about the overall functioning of the liver.

Manual removal of placenta Evacuation of the placenta from the uterus by hand.

Mean Arterial Pressure The average arterial pressure throughout one cardiac cycle, systole, and diastole. MAP is influenced by cardiac output and systemic vascular resistance, each of which is under the influence of several variables.

Metabolic/metabolism The physical and chemical processes that provide energy for cellular processes.

Microbial Analysis A test for pathogens that might cause infection.

Morbidity Likelihood of worsening health. Having a disease or symptoms of a disease. Medical problem caused by a treatment.

Mortality Likelihood of death.

MRI Scan Magnetic resonance imaging (MRI) is a type of scan that uses strong magnetic fields to take images of the inside of the body.

Multi-Professional Team A range of health and social care professionals engaged in the assessment and delivery of care. Working in collaboration with a person-centred ethos, each profession brings a unique and valuable aspect to care. In combination they ensure all aspects of the care needs of people and their families can be considered and supported.

Myopathy Disease of the muscle often leading to muscle wastage or weakness.

Nasal Cannula A device used to deliver supplemental oxygen or increased airflow to a patient or person in need of respiratory help. This device consists of a lightweight tube which on one end splits into two prongs which are placed in the nostrils and from which a mixture of air and oxygen flows.

Non-rebreather Mask Is a type of oxygen mask that can provide high doses of oxygen to spontaneously breathing people. It has a bag reservoir of oxygen from which the person draws oxygen rather than air on inspiration. It ensures there is no re-inhalation of expired air.

Organ Donation The giving of an organ to someone else to help in a transplant operation.

Palliative Care A holistic approach to care delivery for a person and their family living with a life-limiting condition. It aims to ensure quality of life and multi-professional team involvement in care delivery and is integral to all roles across health and social care.

Polyneuropathy Peripheral nerve damage.

Postnatal Up to six weeks following the birth of a baby.

Post-traumatic Stress Disorder (PTSD) An anxiety disorder caused by a stressful life event.

Pre-eclampsia A disorder that generally develops late in pregnancy, after week 20, and is characterized by a sudden onset of high blood pressure, severe swelling of the hands and face, and signs that some organs may not be working normally, including protein in the urine.

Preload the amount the heart fibres stretch prior to contraction of the muscle

Prone Positioning Prone position is a body position in which the person lies flat with the chest down and the back up.

Prophylaxis Prevention of diseases.

Pulmonary Relating to the lungs.

Sedation Administration of sedative drugs, generally to facilitate a medical procedure or diagnostic procedure.

Sepsis A life-threatening organ dysfunction caused by dysregulated host response to infection.

Septic Shock   A subset of sepsis with circulatory and cellular/metabolic dysfunction associated with higher risk of mortality.

Specialist Palliative Care Team   A multi-professional team who have advanced knowledge and skills in palliative care; their involvement is often invited by the main care team and is valuable in the management of complex holistic care needs for the person, their family and supporting care team (including symptom management and psychological care).

Specialist Trainee 6   A doctor in their 6th year of specialty training.

Speech and language therapist (SLT)   A specialist trained to help adults and children manage disorders of speech, language, communication, and swallowing.

Stress-induced Hyperglycaemia   The elevation of blood glucose level above the normal range due to the stress of illness.

Subdural Haematoma   An accumulating mass of blood, usually clotted, or a swelling that is confined to the space between the dura mater and the subarachnoid membrane.

Suction   The collective term that encompasses the measures that are used for clearing the airway of a patient. It involves suctioning, clearing secretions, and maintaining the patency of the airway.

Supine   Sometimes called supine position is when a person is lying on their back with their face upwards.

Swedish Nose   A cap that can be attached to the tracheostomy tube to help maintain humidity.

Syntocinon   A medication that causes the uterus to contract and is administered to prevent or treat excessive bleeding after childbirth.

Systemic   Relating to the main arterial system of the body.

Tachycardia   Fast heart rate

Tetanus   A serious disease caused by a bacterial pathogen that affects the nervous system resulting in painful muscle contractions.

Thrombosis   A blood clot obstructing a blood vessel.

Transparency tracing   A marker is used to trace the outline of a wound directly onto a transparent sterile sheet or grid.

Uterine Artery ligation   A surgical technique to prevent postpartum haemorrhage.

Vaccination   A treatment given to produce immunity against a disease.

Varices   Veins that are enlarged or swollen.

Vasoconstriction   Narrowing of the blood vessels.

Vasodilation   Widening of the blood vessels.

Vasopressors   drugs used to control the vasoconstriction of the blood vessels.

Vortex   Rapidly rotating fluid (blood) which creates a suction in the centre and expels fluid at the periphery.

INDEX

Page numbers in *italics* refer to Figures and Tables and those in **bold** refer to glossary entries. Page numbers followed by (cs) refer to case studies.